AF787533

Marine Natural Products as Anticancer Agents 2.0

Marine Natural Products as Anticancer Agents 2.0

Editors

Celso Alves
Marc Diederich

MDPI • Basel • Beijing • Wuhan • Barcelona • Belgrade • Manchester • Tokyo • Cluj • Tianjin

Editors
Celso Alves
Polytechnic of Leiria
Portugal

Marc Diederich
Seoul National University
Republic of Korea

Editorial Office
MDPI
St. Alban-Anlage 66
4052 Basel, Switzerland

This is a reprint of articles from the Special Issue published online in the open access journal *Marine Drugs* (ISSN 1660-3397) (available at: https://www.mdpi.com/journal/marinedrugs/special_issues/AnticancerAgents2).

For citation purposes, cite each article independently as indicated on the article page online and as indicated below:

LastName, A.A.; LastName, B.B.; LastName, C.C. Article Title. *Journal Name* **Year**, *Volume Number*, Page Range.

ISBN 978-3-0365-7568-1 (Hbk)
ISBN 978-3-0365-7569-8 (PDF)

© 2023 by the authors. Articles in this book are Open Access and distributed under the Creative Commons Attribution (CC BY) license, which allows users to download, copy and build upon published articles, as long as the author and publisher are properly credited, which ensures maximum dissemination and a wider impact of our publications.
The book as a whole is distributed by MDPI under the terms and conditions of the Creative Commons license CC BY-NC-ND.

Contents

About the Editors

Celso Alves

Dr. Celso Alves received his PhD in Marine Science, Technology, and Sea Management (Do*Mar) in 2019 from the University of Aveiro, Portugal. He is a Researcher at the Marine and Environmental Sciences Centre in the Polytechnic of Leiria and an invited assistant Professor at the Polytechnic of Leiria. His scientific work has been focused on the study of plants and marine organisms (e.g., seaweeds, bacteria, fungi, jellyfish, sponges, etc.) as sources of new natural bioactive compounds with the potential for biotechnological and therapeutic applications.

Marc Diederich

Dr. Marc Diederich earned his PhD in molecular pharmacology in 1994 from the University Henri Poincaré Nancy 1, France. After training at the University of Cincinnati, USA, he focused his research on cancer and leukemia cell signaling pathways and gene expression mechanisms triggered by natural compounds with epigenetic, anti-inflammatory, and cell-death-inducing potential. He directs the laboratory for molecular and cellular biology of cancer (LBMCC) in Luxemburg. He was appointed associate Professor of Biochemistry at the College of Pharmacy of Seoul National University in 2012. In 2017, he was tenured and promoted to full professor at SNU. Since 1998, he has been the organizer of the "Signal Transduction" meetings in Luxembourg. Prof. Diederich's research focuses on the development of novel anticancer drugs. As an example, natural marine compounds represent an interesting source of novel leads with potent chemotherapeutic or chemo-preventive properties.

marine drugs

Editorial

Marine Natural Products as Anticancer Agents 2.0

Celso Alves [1,*] and Marc Diederich [2,*]

1 MARE—Marine and Environmental Sciences Centre/ARNET-Aquatic Research Network, ESTM, Polytechnic of Leiria, 2520-630 Peniche, Portugal
2 Department of Pharmacy, College of Pharmacy, Seoul National University, 1 Gwanak-ro, Gwanak-gu, Seoul 08826, Republic of Korea
* Correspondence: celso.alves@ipleiria.pt (C.A.); marcdiederich@snu.ac.kr (M.D.)

Global cancer incidence and death are expected to increase to 28.4 million cases by 2040, despite efforts to understand cancer biology better and to improve its diagnosis and therapy [1]. Inappropriate therapeutic regimens and tumor recurrence due to the development of drug resistance are two major clinical challenges impacting poor patient outcomes [2]. Over the last few decades, the marine environment has become an important source of molecules with potent anticancer properties, exhibiting unusual chemical features and mechanisms of action. Twelve of seventeen drugs of marine origin approved by regulatory entities are used against cancer, and thirty-four of forty compounds in the marine pharmaceuticals pipeline indicate "cancer therapy" [3].

The Special Issue "Marine Natural Products as Anticancer Agents 2.0" (https://www.mdpi.com/journal/marinedrugs/special_issues/AnticancerAgents2, accessed on 11 April 2023) gathered eleven publications, including two reviews and nine research articles, about the anticancer activities of marine natural and/or derived products on in vitro 2D and 3D cellular models, and/or in vivo models of colorectal, breast, lung, myeloma, liver, leukemia, and melanoma cancers. Marine natural and/or derived products addressed herein were obtained from sponges, seaweeds, fungi, and soft corals. Those compounds exhibit great chemical diversity, such as terpenes, alkaloids, fatty acids, phenolics, polysaccharides, and peptides. Some compounds are halogenated. It is also relevant to highlight the key importance of "nature power creativity", evidenced in this Special Issue as a supplier of scaffolds for the synthesis and molecular modeling of new anticancer drugs. Forty-seven analogs were synthesized based on the original structures of natural products of marine origin. These compounds exhibited high specificity and great affinity to interact with biomarkers related to specific intracellular signaling pathways involved in carcinogenesis, including cell cycle, oxidative stress, mitochondrial dysfunction, apoptosis, necrosis, stemness, angiogenesis, migration, and invasion.

Li and co-workers [4] provided a critical review of the application of fucoidans as cancer immunotherapy agents, discussing their action on different immune cells and as co-adjuvants of immunotherapeutic medicines. The prospects and challenges, as well as the current human clinical studies and available registered clinical trials using this type of compound against cancer, were also reported and discussed.

Vasarri and co-workers [5] compiled a critical overview focused on the last five years concerning the ability of marine natural products to prevent cancer cell migration and invasion, events related to the high mortality of patients with solid tumors. Forty-two compounds, including polysaccharides, peptides and proteins, polyphenols, and alkaloids, were identified as possessing migrastatic properties, limiting the pro-metastatic behavior of cancer cells in in vitro and in vivo models. This review provides a valuable guide for the pharmaceutical and scientific community as a starting point to develop new antimetastatic drugs based on the reported marine natural products.

The research and development of new drugs to reinforce the available therapeutic options will be crucial to improve the effectiveness of current cancer therapeutic regimens.

Citation: Alves, C.; Diederich, M. Marine Natural Products as Anticancer Agents 2.0. *Mar. Drugs* **2023**, *21*, 247. https://doi.org/10.3390/md21040247

Received: 11 April 2023
Accepted: 14 April 2023
Published: 17 April 2023

Copyright: © 2023 by the authors. Licensee MDPI, Basel, Switzerland. This article is an open access article distributed under the terms and conditions of the Creative Commons Attribution (CC BY) license (https://creativecommons.org/licenses/by/4.0/).

Thus, the efforts to discover new chemical entities from natural origins that can inspire the development of new anticancer drugs, including synthesis and/or semi-synthesis approaches, are of the utmost relevance.

Sala and collaborators [6] isolated two novel free porphyrins, isabellin A and B, and the known compounds corallistin D and deuteroporphyrin IX from the marine sponge *Isabella* sp., previously collected in the hard substrate off Zuytdorp, Western Australia. The new free porphyrin, isabellin A, exhibited a marked cytotoxic effect on the NS-1 malignant myeloma cell line, similar to the positive control sparsomycin. Mohamed and co-authors [7] isolated five oxygenated cembrenoids, sarcoconvolutum A–E, from the soft coral *Sarcophyton* sp. collected in the Egyptian Red Sea. The cembrene diterpene sarcoconvolutum E exhibited the highest cytotoxicity on A549 (IC_{50}: 49.70 μg/mL) and HSC-2 (IC_{50}: 53.17 μg/mL) malignant cells derived from lung adenocarcinoma and squamous cell carcinoma of the oral cavity, respectively.

On the other hand, Patel and co-workers [8] explored the chemical structure of clavatadines, previously isolated from the marine sponge *Suberea clavate*, as a scaffold for developing new anticancer drugs. The authors synthesized a library of thirty-two pirocyclic clavatadine analogs, displaying a CC_{50} range between 0.4 and 12.3 μM on A-375 melanoma cells. The highest selectivity was exhibited by analogs 29 and 37, which activate caspases 3/7, key biomarkers of apoptosis. Lu and collaborators [9] also designed and semi-synthesized a series of fifteen derivatives of brefeldin A, a macrolactone biosynthesized by the marine fungus *Penicillium* sp. (HS-N-29), previously isolated from the medicinal mangrove *Acanthus ilicifolius*. Analog 7 (brefeldin A 7-*O*-2-chloro-4,5-difluorobenzoate) exhibited the smallest IC_{50} value (0.84 μM) on the human chronic myelogenous leukemia K562 cancer cell line. The mechanism of action underlying its cytotoxicity seems to be related to the blockage of the cell cycle, induction of apoptosis, inhibition of BCR-ABL phosphorylation, and downregulation of the expression of signaling molecules of the AKT pathway, including mTOR and p70S6K. Suksamai and collaborators [10] synthesized 5-*O*-(*N*-Boc-L-alanine)-renieramycin T (OBA-RT) from renieramycin T, an alkaloid commonly found in sponges and nudibranchs. OBA-RT can suppress cancer stem cell (CSC) activity and induce apoptosis in malignant lung cells, inhibiting Ak, which plays a key role in regulating CSC maintenance.

Alves and colleagues [11] studied the cytotoxic properties of three bromoditerpenes isolated from the red seaweed *Sphaerococcus coronopifolius*, named 12*R*-hydroxy-bromosphaerol, 12*S*-hydroxy-bromosphaerol, and bromosphaerol. Bromo groups, in their structure, characterize these terpenes due to bromine substitution, a rare chemical feature among secondary metabolites. The compounds displayed increased hydrogen peroxide production and induced apoptosis of MCF-7 cells derived from breast adenocarcinoma.

The anticancer activities of peptides (1–12), extracted and purified from the brown seaweed *Laminaria japonica* (LJPs), were evaluated through in vitro and in vivo models of liver cancer [12]. The LJP-1 peptide exhibited the highest anticancer activity, decreasing tumor growth in in vivo models. According to the evidence reported by Wu and co-workers [12], its mechanism of action seems to be related to the induction of cell death by caspase-dependent apoptosis, partly by inhibiting PI3K and MAPK signaling pathways and regulating the expression of cell cycle checkpoint proteins.

The development of resistance to anticancer drugs seriously threatens cancer treatment success. Distinct strategies have been designed to overcome these challenges, including drug synergism. Su and collaborators [13] explored the potential of a novel resolvin, 7*S*,15*R*-dihydroxy-16*S*,17*S*-epoxy-docosapentaenoic acid (diHEP-DPA), synthesized by cyanobacterial lipoxygenase from docosa–hexaenoic acid (DHA) to overcome the chemoresistance to 5-fluorouracil (5-FU) of colorectal cancer cells (CRCs) using in vitro and in vivo models. The new resolvin suppressed key events related to chemoresistance to 5-FU resulting from prolonged exposure, such as the enrichment of CSCs, the infiltration of tumor-associated macrophages, and the epithelial–mesenchymal transition in colorectal tumors. This evidence suggests that the therapeutic application of diHEP-DPA in combination with 5-FU-based chemotherapeutics against colorectal cancer is potentially effective.

Angiogenesis is the biological process responsible for forming new blood vessels, which play a key role in tumor growth, maintenance, and metastasis, being a valid target for tumor therapeutics. Dong and collaborators [14] evaluated the anti-angiogenesis activity of bis(2,3,6-tribromo-4,5-dihydroxybenzyl) ether (BTDE), a bromophenol previously isolated from the red seaweed *Rhodomela confervoides*. BTDE inhibited migration, invasion, tube formation, and the activity of matrix metalloproteinase 9 of human umbilical vein endothelial cells. It also prevented the migration, invasion, and vasculogenic mimicry formation of A549 lung adenocarcinoma cells. In vivo, BTDE blocked intersegmental vessel formation in zebrafish embryos.

Altogether, the eleven scientific papers published in this Special Issue provide an exciting overview of marine natural products as potential anticancer agents.

As Guest Editors, we acknowledge the efforts provided by all researchers and reviewers that participated in this Special Issue, the editorial board, and the *Marine Drugs* editorial office for their support and assistance. Special thanks go to Dr. Grace Qu.

Funding: Marc Diederich was supported by the National Research Foundation (NRF) by the MEST of Korea for Tumor Microenvironment Global Core Research Center (GCRC) grant (grant number NRF 2011-0030001), by the Seoul National University Research Grant (Funding number: 800-20160150) and by the Creative-Pioneering Researchers Program through Seoul National University (SNU) (Funding number: 370C-20160062). Research at SNU is also supported by the National Research Foundation (NRF) (Grant Number 2022R1A2C101314111). Support from the BrainKorea21 FOUR program is acknowledged. Marc Diederich is supported by the "Recherche Cancer et Sang" foundation, the "Recherches Scientifiques Luxembourg" association, the "Een Häerz fir kriibskrank Kanner" association, the Action LIONS "Vaincre le Cancer" association, and Télévie Luxembourg. C.A. acknowledges the support by the Portuguese Foundation for Science and Technology (FCT) through the Strategic Projects granted to MARE—Marine and Environmental Sciences Centre (UIDP/04292/2020 and UIDB/04292/2020), Associate Laboratory ARNET (LA/P/0069/2020), and through the NEURONS4 (2022.09196.PTDC), MArTics (FCT/DRI/CAPES 2019.00277.CBM) and NEURONS (FCT/DRI/PNAAE 2021.09608.CBM) projects.

Conflicts of Interest: The authors declare no conflict of interest.

References

1. Sung, H.; Ferlay, J.; Siegel, R.L.; Laversanne, M.; Soerjomataram, I.; Jemal, A.; Bray, F. Global Cancer Statistics 2020: GLOBOCAN Estimates of Incidence and Mortality Worldwide for 36 Cancers in 185 Countries. *CA Cancer J. Clin.* **2021**, *71*, 209–249. [CrossRef] [PubMed]
2. Wang, N.; Ma, T.; Yu, B. Targeting epigenetic regulators to overcome drug resistance in cancers. *Signal Transduct. Target. Ther.* **2023**, *8*, 69. [CrossRef] [PubMed]
3. Mayer, A.M.S. The Global Marine Pharmaceuticals Pipeline. Available online: https://www.marinepharmacology.org/about (accessed on 5 April 2023).
4. Li, Y.; McGowan, E.; Chen, S.; Santos, J.; Yin, H.; Lin, Y. Immunopotentiating Activity of Fucoidans and Relevance to Cancer Immunotherapy. *Mar. Drugs* **2023**, *21*, 128. [CrossRef] [PubMed]
5. Vasarri, M.; Barletta, E.; Degl'Innocenti, D. Marine Migrastatics: A Comprehensive 2022 Update. *Mar. Drugs* **2022**, *20*, 273. [CrossRef] [PubMed]
6. Sala, S.; Moggach, S.A.; Nealon, G.L.; Fromont, J.; Gomez, O.; Vuong, D.; Lacey, E.; Flematti, G.R. Type-I Hemins and Free Porphyrins from a Western Australian Sponge *Isabella* sp. *Mar. Drugs* **2023**, *21*, 41. [CrossRef] [PubMed]
7. Mohamed, T.A.; Elshamy, A.I.; Abdel-Tawab, A.M.; AbdelMohsen, M.M.; Ohta, S.; Pare, P.W.; Hegazy, M.-E.F. Oxygenated Cembrene Diterpenes from *Sarcophyton convolutum*: Cytotoxic Sarcoconvolutum A–E. *Mar. Drugs* **2021**, *19*, 519. [CrossRef] [PubMed]
8. Patel, P.A.; Bruun, T.; Ilina, P.; Mäkkylä, H.; Lempinen, A.; Yli-Kauhaluoma, J.; Tammela, P.; Kiuru, P.S. Synthesis and Cytotoxicity Evaluation of Spirocyclic Bromotyrosine Clavatadine C Analogs. *Mar. Drugs* **2021**, *19*, 400. [CrossRef] [PubMed]
9. Lu, X.-X.; Jiang, Y.-Y.; Wu, Y.-W.; Chen, G.-Y.; Shao, C.-L.; Gu, Y.-C.; Liu, M.; Wei, M.-Y. Semi-Synthesis, Cytotoxic Evaluation, and Structure - Activity Relationships of Brefeldin A Derivatives with Antileukemia Activity. *Mar. Drugs* **2022**, *20*, 26. [CrossRef] [PubMed]

10. Suksamai, D.; Racha, S.; Sriratanasak, N.; Chaotham, C.; Aphicho, K.; Lin, A.C.K.; Chansriniyom, C.; Suwanborirux, K.; Chamni, S.; Chanvorachote, P. 5-*O*-(*N*-Boc-L-Alanine)-Renieramycin T Induces Cancer Stem Cell Apoptosis via Targeting Akt Signaling. *Mar. Drugs* **2022**, *20*, 235. [CrossRef] [PubMed]
11. Alves, C.; Silva, J.; Pintéus, S.; Guedes, R.A.; Guedes, R.C.; Alvariño, R.; Freitas, R.; Goettert, M.I.; Gaspar, H.; Alfonso, A.; et al. Bromoditerpenes from the Red Seaweed *Sphaerococcus coronopifolius* as Potential Cytotoxic Agents and Proteasome Inhibitors and Related Mechanisms of Action. *Mar. Drugs* **2022**, *20*, 652. [CrossRef] [PubMed]
12. Wu, Y.; Li, Y.; Guo, W.; Liu, J.; Lao, W.; Hu, P.; Lin, Y.; Chen, H. *Laminaria japonica* Peptides Suppress Liver Cancer by Inducing Apoptosis: Possible Signaling Pathways and Mechanism. *Mar. Drugs* **2022**, *20*, 704. [CrossRef] [PubMed]
13. Su, Y.; Choi, H.S.; Choi, J.H.; Kim, H.-S.; Jang, Y.-S.; Seo, J.-W. 7*S*,15*R*-Dihydroxy-16*S*,17*S*-epoxy-docosapentaenoic Acid Overcomes Chemoresistance of 5-Fluorouracil by Suppressing the Infiltration of Tumor-Associated Macrophages and Inhibiting the Activation of Cancer Stem Cells in a Colorectal Cancer Xenograft Model. *Mar. Drugs* **2023**, *21*, 80. [CrossRef] [PubMed]
14. Dong, S.; Chen, Z.; Wang, L.; Liu, Y.; Stagos, D.; Lin, X.; Liu, M. Marine Bromophenol Bis(2,3,6-Tribromo-4,5-Dihydroxybenzyl) ether Inhibits Angiogenesis in Human Umbilical Vein Endothelial Cells and Reduces Vasculogenic Mimicry in Human Lung Cancer A549 Cells. *Mar. Drugs* **2021**, *19*, 641. [CrossRef] [PubMed]

Disclaimer/Publisher's Note: The statements, opinions and data contained in all publications are solely those of the individual author(s) and contributor(s) and not of MDPI and/or the editor(s). MDPI and/or the editor(s) disclaim responsibility for any injury to people or property resulting from any ideas, methods, instructions or products referred to in the content.

marine drugs

MDPI

Review

Immunopotentiating Activity of Fucoidans and Relevance to Cancer Immunotherapy

Yani Li [1], Eileen McGowan [1,2,3,4], Size Chen [2,3,4,5], Jerran Santos [6], Haibin Yin [7] and Yiguang Lin [1,2,3,4,5,7,*]

1 School of Life Science, Faculty of Science, University of Technology Sydney, P.O. Box 123, Broadway, NSW 2007, Australia
2 Department of Immuno-Oncology, First Affiliated Hospital of Guangdong Pharmaceutical University, Guangzhou 510080, China
3 Guangdong Provincial Engineering Research Center for Esophageal Cancer Precision Therapy, Guangdong Pharmaceutical University, Guangzhou 510080, China
4 Key Laboratory of Cancer Immunotherapy of Guangdong High Education Institutes, Guangdong Pharmaceutical University, Guangzhou 510080, China
5 Guangdong Provincial Key Laboratory of CAR-T Cell Therapy Associated Adverse Effect Monitoring, Guangdong Pharmaceutical University, Guangzhou 510080, China
6 Advanced Tissue Engineering and Stem Cell Biology Group, Faculty of Science, University of Technology Sydney, P.O. Box 123, Broadway, NSW 2007, Australia
7 Research & Development Division, Guangzhou Anjie Biomedical Technology Co., Limited, Guangzhou 510535, China
* Correspondence: yiguang.lin@hotmail.com

Abstract: Fucoidans, discovered in 1913, are fucose-rich sulfated polysaccharides extracted mainly from brown seaweed. These versatile and nontoxic marine-origin heteropolysaccharides have a wide range of favorable biological activities, including antitumor, immunomodulatory, antiviral, antithrombotic, anticoagulant, antithrombotic, antioxidant, and lipid-lowering activities. In the early 1980s, fucoidans were first recognized for their role in supporting the immune response and later, in the 1990s, their effects on immune potentiation began to emerge. In recent years, the understanding of the immunomodulatory effects of fucoidan has expanded significantly. The ability of fucoidan(s) to activate CTL-mediated cytotoxicity against cancer cells, strong antitumor property, and robust safety profile make fucoidans desirable for effective cancer immunotherapy. This review focusses on current progress and understanding of the immunopotentiation activity of various fucoidans, emphasizing their relevance to cancer immunotherapy. Here, we will discuss the action of fucoidans in different immune cells and review how fucoidans can be used as adjuvants in conjunction with immunotherapeutic products to improve cancer treatment and clinical outcome. Some key rationales for the possible combination of fucoidans with immunotherapy will be discussed. An update is provided on human clinical studies and available registered cancer clinical trials using fucoidans while highlighting future prospects and challenges.

Keywords: fucoidan; seaweed; immunopotentiation; immunomodulatory; immunotherapy; cancer treatment; cytokines

Citation: Li, Y.; McGowan, E.; Chen, S.; Santos, J.; Yin, H.; Lin, Y. Immunopotentiating Activity of Fucoidans and Relevance to Cancer Immunotherapy. *Mar. Drugs* **2023**, *21*, 128. https://doi.org/10.3390/md21020128

Academic Editors: Celso Alves and Marc Diederich

Received: 31 December 2022
Revised: 5 February 2023
Accepted: 11 February 2023
Published: 15 February 2023

Copyright: © 2023 by the authors. Licensee MDPI, Basel, Switzerland. This article is an open access article distributed under the terms and conditions of the Creative Commons Attribution (CC BY) license (https://creativecommons.org/licenses/by/4.0/).

1. Introduction

Fucoidans are proving to be promising pharmaceutical agents, widely cited as exhibiting antitumor, immunomodulatory (immunopotentiating), anti-inflammatory, and other pharmacological properties [1–8]. These extracts contain exceedingly large amounts of vitamins and minerals, and, therefore, for many years, they have been used as safe dietary supplements to support and improve human immunity [9]. Fucoidan extracts, as soluble dietary fibers, play critical roles in providing nourishment with therapeutic benefits in the prevention of disease and cancer treatment [3,9]. Due to the medicinal benefits of fucoidans, they have been used successfully as a natural source of iodine to treat thyroid complaints in several Asian and Western countries [10]. Although registered as a Food and Drug

Administration (FDA)-approved safe food supplement with multiple beneficial effects, the FDA has not approved therapeutic fucoidan products for clinical use. The underlying problems and obstacles associated with the clinical use of fucoidan(s) is discussed in this review, with particular focus on the immunopotentiating activity of fucoidans and their relevance to cancer immunotherapy.

Fucoidans were first isolated from the extracellular mucus matrix of brown macroalgae, class Phaeophycceae, species *Fucus vesiculosus, Asophyllum nodosum, Laminaria digiata,* and *Laminaria saccharina,* in 1913, by the Swedish professor Hareld Kylin at Uppsala University [11–13]. The name fucoidan was initially used as a general term referring to a variety of high-molecular weight sulfated polysaccharides derived from fibrillar cell walls and mucous matrices of diverse species of brown macroalgae [14]. Until relatively recently, the International Union of Pure and Applied Chemistry (IUPAC) based the fucoidan nomenclature on the generic sulfated fucan structure—a polysaccharide with a backbone structure based on sulfated L-fucose residues, with the main structure consisting of a minimum of 10 monosaccharides [15]. Hence, the names fucoidan, fucoidans, and sulfated fucans have been used synonymously in the literature, distinct from fucans and fucosans. Recently, in 2017, the term fucoidan(s) from brown algae was revised, and now is clearly established to refer to heteropolymers with more diverse backbones [14].

The bioactivities of these versatile marine-origin heteropolysaccharides differ depending on the seaweed species and environmental growth conditions. There are approximately 250 genera and 1500–2000 species of brown algae, and chemical composition, structure of fucoidans, and bioactivity differ from species to species [16]. Fucoidan extracts from various species of brown seaweed consist of different amounts of monosaccharide compositions, including fucose, mannose, galactose, glucose, and xylose [17]. The proportion of these monosaccharides within each fucoidan influences its capability to induce a particular pharmacological activity. For example, *Fucus vesiculosus* fucoidan shows a strong 1,1-diphenyl-2-picrylhydrazyl (DPPH) radical scavenging activity [17] and *Ascophyllum nodosum* fucoidan promotes T cell proliferation [18]. Hence, it is important to be aware that the source of a fucoidan plays a critical role in inducing its pharmacological activities, and, therefore, throughout this review we have identified the source, molecular weight of the fucoidan, and subsequent fraction isolates when it has been specified in the literature. Methods of extraction are also major factors affecting the structural composition and bioactive properties of fucoidans both within and between brown algae species (discussed in Section 2).

All these factors mentioned contribute to the difficulty in determining the type of fucoidan and the effective dose of a specific fucoidan for use in preclinical and clinical studies. Fucoidan derivatives or variants, where the molecular weight of fucoidan has been substantially reduced to as little as two or three monosaccharides, have been shown to lack the immune ability (activation) of a high molecular weight fucoidan (HMWF) [19]. Highly purified fucoidan fractions, defined as low molecular weight fucoidans (LMWFs), also fall below the standard IUPAC definition of a fucoidan with reduced or altered bioactivity. Hence, the molecular weight and bioactivity of fucoidans and their variants used in preclinical studies influence efficacy and are important discussion points in this review.

Cancer immunotherapy, including immune checkpoint inhibitors (ICI) and adoptive T cell transfer therapy (such as CAR-T cell therapy), has revolutionized cancer treatment and achieved an unprecedented clinical outcome in the treatment of homological malignancies. However, significant challenges remain ahead in the treatment of solid tumors using these approaches. Effective treatment of solid tumor requires preferential activation of CTL-mediated cytotoxicity against cancer cells. To overcome these seemingly intractable obstacles, more 'powerful' immune cells or CAR-T cells with enhanced antitumor efficacy are required [20]. To improve ICI efficacy, combinations with additional therapeutics, such as fucoidans, may be a viable approach [18]. Fucoidans are natural polysaccharides that have antitumor properties and immunopotentiating effects with low toxicity in both animal models and humans. These polysaccharides are strong agonists of TLR4, which induces the activation of DCs in humans. Therefore, fucoidans could be desirable candidates for use in enhancing cancer immunotherapy [21].

Although fucoidans are promising antitumor candidates in cancer therapy, their efficacy will be highly dependent on the species type and the extraction methods of the fucoidan compounds. Fucoidans as adjuvants have been found to enhance the efficacy of ICIs in the treatment of melanoma [18,22] and metastatic lung cancer [23]. As such, fucoidans, used in combination with other cancer immunotherapy drugs, have made significant progress in the field of cancer. In clinical studies, fucoidan (*Undaria pinnatifida*), co-administered with 20 mg of tamoxifen to treat patients with breast cancer, demonstrated increased treatment efficacy and adverse effects were not detected (ACTRN12615000673549) [24], suggesting that fucoidans could be co-administered with other hormonal therapeutic drugs and act as efficacious adjuvants. However, detailed immunomodulatory mechanisms of fucoidans are elusive and have not been fully elucidated. Hence, this review aims to provide comprehensive information on the immunomodulatory mechanisms of fucoidans, including the association between fucoidan and inflammatory cytokines and signaling pathways to emphasize the potential of fucoidans in modern cancer immunotherapies. Finally, we discuss current clinical studies and the clinical efficacy of fucoidans in cancer treatments, especially focusing on cancer immunotherapy.

2. Overview of Fucoidans

2.1. Structural Characteristics of Fucoidans

The structure and composition of fucoidans vary depending on the source [25], marine species [8,14,25–30], harvest season [6,31], and extraction methods (Table 1) [6,29,31]. When harvested from various sources and species at different times of the year, fucoidans have been shown to have distinct structural characteristics [14,25–30], and the compositional properties are often varied when derived using different extraction methods, which have been extensively reviewed in several species [14,25–30]. In particular, extraction methods and sources are the two critical factors that influence the proportions of monosaccharides contained within different fucoidan extracts (Table 1) [32–34], leading to the inducement of different immune activities. For example, previous studies have shown that fucoidan extracts from *Ecklonia cava, Ascophyllum nodosum, Undaria pinnatifida, Laminaria japonica*, and *Fucus vesiculosus* induced T cell activation [23], promoted T cell proliferation [18], dendritic cell (DC) maturation [35], macrophages [36], and activation of natural killer cells (NK), respectively. Although fucoidans have no universal structure, the fucoidan extracted from *Fucus vesiculosus*, known as bladderwrack, has the most straightforward and typical fucoidan chemical structure among all species of brown seaweed. Patankar et al. (1993) reported that fucoidan derived from *Fucus vesiculosus* has a base of repeating $\alpha(1\rightarrow3)$-linked α-L-fucopyranose units with a substituted sulfate group at the C-4 position on the chain and fucose enabling branching points within the chain [29,37,38]. Subsequently, two additional structural models of fucoidan have been reported: (1) an alternated $(1\rightarrow4)$-linked α-L-fucopyranose units [29,34,39,40]; (2) an alternated $(1\rightarrow3)$ and $\alpha(1\rightarrow4)$-linked sulfated L-fucopyranose [4,29,40–42]. As previously mentioned, fucoidans are heteropolysaccharides that consist primarily of abundant L-fucose residues and sulfate groups, but they also contain traces of monomers, such as galactose, uronic acid, xylose, mannose, glucose, and glucuronic acid [12,29,39,41–44]. Previous characterization demonstrated variations in monosaccharide composition, molecular weight, types of glycosidic linkages, the presence of branching, and the degree of sulfation [32,43,45,46]. The importance of understanding these structural and compositional variations is that they can have varying impacts on therapeutic effects in cancer treatment and other inflammatory-based diseases.

The pharmacological effects of fucoidan vary with their molecular weight. Although the IUPAC definition of fucoidan is a minimum of 10 monosaccharides, fractional derivatives are commonly used to assess fucoidan bioactivity [47]. Fucoidans are usually classified as being either a low molecular weight fucoidan (LMWF) or high molecular weight fucoidan (HMWF), as the pharmacological effects of fucoidans vary with their molecular weight. Generally, LMWF refers to molecular weight < 10 kDa, while HMWF refers to a fucoidan with a molecular weight > 10,000 kDa, and medium molecular weight is 10–10,000 kDa [33,48]. However, other standards of classification are also used. For example, HMWF means a fucoidan with an average molecular weight of 300 kDa or more, while a fucoidan with an average MW < 300 kDa is considered LMWF [49].

Table 1. Fucoidans from various algae.

Name of Algae	Place of Collection	Extraction Method	Yield (%)	Monosaccharide Composition (%)	Molecular Weight (kDa)	Ref.
Ascophyllum nodosum	ND	Acid hydrolysis, centrifugal partition, chromatography.	ND	Fuc: ND.	ND.	[50]
Cladosiphon navae-caledoniae	Daiichi Sangyo Corporation (Osaka, Japan)	ND	HMWF: 85, LMWF: 72	ND LMWF: Fuc: 73, xyl: 12, man: 7	LMWF: <500.	[33]
Fucus serratus, Fucus vesiculosus, Ascophyllum nodosum	Coast of Aberystwyth at low tide, UK	$CaCl_2$ extraction	6.0 wt, 9.8 wt, 8.0 wt	fuc:18–28 wt, sulphate: 30–40 wt; fuc: 26–39 wt, sulphate: 9–35 wt; fuc: 35–46 wt, sulphate: 6–22 wt.	1608; 1364 1374	[31]
Fucus vesiculosus	Purchased from Sigma	ND	ND	Fuc: 97, gal: ND, xyl: ND.	100	[37]
Fucus vesiculosus	Fucoidan extract 1 (FE1): from Marinova; FE2 and FE3 from Sigma-Aldrich	ND	FE1: 52.5 FE2: 52.2 FE3: 50.5	FE1: Fuc: 73.1, xyl: 8.0, man: 1.3, gal: 3.5, glu: 0.7. FE2: Fuc: 79.1 xyl: 3.9, man: 0.8, gal: 5.5, glu: 0.8. FE3: Fuc: 71.2, xyl: 5.3, man: 1.5, gal: 5.4, glu: 1.3.	FE1: 91 FE2: 60 FE3: 42	[32]
Fucus evanescens	Littoral of Iturup island (Kuril Islands)	$CaCl_2$ extraction	Fraction F1: 3.9, Fraction F2: 2.6, Fraction F3: 21.4, Fraction F4: 47.4 Fraction F5: 4.5	F1: fuc: 35.4, xyl: 6.1, man: 0.8, glu: 4.0. F2: fuc: 10.7, xyl: 17.4, gal: 3.0, man: 3.7, glu: 1.1. F3: fuc: 33.2, xyl:8.1, gal:4.5, man: 3.5 F4: fuc: 58.7, xyl: 1.6, gal: 1.6. F5: fuc: 34.0, xyl: 3.8, gal: 3.4.	ND.	[51]
Laminaria Saccharina, Laminaria digitata, Cladosiphon okamuranus, Fucus evanescens, Fucus vesiculosus, Fucus serratus, Fucus distichus, Fucus spiralis, Ascophyllum nodosum	ND	$CaCl_2$ extraction	ND	Fuc: 36.7 (*w*/*w*), xyl: 1.2 (*w*/*w*), man: 1.0 (*w*/*w*), glu: 2.2 (*w*/*w*), gal: 4.6 (*w*/*w*). Fucose: 30.1 (*w*/*w*), xyl: 1.9 (*w*/*w*), man: 1.7 (*w*/*w*), glu: 1.4 (*w*/*w*), gal: 6.3 (*w*/*w*). Fuc: 30.9 (*w*/*w*), xyl: 0.7 (*w*/*w*), glu: 2.2 (*w*/*w*). Fuc: 58.7 (*w*/*w*), xyl: 1.6 (*w*/*w*), gal: 1.6 (*w*/*w*). Fuc: 26.1 (*w*/*w*), xyl: 2.4 (*w*/*w*), man: 3.1 (*w*/*w*), glu: 2.2 (*w*/*w*), gal: 5.0 (*w*/*w*). Fuc: 24.8 (*w*/*w*), xyl: 2.4 (*w*/*w*), man: 2.1 (*w*/*w*), glu: 2.0 (*w*/*w*), gal: 4.8 (*w*/*w*). Fuc: 40.8 (*w*/*w*), xyl: 0.8 (*w*/*w*), gal: 0.8 (*w*/*w*). Fuc: 33.0 (*w*/*w*), xyl: 2.8 (*w*/*w*), man: 1.4 (*w*/*w*), glu: 1.2 (*w*/*w*), gal: 3.0 (*w*/*w*). Fuc: 26.6 (*w*/*w*), xyl: 4.4 (*w*/*w*), man: 2.6 (*w*/*w*), glu: 1.1 (*w*/*w*), gal: 4.7 (*w*/*w*).	200–500	[34]

Table 1. *Cont.*

Name of Algae	Place of Collection	Extraction Method	Yield (%)	Monosaccharide Composition (%)	Molecular Weight (kDa)	Ref.
Laminaria hyperborea	ND	ND	ND	Fuc: 97.8, gal: 2.2, glu: ND.	469.2	[45]
Undaria pinnatifida	Great Barrier Island, Port Underwood New Zealand	$CaCl_2$ extraction	Increased from July (25.4–26.3) to September (57.3–69.9).	Crude fucoidan (F0): L-fuc: 39.24, D-gal: 26.48, D-xyl: 28.85, D-man: 5.04, α-D-glu: 0.95. Commercial fucoidan: L-fuc: 87.12, D-gal: 5.69, D-xyl: 4.85, D-man: 1.39, α-D-glu: 0.94. Fucoidan fraction F1: L-fuc: 48.51, D-gal: 37.86, D-xyl: 3.74, D-man: 6.97, α-D-glu: 2.91. F2: L-fuc: 53.21, D-gal: 42.12, D-xyl: 1.15, D-man: 2.24, α-D-glu: 1.28. F3: L-fuc: 59.71, D-gal: 28.74, D-xyl: 1.58, D-man: 7.19 α-D-glu: 2.77.	F0: 171 F1: 81 F2: 22 F3: 27	[6]
Undaria pinnatifida	Five fucoidans purchased from Sigma Aldrich, Anhui Minmetals Development I/E Co. Ltd., Matakana SuperFoods, Glycomix UK, and Leili Ltd	$CaCl_2$ extraction	*Undaria pinnatifida* fucoidan (S): ≥95, Crude fucoidan (S1): ND, S2: 75.5 S3: ND, S4: 75 S5: ND	Fucoidan(S): fuc: 27.44, gal: 25.34, Fraction S1: fuc: 19.50, gal: 21.20. Fraction S2: glu: 96.71, Fraction S3: fuc: 13.83, gal: 13.24. Fraction S4: fuc: 20.35, gal: 19.26 2.79. Fraction S5: fuc: 19.23, gal: 21.00, glu: 6.38.	S: 440 S1: 440–2000 S2: <2000 S3: 38.9–440 S4: 35.2–440 S5: >2	[52]
Undaria Pinnatifida	From Sigma Aldrich	$CaCl_2$ extraction	*Undaria pinnatifida* fucoidan: ≥95 LMWF: ND	ND.	ND LMWF: <10	[48]
Undaria Pinnatifida Fucus vesiculosus	Port Underwood, New Zealand	$CaCl_2$ extraction	Sporophyll derived from farm 327: 69, Sporophyll derived from farm 106: 57.28	Crude fucoidan (F0): fuc: 39.24, xyl: 28.85, gal: 26.48, man: 5.04, glu: 0.95, F1: fuc: 48.51, xyl: 3.74, gal: 37.86, man: 6.97, glu: 2.91. F2: fuc: 53.21, xyl: 1.15, gal: 42.12, man: 2.24, glu: 1.28. Fraction F: fuc: 59.71, xyl: 1.58, gal: 28.74, man: 7.19, glu: 2.77, Fucoidan (Sigma): fuc: 87.12, xyl: 4.85, gal: 5.69, man: 1.39, glu: 0.94.	F0: >150 F1: 81, F2: 22 F: 27 54	[53]

Abbreviations are as follows: ND, not detailed; HMWF, high molecular weight fucoidan; LMWF, low molecular weight fucoidan; gal, galactose; fuc, fucose; xyl, xylose; man, mannose; glu, glucose.

2.2. Pharmacological Actions of Fucoidans

Fucoidans have been shown to exhibit a variety of beneficial pharmacological effects, including antitumor [5,54–58], anti-inflammatory [3–5], immunomodulatory [4,5] antioxidant [6–8], anticoagulant [5,59–62], antithrombotic [5,63,64], antiangiogenic [5,56,65–69], and antiviral [70–75].

The antitumor effects of fucoidans have been extensively investigated in vitro in various tumor cell lines, especially in lung and breast cancer cell lines [1,76,77], and in vivo in animal models [78]. The antitumor mechanisms of fucoidans in these tumor cells (e.g., A549, MCF-7) include cell cycle arrest at the sub-G_1/G_1 phase [79–82], caspase-dependent apoptosis [80,81,83], regulation of specific apoptotic proteins (e.g., poly [ADP-ribose] polymerase 1 (PARP1) [84–86], protein kinase RNA-like endoplasmic reticulum kinase (PERK), B-cell lymphoma 2 (Bcl-2) [84], BAX [84,87], and caspases -3, -8, and -9 [80,84,86]). Increasing evidence has shown that fucoidans are capable of exhibiting direct and indirect inhibitory effects on tumor cells by regulating several important signaling pathways, such as extracellular signal-regulated kinase 1/2 (ERK1/2) [56,84,88], phosphoinositide 3-kinase-Akt (PI3K/Akt) [84,88], p38 mitogen-activated protein kinase (p38 MAPK) [84], and mammalian target of rapamycin (mTOR) pathways [87,88].

In the in vitro study by Miyamoto et al. (2009) [80], they found that fucoidan (*Cladosiphon okamuranus*) was cytotoxic to MCF-7 cells and resulted in a significant increase in the number of apoptotic MCF-7 cell bodies, with condensation of chromatin and DNA fragmentation at the sub-G_1 phase of the cell cycle [80]. They then demonstrated that cell cycle arrest at the sub-G_1 phase was accompanied by activation of caspases (caspase 7, -8, -9) and PARP cleavage in fucoidan-treated MCF-7 cells at a concentration of 1000 μg/mL [80]. These results suggest that fucoidan (*Cladosiphon okamuranus*) induces apoptosis through activating specific caspases (e.g., caspase-7, -8, -9) and interacts with apoptotic proteins (e.g., PARP) to induce apoptosis in MCF-7 cells at a high concentration (e.g., 1000 μg/mL). In another in vitro study, Zhang et al. showed that fucoidan (Mozuku, *Cladosiphon novaecaledoniae*) caused an accumulation of apoptotic MCF-7 cells at the G_1 phase of the cell cycle [79], and these apoptotic MCF-7 cells presented with shrunken nuclei and fragmented chromatin [79]. They found that fucoidan (Mozuku, *Cladosiphon novaecaledoniae*) was cytotoxic to MCF-7 cells and inhibited 60% of MCF-7 cell growth at a concentration of 820 μg/mL [79]. Banafa et al. showed, in vitro, that fucoidan (*Fucus vesiculosus*) could induce apoptosis in MCF-7 cells through inducing cell cycle arrest at the G_1 phase by downregulating the expression levels of cyclin D1 and CDK-4 in MCF-7 cells [83]. They also revealed that fucoidan (*Fucus vesiculosus*) could induce apoptosis by downregulating the anti-apoptotic protein of Bcl-2 and upregulating the pro-apoptotic protein of Bax in fucoidan-treated MCF-7 cells [83]. In addition, they demonstrated that treatment with fucoidan (*Fucus vesiculosus*) could activate caspase-8 and increase cytochrome C release in MCF-7 cells [83], supporting the theory that a caspase-dependent pathway may lead to apoptotic protein cleavage, such as Bid cleavage [83]. Furthermore, a more recent in vitro study by Abudabbus et al. (2017) showed that commercial fucoidan (*Fucus vesiculosus*) caused cell cycle arrest at the sub-G_1/G_1 phase with activation of caspases 3, -7, and -9 [81]. Overall, these results suggest that the fucoidan (e.g., *Cladosiphon novaecaledoniae*, *Fucus vesiculosus*)-induced apoptosis involves the activation of caspases (caspase 3, -7, -8, -9) and cell cycle arrest at the G_0/G_1 phase in MCF-7 cells.

The molecular weight of fucoidan also influences its potential to induce apoptosis in MCF-7 and MDA-MB-231 cell lines. In a recent in vitro study conducted by Lu et al. (2018), they demonstrated that a LMWF from New Zealand *Undaria pinnatifida* was cytotoxic and exhibited maximum anti-proliferative effects in both MCF-7 and MDA-MB-231 cells at concentrations of 200 μg/mL and 300 μg/mL, respectively [52]. They also demonstrated that this LMWF (New Zealand *Undaria pinnatifida*) significantly increased the total caspase in MDA-MB-231 cells at a concentration of 300 μg/mL [52]. Notably, the concentration of fucoidan used in the study was much lower than in the previous studies by Zhang et al. (2013) [89], Miyamoto et al. (2009) [80], and Banafa et al. (2013) [83]. Therefore, these results suggest that the effective concentration of fucoidan used to induce apoptosis in breast cancer cell lines (MCF-7, MDA-MB-231) varies significantly.

Regardless of the species of fucoidan, all fucoidans tested inhibited A549 cell growth and proliferation by adjusting their concentrations in both in vitro and in vivo studies. An in vitro study conducted by Boo et al. (2011) showed that fucoidan (*Undaria pinnatifida*) significantly inhibited A549 cell growth leading to the accumulation of apoptotic A549 cell bodies at the sub-G_1 phase of the cell cycle at a concentration of 200 μg/mL [84]. These apoptotic A549 cell bodies presented with chromatin condensation, membrane blebbing, and cell shrinkage [84]. Boo et al. (2011) also demonstrated that fucoidan (*Undaria pinnatifida*) could induce apoptosis by activating caspase-9, decreasing pro-caspase-3, and then inducing PARP cleavage in A549 cells at a concentration of 200 μg/mL [84]. Furthermore, they revealed that fucoidan-induced A549 cell apoptosis is also associated with downregulation of antiapoptotic Bcl-2 proteins and upregulation of pro-apoptotic BAX proteins at a concentration of 200 μg/mL [84]. In addition, they also demonstrated that fucoidan (*Undaria pinnatifida*) activated the ERK1/2 signaling pathway [84], whilst inhibiting the p38 MAPK and PI3K/Akt signaling pathways [84], suggesting that fucoidan (*Undaria pinnatifida*) induces apoptosis in A549 cells through regulating the MAPK-based signaling pathways (ERK1/2, p38 MAPK, and PI3K/Akt). In particular, this was the first in vitro study in which researchers confirmed that fucoidan-induced apoptosis is associated with the regulation of apoptotic proteins (e.g., PARP, Bcl-2, Bax), signaling pathways (e.g., ERK1/2, p38 MAPK, PI3K/Akt), and specific caspases (e.g., caspase-9, pro-caspase-3) in A549 cells [84]. Similarly, an in vitro study by Hsu et al. (2017) demonstrated that commercial fucoidan (*Fucus vesiculosus*) induced cell cycle arrest at the sub-G_1/G_1 phases by upregulating p21 gene expressions in A549 cells at a concentration of 200 μg/mL and induced apoptosis by activating PARP proteins and caspase-3 in A549 cells at a concentration of 400 μg/mL [86]. They also reported that the commercial fucoidan (*Fucus vesiculosus*) could induce apoptosis through inducing an ER stress response by activating the PERK/ATF4/CHOP pathways [86]. These results suggest that fucoidan induces A549 cell apoptosis not only through regulating apoptotic proteins (e.g., PARP, Bcl-2, Bax), genes (e.g., p21) and caspases (e.g., caspase-9 and -3), but also by regulating extrinsic signaling pathways, such as the PERK/ATF4/CHOP pathways.

Furthermore, similar results were also obtained in in vitro studies by Lee et al. (2012) and Hsu et al. (2018) [85]. Lee et al. (2012) demonstrated that commercial fucoidan (*Fucus vesiculosus*) inhibited cell proliferation of A549 cells at a concentration of 400 μg/mL [88], and Hsu et al. (2018) demonstrated that fucoidan treatment could significantly inhibit A549 cells at concentrations of 200 and 400 μg/mL (IC_{50} = 10 μM) [85]. Lee et al. (2012) found that commercial fucoidan (*Fucus vesiculosus*) could suppress MMP-2 activity, migration, and invasion of A549 cells at a concentration of 200 μg/mL, and also revealed that commercial fucoidan (*Fucus vesiculosus*) could inhibit MMP-2 expression, metastasis, and invasion by inhibiting phosphorylation levels of the ERK1/2 and PI3K-Akt-mTOR pathways and its downstream targets 4E-BP1 and p70S6K at a concentration of 200 μg/mL [88]. Thus, these results suggest that fucoidan inhibits the MMP-2 activity by regulating the ERK1/2 and/or PI3K-Akt pathways but may only partially involve the mTOR pathway. These results also indirectly indicate that commercial fucoidan (*Fucus vesiculosus*) inhibits A549 cell growth and proliferation by downregulating the PI3K-Akt-mTOR and ERK1/2 signaling pathways in a concentration range of 200–400 μg/mL. Furthermore, the in vitro study by Chen et al. (2021) also demonstrated that fucoidan inhibits A549 cell proliferation by decreasing the level of protein expression of p-mTOR and downstream proteins p-S6K, p-P70S6K, and p-4EBP1 in the mTOR pathway [87]. They also demonstrated that fucoidan induces apoptosis by reducing the expression levels of anti-apoptotic Bcl-2 proteins and increasing the expression levels of pro-apoptotic BAX proteins in A549 cells [87]. These results reinforce that fucoidan-induced apoptosis in A549 cells is associated with the balance of the Bcl-2/Bax ratio, and the regulation of the ERK1/2 and PI3K-Akt-mTOR pathways. Taken together, these results substantiate the theory that the balance of the apoptotic protein ratio and the activation of signaling pathways are essential for fucoidan to induce apoptosis in A549 tumor cells.

More importantly, the in vivo study by Chen et al. (2021) also demonstrated that fucoidan (*unknown source*) significantly inhibits the volumes and weights of A549 cells in xenograft mice after oral intake of fucoidan (25 mg/kg) for 14 days [87], and the expression value of Ki67 was also lower in the fucoidan-fed group than in the control group [87]. These results are consistent with a previous in vivo study conducted by Chen et al. (2016). This study also showed that fucoidan reduced approximately 23.3% and 40.3% of the mean tumor volume and weight at 0.5 mg/kg and 10 mg/kg, respectively, in the tumor xenograft model A549 [90], and also confirmed that the expression value of Ki67 was lower than in the control group [90]. These results support the theory that fucoidan directly induces A549 cell apoptosis in an in vivo model. The anti-inflammatory and immunomodulatory effects of fucoidan are interlinked with the antitumor effects. An overview of these effects is presented here, and a more detailed discussion is given in later sections. Upon exposure to pathogen-associated molecular patterns (PAMP), viruses and bacteria, innate (e.g., macrophages, dendritic cells (DC), natural killer (NK) cells), and adaptive immune cells (e.g., CD4+ helper and CD8+ cytotoxic T cells), are activated in response to inflammation [2,3]. The development of lung and breast carcinomas is associated with the activation of some vital pro-inflammatory biomarkers, including cytokines (e.g., TNF-α, IL-1, IL-6, IL-12), chemokines, cyclooxygenase-2 (COX-2), prostaglandins, C-reactive protein (CRP) [91], inducible nitric oxide synthase (iNOS) and nitric oxide (NO), which facilitate tumor initiation and progression [3,92]. Many previous studies have reported that fucoidan regulates these biomarkers and MAPK signaling pathways to induce anti-inflammatory and immunomodulatory effects in immune cells [18,23,93–97]. Furthermore, the upregulated expression of these biomarkers activates intrinsic and extrinsic signaling pathways, such as the NF-κB and MAPK pathways [3,98]. Therefore, regulating the expression of these pro-inflammatory biomarkers is critical to overall disease control and management.

Some studies demonstrating the anti-inflammatory effects of fucoidans are presented here for discussion. In an in vitro study, Jeong et al. (2017) reported that fucoidan (*Fucus vesiculosus*) was non-cytotoxic to RAW264.7 murine macrophages at 100 µg/mL and attenuated the production of pro-inflammatory cytokines of TNF-α and IL-1β in RAW264.7 murine macrophages treated with liposaccharide (LPS) [96]. These results are consistent with the findings presented in a recent in vitro study where they showed that a particular fucoidan (*Saccharina japonica*) fraction (LJSF4) induced a strong inhibitory effect on the production of pro-inflammatory cytokines, including TNF-α, IL-1β, and IL-6 [97]. These results strengthen the argument that fucoidan, regardless of its species derivation, has the ability to induce anti-inflammatory effects in RAW264.7 macrophages. Furthermore, Lee et al. (2012) found that three *Ecklonia cava* fucoidan fractions (F_1, F_2, F_3) were not toxic to the RAW 264.7 macrophages at a concentration of 12.5–100 µg/mL and could significantly inhibit NO production, iNOS, COX-2 mRNA expression level, and pro-inflammatory cytokines (TNF-α, IL-1β, and IL-6) in LPS-treated RAW264.7 macrophages [99], where the F_3 fraction had the highest inhibitory effects on NO production [99]. These results suggest that there may be an association between the inhibition of the iNOS/NO pathway and attenuation of pro-inflammatory cytokines (TNF-α, IL-1β, and IL-6), but more studies are required to verify whether there is a connection between these two stimuli. Furthermore, the investigations by Fernando et al. (2017) also showed similar results; they found that the F2,4 fraction (*Chnoospora minima* fucoidan) was non-cytotoxic to LPS-treated RAW264.7 macrophages and exhibited a maximum inhibition in NO production, while the mRNA expression of pro-inflammatory cytokines (TNF-α, IL-1β, IL-6) was decreased in LPS-treated RAW264.7 macrophages at a concentration of 50 µg/mL [100]. Sanjeewa et al. (2018) reported that the *Sargassum horneri* fucoidan f4 fraction (36.86% fuc and 18.47% sulfate contents) exhibited the maximum inhibitory effects on NO production and significantly inhibited the mRNA expression levels of the pro-inflammatory cytokines of TNF-α and the PEG_2 enzyme in LPS-treated RAW264.7 murine macrophages without causing any toxicities [101], but only slightly inhibited IL-6 production [101]. They also demonstrated that the f4 fraction could dose-dependently inhibit the expression of the iNOS and COX-2 proteins [101], as well as inhibit the phosphorylation of IκB-α and p-I κB-α [101]. These results suggest that the *Sargassum horneri* fucoidan f4 fraction induces anti-inflammatory effects in LPS-treated RAW264.7 macrophages through the NF-κB pathway [101].

Sanjeewa et al. (2017) demonstrated that a crude fucoidan extracted from *Sargassum horneri* had no cytotoxicity to RAW264.7 murine macrophages and exhibited a maximum suppressive effect on NO production in LPS-treated RAW264.7 murine macrophages [102]; it also reduced the secretion of pro-inflammatory cytokines TNF-α and IL-1β and downregulated the expression levels of iNOS and COX-2 proteins in RAW264.7 murine macrophages treated with LPS [102]. More importantly, they also showed that CCP fucoidan (*Sargassum horneri*) (100 μg/mL) induced anti-inflammatory effects in RAW264.7 murine macrophages treated with LPS by inhibiting the translocation of NF-κB p50 and p65 to the nucleus and downregulation of phosphorylation of p38 and ERK1/2 that was shown to increase with LPS stimulation in RAW264.7 macrophages [102].

Fucoidan has also been shown to act as a pro-inflammatory cytokine modulator in other types of cells, including mesenchymal stem cells (MSCs) [103], THP-1 monocytes [104], human peripheral blood mononuclear cells (PBMC) [105], porcine peripheral blood polymorphonuclear cells (PMN) [106], and human intestinal epithelial cells (Caco-2 cells) [107], indicating that fucoidan is capable of inducing anti-inflammatory effects in a broad range of cells. In an earlier in vitro study, Hwang et al. (2016) reported that LMWF (*Sargassum hemiphyllum*) induced anti-inflammatory effects in Caco-2 cells by downregulating LPS-induced TNF-α and IL-1β [107], which is in line with the findings from another in vitro study conducted by Ahmad et al. (2021) [105]; they demonstrated that fucoidan (*Undaria pinnatifida*) induced significant inhibitory effects on the pro-inflammatory cytokines of TNF-α and IL-6 in LPS-treated human PBMC cells [105]. However, the expression of IL-1β was only slightly reduced in this study [105], suggesting that fucoidan (*Undaria pinnatifida*) is less effective in reducing the expression of IL-1β in LPS-treated human PBMC cells as compared to the potency of the other two pro-inflammatory cytokines, namely TNF-α and IL-6. Furthermore, they also showed that fucoidan (*Fucus vesiculosus*) significantly inhibited three pro-inflammatory cytokines, namely TNF-α, IL-1β, and IL-6, in LPS-treated human PBMC [105]. Taken together, these results support the theory that *Fucus vesiculosus* fucoidan has a greater capability than *Undaria pinnatifida* fucoidan to exhibit inhibitory effects on pro-inflammatory cytokines, namely TNF-α, IL-1β, and IL-6, in LPS-treated human PBMC cells. It also indirectly indicates that *Fucus vesiculosus* fucoidan may have a greater cytotoxic level than *Undaria pinnatifida* fucoidan in LPS-treated human PBMC cells. *Macrocystis pyrifera* fucoidan and fractionated *Macrocystis pyrifera* fucoidan (5–30 kDa) also significantly inhibited pro-inflammatory cytokines TNF-α in LPS-treated THP-1 cells [105]. Furthermore, Kim et al. (2018) reported that fucoidan has a negative effect on inhibiting the production of TNF-α in PBMC [106]; this was found in the process of suppressing excessive phagocytosis of porcine peripheral blood PMN [106]. However, the mRNA expression level of TNF-α was reduced by adding fucoidan to LPS-stimulated PBMCs [106]. These results are in line with those reported in MSCs [103], they found that after coculture of MSCs treated with fucoidan with LPS-stimulated macrophages, the level of pro-inflammatory cytokines of TNF-α decreased, suggesting that MSCs treated with fucoidan are capable of inhibiting the production of TNF-α in LPS-stimulated macrophages. Another important in vitro study designed three fucoidan/chitosan nanoparticles for the topical delivery of methotrexate [104]. To assess the anti-inflammatory effect of this compound, Barbosa et al. (2019) characterized the fucoidan/chitosan (F/C) nanoparticles into three groups based on the weight ratio of fucoidan and chitosan, named 1F/1C, 3F/1C, and 5F/1C [104]. According to their findings, the 5F/1C nanoparticle contained a large amount of fucoidan and showed the highest inhibitory effects on the production of pro-inflammatory cytokines, namely TNF-α, IL-1, and IL-6, in human THP-1 monocytes [104], suggesting that the fucoidan content in the 5F/1C nanoparticle plays an important role in inducing anti-inflammatory effects in human

THP-1 monocytes. These outcomes allow us to envisage the possibility of fucoidan being used as an anti-inflammatory agent in the treatment of inflammatory diseases, especially when developed as a nanoparticle.

All these results further strengthen the concept that fucoidan may induce its anti-inflammatory effects by inhibiting pro-inflammatory cytokine secretion and mRNA expression levels of pro-inflammatory cytokines (TNF-α, IL-1β, and IL-6) in LPS-stimulated immune cells including RAW264.7 murine macrophages [96,97,99,101,102,108], Caco-2 cells [107], THP-1 cells [105], human PBMC, porcine peripheral blood PMNs, and MSCs. More importantly, macrophages appear to play an essential role in the initial stages of the anti-inflammatory effects of fucoidan. However, Obluchinskaya et al. (2022) demonstrated that *Fucus vesiculosus* fucoidan extracts (FV1 and FV3) containing a high polyphenol content (135.9 PhE/g DW) induced a greater radical scavenging activity than four other seaweeds (*Saccharina japonica, Fucus distichus, Fucus serratus,* and *Ascophyllum nodosum*) [17], suggesting that the chemical composition in fucoidans may also influence its capability to induce anti-inflammatory effects.

Fucoidan antioxidant effects have been shown to prevent disruptions caused by the excessive accumulation of amyloid-β and reactive oxygen species (ROS) in the human body [109]. Several previous in vitro studies have demonstrated that fucoidans can act as ROS scavengers by removing free hydroxyl radicals and superoxide radicals [110,111]. The antithrombotic and anticoagulant effects of fucoidans are demonstrated primarily by prolonged activated partial thromboplastic time (APTT), prothrombin time (PT), and thrombin time (TT) [60], indicating that fucoidans can exhibit inhibitory effects on several intrinsic factors (e.g., II, V, VIII, IX, XI, XII) and extrinsic pathways to induce antithrombotic and anticoagulant effects in in vitro studies [62,109]. Fucoidans have also been shown to help relieve symptoms of various viral diseases, including severe acute respiratory syndrome coronavirus 2 (SRAS-CoV-2) [75], I-type influenza virus [73], human immunodeficiency virus 1 (HIV-1) [70], and herpes simplex virus (HSV) [72], by inhibiting virus attachment to host cells or directly inhibiting specific viral-related antigen productions. Fucoidans have also been shown to inhibit angiogenesis by regulating vascular endothelial growth factors (VEGF), fibroblast growth factor 2 (FGF-2), matrix metalloproteinases (MMPs), and chemokines (e.g., CXCL12) [67,109].

2.3. Pharmacokinetics of Fucoidans

The absorption of fucoidans is dependent on their source and structure. Several studies have investigated fucoidan absorption using the ELISA method and suggested that the molecular weight of a fucoidan may influence its absorption and excretion [112]. However, this observation is not entirely consistent with those obtained from other relevant in vivo and human clinical studies [113–120]. They suggested that the dosage, species, and structure of a fucoidan would also contribute to the variation in absorption and elimination [113–117]. Zhao et al. reported that oral administered LMWF (*Laminaria japonica*) reached the highest concentration in rat plasma at 15 h [113], which was faster than LMWF (*Laminaria japonica*, MW = 35 kDa) at the same oral dose [113]. The results suggest that the molecular weight of fucoidan below 10 kDa with a high oral dose would help to increase the absorbed amount of fucoidan in a relatively short timeframe (15 h vs. 25 h). It also indicated that the molecular weight of fucoidan ranging from 10–40 kDa has a long absorption time in rat plasma. Others showed that oral administration of LMWF (*Laminaria japonica*) in rat plasma reached the C_{max} in under 2 h [114,115], which has a shorter absorption time after oral administration. When Zhao et al. (2016) used a higher oral dose of fucoidan (oral dose = 400 mg/kg and 800 mg/kg) in rats, the time to take to reach C_{max} was much longer. Thus, the oral dose of LMWF could also be a critical factor affecting the pharmacokinetics of fucoidan in rats. Furthermore, Pozharitskaya et al. demonstrated that the fucoidan concentration (*Fucus vesiculosus*), in the plasma of rats reached a maximum level (0.125 μg/g) at 4 h after intragastric administration. These results were not entirely consistent with those obtained from human clinical studies. A human study showed that the plasma concentration of fucoidan (*Cladosiphon okamuranus*, molecular weight = 66 kDa, dose = 1 g) reached the maximum level in 7 out of 10 samples (serum: up to 100 ng/mL) at 6 h after 1 g of fucoidan administered to healthy volunteers, and only one sample reached the highest concentration (approximately 62 ng/mL) at 9 h [116]. These results indicate that the human intestinal absorption rate of fucoidan varies between individuals. They also found that the concentration of fucoidan was elevated in urine (up to 1000 ng/mL) after oral administration [116], but the molecular weight of fucoidan was reduced to 1.8–3.1 kDa in urine [116]. These results indicate that orally administered LMWF has a higher absorption and elimination rate than intragastrical administered HMWF, suggesting that the molecular weight of fucoidan could be a critical factor influencing the pharmacokinetics of fucoidan in the body. Fucoidan species is less likely to be a factor affecting the pharmacokinetics of fucoidan, suggesting that LMWF from *Fucus vesiculosus* or *Cladosiphon okamuranus* is capable of being developed and used for therapeutic purposes.

The pharmacokinetics of fucoidan is also influenced by the route of administration. A LMWF (*Laminaria japonica,*) reached the C_{max} (110.53 μg/mL) in 5 min after I.V. injection [118], but oral administered LMWF (*Laminaria japonica,*) was detected at 2 h after intragastric administration [118]. Similar results were also obtained from a recent study by Bai et al. (2020); they demonstrated that the fluorescein isothiocyanate labeled (FITC) fucoidan (*Fucus vesiculosus*, MW = 107.8 kDa, I.V. injection dose = 50 mg/kg) reached the C_{max} (66.37 μg/g) in mouse plasma at 30 min and was not detectable in the blood after 4 h [120]. They also showed that FITC fucoidan could circulate to other organs in mice, such as the lung (C_{max} = 110.92 μg/g at 4 h), liver (C_{max} = 284.7 μg/g at 0.5 h), spleen (C_{max} = 77.79 μg/g at 6 h), and kidney (C_{max} = 1092.31 μg/g at 4 h) [120]. Data on pharmacokinetics in humans is still limited.

2.4. Biomedical Usages of Fucoidans

Fucoidans are important pharmaceutical candidates in cancer therapy because of their high nutritional and biomedical value. Fucoidans have been classified as a dietary supplement that is generally recognized as safe by the FDA and is recognized as a safe food ingredient [42,121,122]. Prior to becoming an FDA-approved food supplement in 2017 and commercially available on the market, seaweed has been widely used as a functional food and as an established ingredient in local cuisine in several Asian countries, including China, Japan, and Korea [55]. During the 16th to 18th centuries, seaweed was discovered to have medicinal benefits in the treatment of goiter, psoriasis, asthma, several thyroid deficiencies, and skin diseases in China, France, and the United States [10]. In addition, fucoidan derived from *Fucus vesiculosus* has been used in a variety of combination products in European countries, including (1) homeopathic medical products in Austria; (2) laxatives in Belgium and Poland; (3) an authorized iodine supplement in Denmark; (4) an adjuvant in slimming diets in France, Spain, and the United Kingdom, and (5) as a traditional herbal remedy to treat obesity and rheumatic pain in the United Kingdom [10]. Fucoidan, as a nutritional supplement, is administered primarily through oral tablets and liquid administration. On the other hand, fucoidan is currently used as an ingredient in cosmetic and nutraceutical products.

3. Immunopotentiating Effects of Fucoidans

Fucoidan was first observed to support the immune response in the early 1980s [123]. The effect of fucoidans on immune potentiation emerged in the 1990s [124,125]. Over the past two decades, research into the immunomodulatory (immunopotentiating) effects of fucoidans has expanded significantly.

3.1. Overall Effects of Fucoidans on the Immune System

Fucoidans have now been shown to have immunopotentiating effects on both the adaptive and innate immune response (Figure 1). The immunopotentiating effects of fucoidan have been identified in studies using T cells [2,126,127], macrophages [2,36,128], DC (DCs) [94,127], and natural killer cells (NK) [72,127,129,130]. Toll-like receptors (TLRs) and scavenger receptor type A (SR-A) receptors are the two critical controllers in fucoidan-activated DCs [35,131,132]. Pro-inflammatory cytokines, such as TNF-α, IFN-γ, and interleukin 6 (IL-6), have been proposed as a mechanism to regulate fucoidan-activated macrophages and NK cells to induce antitumor immunity dependent on dose and molecular weight [35,95,133].

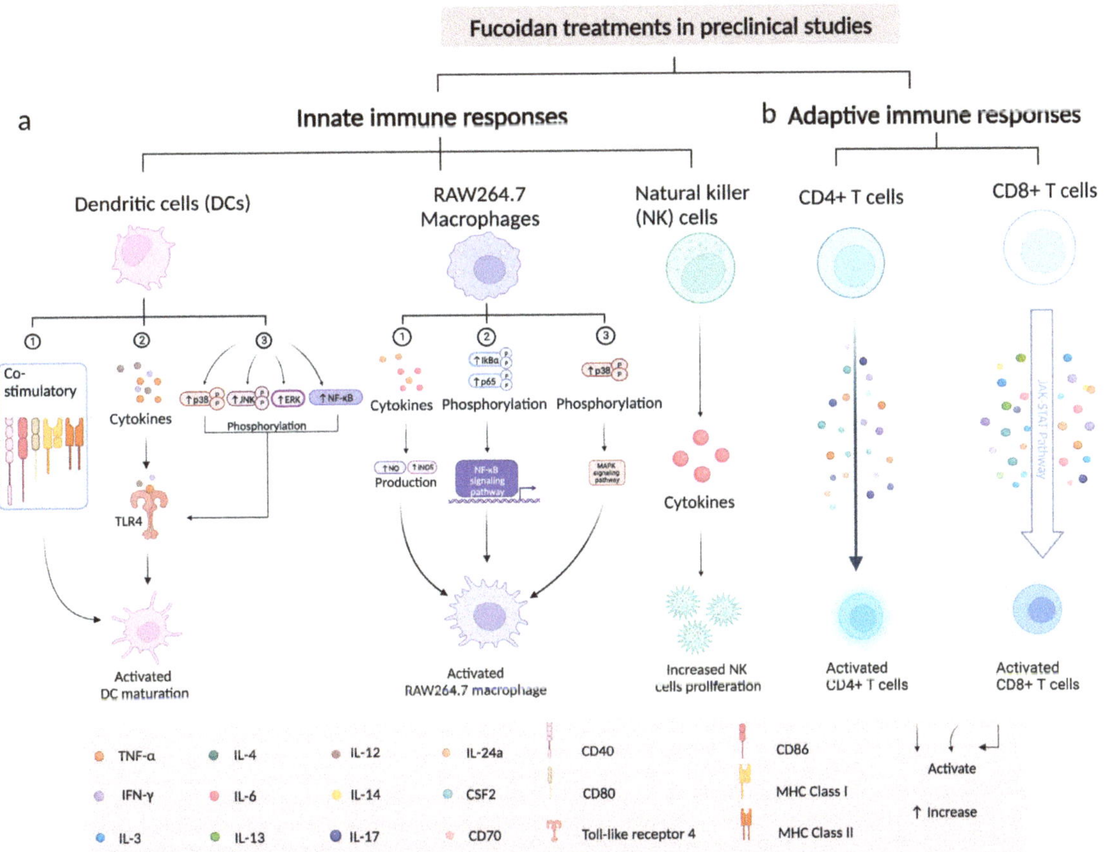

Figure 1. Effects of fucoidans on different types of immune cells. (**a**) Effect of fucoidans on innate immune responses through DC, RAW264.7 murine macrophages, and NK cells; (**b**) effect of fucoidans on adaptive immune responses via CD4+ and CD8+ T cells (this figure was created with BioRender.com, accessed on 5 February 2023).

3.2. Immunological Effect of Fucoidans on T Cells

Fucoidan immunomodulatory effects are preferentially studied using T cells, particularly when investigating its antitumor immunity. However, studies investigating the direct effect of fucoidans on T cells are relatively limited. So far, there has been no study examining the effect of fucoidan on CAR-T cells.

Fucoidan antitumor immune responses have been studied in both in vivo and in vitro models [4,94,132,134]. When co-cultured CD8+ T cells and human breast cancer cells (MCF-7) were used to investigate the immune response of fucoidan, it was discovered that the number of CD8+ T cells and interferon-γ (IFN-γ) was doubled in the fucoidan-treated group compared to the control [93]. However, when NY-ESO-1-specific CD8+ T cells were stimulated by fucoidan (*Fucus vesiculosus*)-treated DCs, interferon-γ (IFN-γ) secretion was higher than in the CD8+ T cells group [93], suggesting that fucoidan can activate NY-ESO-1-specific CD8 + T cells by increasing IFN-γ production. Similar results were also obtained from a separate study, which demonstrated that fucoidan promotes both CD4+ and CD8+ T cell responses by upregulating the pro-inflammatory cytokines of Th1 and Tc1 cells, namely IFN-γ and TNF-α [94]. However, because this immune response depends on IL-12 production, fucoidan may be able to enhance Th1 and Tc1 immune responses if it increases IL-12 production in the presence of Th1 and Tc1 cells. Furthermore, this study also demonstrated that fucoidan could be used as an adjuvant to enhance T cell responses by upregulating the production of IFN-γ, as well as increasing CD44+ CD4 cell and memory T cell proliferation [94]. These findings suggest that fucoidan induces direct immune responses in CD4 and CD8 T cells acting as an adjuvant to boost T cell immune responses.

Yang et al. demonstrated that fucoidans from *Ascophyllum nodosum* and *Fucus vesiculosus* directly promote T cell proliferation and activation through upregulating IFN-γ and TNF-α secretion in CD8+ T cell populations [18]. Furthermore, gene set enrichment analysis (GSEA) revealed that some representative genes within the JAK/STAT pathway were increased in the fucoidan treatment group, including IL-3, IL-6, IL-13, IL-14, IL-24a, CSF2, and CD70 indicating that fucoidan improves CD8+ T cell activation and proliferation via the JAK/STAT pathway [18]. More importantly, they found that the T cell receptor (TCR) complex played a critical role in promoting the activation and proliferation of CD8+ T cells and that it interacted with the TCR/CD3 complex to enhance T cell activation [18], which has a significant advantage in the discovery of new molecular mechanisms of fucoidan-induced immunomodulatory effects. These results are partially consistent with another study in which the treatment with intranasal fucoidan (*Ecklonia cava*) treatment increased the level of IFN-γ and TNF-α in mLN CD8 and CD4 T cells in both C57BL/6 and BALB/c micc [23]. This study explored a new route of administration of fucoidan in mice whilst also showing that fucoidan (*Ecklonia cava)* can activate T cells and enhance T cell proliferation by increasing the production levels of IFN-γ and TNF-α [23]. Lee et al. showed that *Undaria pinnatifida* fucoidan-rich extract significantly increased CD4+ and CD8+ T cells proliferation in cyclophosphamide (CP)-treated immunosuppressed mice via increasing the expression levels of cytokines (IFN-γ, TNF-α) and plasma antibodies (TgM, total IgG) [135]. These results suggest that IFN-γ and TNF-α are the two critical effectors involved in fucoidan-induced immunological effects in CD4+ and CD8+ T cells, specifically in T cell activation and proliferation. In particular, this new discovery regarding the different effects of fucoidan administration needs to be further investigated, especially its immunomodulatory effects on T cells using the dominant fucoidan species, *Fucus vesiculosus*. Combined, these experimental results demonstrate that fucoidan has potent immunomodulatory effects on T cells.

Fucoidan can also induce indirect immune responses in T cells. LMWF (*Undaria pinnatifida*) has been shown to induce indirect immune responses in CD4+ and CD8+ T cells through DCs [35], as DCs treated with LMWF activated T cells and significantly increased CD4+ and CD8+ T cell proliferation, indicating that DCs treated with LMWF play a critical role in T cell activation and proliferation.

Table 2 summarizes the immune cells and cytokines involved in the mechanism of immunopotentiation of fucoidans.

Table 2. The immunomodulatory effects of fucoidans on different types of immune cells.

Fucoidan Sources	Immune Cells	Involved Cytokines	Research Methods	Effects of Fucoidan	Ref.
Fucus vesiculosus	CD4+ T cells, CD8+ T cells, dendritic cells	IFN-γ, TNF-α, IL-12, IL-6, IL-12p40	In vivo	Upregulated the production of IFN-γ and TNF-α in the presence of Th1 and Tc1 cells, to promotes CD8+ and CD4+ T cell responses. Induced maturation of DCs by upregulating TNF-α, IL-6, and IL-12p40 in spleen DCs. Increased the cell proliferation of CD44+ CD4 and memory T cells. Acts as an adjuvant to boost T cell immune responses.	[94]
Fucus Vesiculosus, Ascophyllum nodosum	CD4+ T cells, CD8+ T cells	IFN-γ, TNF-α, IL-3, IL-6, IL13, IL-14, L-24a, CSF2, CD70	In vivo, In vitro	Promoted T cell proliferation and activation through upregulating IFN-γ and TNF-α secretion in CD8+ T cell populations. Promoted T cell proliferation via the JAK/STAT pathway. Interacted with TCR/CD3 complexes to enhance T cell activation. Co-administration with PD-1 antibody reduced tumor size and weight in mice. Co-administration with PD-1 antibody increased the ratio of CD8+ and CD4+ T cells in the spleen.	[18]
Fucus vesiculosus	CD8+ T cells, dendritic cells	IFN-γ	In vivo	Increased the cell proliferation of CD8+ T cells and also upregulated the production of IFN-γ. Inhibited SR-A in DCs by increasing the binding of NY-ESO-1 to DCs. In co-culture fucoidan-treated DCs with CD8+ T cells, serum IFN-γ increased.	[93]
Ecklonia cava	CD8+ T cells, CD4+ T cells	IFN-γ, TNF-α	In vivo	Activated T cells and enhanced T cell proliferations by increasing serum IFN-γ and TNF-α. Co-administration with PD-1 antibody prolonged survival in metastatic lung cancer. Acted as an adjuvant to enhance the therapeutic efficacy of immunotherapy.	[23]
Undaria pinnatifida	CD8+ T cells, CD4+ T cells, dendritic cells, CD11b+ macrophages, CD3-CD19-CD49b+ NK cells	TNF-α, IL-12, IL-6, TLR4, CD40, CD86, MHC I, MHC II, ERK, JNK, p38, p-iκB, p-NF-κB p65	In vivo, In vitro	The LMWF-treated DCs activated T cells. The LMWF-treated DCs significantly increased CD4+ and CD8+ T cell proliferation. Activated the maturation of DCs by upregulating TLR4, CD40, CD86, MHC I, and MHC II. Activated the maturation of DCs by activating the TLR4, MAPK, and NF-κB signaling pathways. Activated the TLR4 signaling pathway by upregulating the phosphorylation of ERK, JNK, p38, and p-iκB while downregulating the level of p-NF-κB p65. Enhanced CD11b+ macrophage and CD3-CD19-CD49b+ NK cell proliferation by upregulating IL-6. Restored CTX-induced immunosuppression.	[35]
Fucus vesiculosus	Dendritic cells	IL-12, NF-α, FN-γ	In vitro	Activated the maturation of DCs by upregulating TNF-α, IFN-γ, and IL-12.	[131]
Laminaria Japonica, Laminaria cichoriodes, Fucus evanescens	HEK293 (human embryonic kidney cells)	NF-κB, TLR2, TLR4	In vitro	Activated the NF-κB by interacting with human TLR2 and TLR4.	[134]
Fucus vesiculosus, Undariia pinnatifidat, Macrocystis pyrifera	Human peripheral blood mononuclear cells (PBMCs)	IFN-γ	In vitro	Promoted activation and proliferation of PBMCs. Reached the highest PBMC activation by increasing maximum IFN-γ secretion. Increased IFN-γ secretion after co-culture of Nivolumab-treated PBMCs and PC3 cells in the presence of anti-CD3. Fucoidan reached the highest activation level of PBMCs through increasing maximum IFN-γ secretion at the concentration of 10 μg/mL and 50 μg/mL. Inhibited PC3 proliferation.	[136]

Table 2. *Cont.*

Fucoidan Sources	Immune Cells	Involved Cytokines	Research Methods	Effects of Fucoidan	Ref.
Fucus evanescens	Human peripheral blood dendritic cells	TNF-α	In vivo	Induced PBDC maturation and increased TNF-α.	[132]
Fucus vesiculosus	M2 macrophages	TNF-α, IL-6, CCL22	In vitro	Inhibited TNF-α and IL-6. Downregulated CCL22 chemokine by inhibiting p65-NF-κB phosphorylation.	[133]
Undaria pinnatifida	RAW 264.7 macrophages	TNF-α, IL-6, NO, iNOS, p38, κB-α, p65	In vitro	Increased the expression of IL-6 and TNF-α. Enhanced NO and iNOS production. Activated the NF-κB signaling pathway by upregulating the phosphorylation levels of IκB-α and p65. Activated the MAPK signaling pathway by increasing p38 phosphorylation.	[95]
Unknown	RAW 264.7 macrophages	iNOS, NO, p38, SR-A	In vitro	Activated iNOS and increased NO production through the NF-κB and MAPK signaling pathways.	[137]
Undaria pinnatifida sporophyllus, Fucus vesiculosus	Spleen cells, B lymphocytes	IFN-γ, NO, CD25, CD69	In vitro	Enhanced spleen cell proliferation and viability. Increased the expression of CD19, IFN-γ and NO on spleen cells. Increased a higher expression level of CD25 and CD69 on B lymphocytes. Increased the level of CD25 and CD69 on B lymphocytes. Increased spleen cell proliferation and viability. Reduced necrotic spleen cell populations.	[138]

3.3. Immunological Effect of Fucoidan on Dendritic Cells

In early studies, DCs were considered to be a potential target for the immunomodulatory capacity of fucoidan [131]. The DCs are critical mediator cells that interact with fucoidan to activate pattern recognition receptors (PRR), resulting in T cell priming and acquired immunity [139]. Toll-like receptors (TLRs) and scavenger receptors (SRs) have emerged as critical regulators that can interact with DC and fucoidan to influence innate and adaptive immunity [94,139,140]. Fucoidan can activate DC maturation by increasing specific surface molecules, such as CD40, CD86, MHC class I and class II, or cytokines, including IL-12 [94], TNF-α [132] and IFN-γ, in the host [131].

3.3.1. Fucoidan Activates the Maturation of DCs via Toll-like Receptors

The TLRs are essential receptors for initiating DCs and triggering primary immune responses and are typically involved in the recognition of potential pathogens and the activation of DCs [139]. Activation of TLRs can alter the ability of DCs to interact with T cells by regulating three types of signals delivered by DC to promote T cell expansion and differentiation into effectors: (1) antigen-specific signal 1; (2) co-stimulatory 'signal 2' proteins, such as CD40, CD80, and CD 86; (3) cytokines, such as TNF-α and INF-γ [139,141]. As previously reported, LMWF from *Undaria pinnatifida* stimulated the maturation of DCs by activating the toll-like receptor 4 (TLR4), and its downstream MAPK and NF-κB signaling pathways markedly increasing the expression of CD40, CD86, MHC I, and MHC II molecules [35].

Another LMWF fucoidan (*Ecklonia cava*) has also been shown to promote similar activation of DCs by increasing the levels of CD40, CD80, CD86, and MHC class I and II molecules in fucoidan-treated mice, upregulating the production of several pro-inflammatory cytokines, such as IL-6, IL-12, and TNF-α [130]. In this study, the LMWF-mediated DC maturation process is activated through the TLR4 signaling pathway. Mechanistically, fucoidan activated the TLR4 signaling pathway by upregulating the phosphorylation level of ERK, JNK, p38, and p-iκB while downregulating the level of p-NF-κB p65 [35]. This discovery supports the role of TLR4 as a critical mediator in fucoidan-activated DC maturation and cytokine production.

Fucoidan (*Fucus vesiculosus*) also contributed to activation of the maturation of human monocyte-derived DCs [131], as well as the upregulation of the expression of co-stimulatory molecules of DCs, promoting the secretion of cytokines, namely TNF-α, IL-12 and IFN-γ [131].

It is worth noting that different sources of fucoidan used in the above studies could lead to the activation of DCs, implying that the actual source of fucoidan may not be a critical factor. One common feature of LMWFs was that in all experiments they were shown to be endotoxin-free, which differ from HMWFs that potentially were contaminated with endotoxin.

3.3.2. Fucoidans Activate the Maturation of DCs via Scavenger Receptor Type A (SR-A)

Fucoidans inhibited SR-A in DCs by significantly increasing the binding of NY-ESO-1 to DCs. The DCs treated with fucoidan (species data not shown) exhibited a more mature phenotype than the DCs without fucoidan treatment [93]. This result indicates that SR-A is a critical factor that may influence DC maturation. Fucoidan (*Fucus evanescens*) was shown to indirectly induce human peripheral blood dendritic cell maturation (PBDC) and increase TNF-α production [132]. Therefore, fucoidan (*Fucus evanescens*)-medicated DC maturation can be blocked if fucoidan is pretreated with a TNF-α-neutralizing antibody [132]. Furthermore, a consistent result was obtained in a later in vivo study, in which they not only demonstrated that fucoidan (*Fucus vesiculosus*) could induce maturation in mouse DCs and induce upregulation of TNF-α, but also showed that fucoidan (*Fucus vesiculosus*) increased the production of IL-6 and IL-12 in spleen DCs [94]. These findings imply that fucoidan is a viable candidate for induced antitumor immune responses by regulating the levels of IFN-γ, TNF-α, or other specific interleukins, such as IL-6 and IL-12 levels.

3.4. Immunological Effect of Fucoidan on Macrophages

The immunomodulatory effect of fucoidan via macrophages is strongly associated with the production of pro- and anti-inflammatory cytokines, such as interleukin 6 (IL-6) [36,95], TNF-α [36,95,128], nitric oxide (NO) [128,137], and inducible nitric oxide synthase (iNOS) [95,128,142].

In the innate and adaptive immune systems of mammals, macrophages are the first line of defense against pathogens and tumors [95]. Macrophages have been shown to interact with fucoidan to inhibit tumor initiation, progression, and metastasis within the malignant tumor microenvironment (TME) [133,143]. A recent study demonstrated that LMWF from *Undaria pinnatifida* markedly increased the number of macrophages in splenocytes with elevated levels of IL-6 secretion [35], implying that fucoidan-mediated IL-6 secretion may play an essential role in macrophage activation.

Fucoidan has been shown to induce immunomodulatory effects after being treated with M2 macrophages by suppressing cytokines (IL-6 and TNF-α), and downregulating CCL22 chemokine by inhibiting p65-NF-κB phosphorylation [95,133]. However, different results were found in a different study where they demonstrated that LMWF-treated RAW264.7 macrophages increased the expression of pro-inflammatory mediators of IL-6 and TNF-α [95], as well as enhancing NO and iNOS production [95]. Furthermore, LMWF also activated the NF-κB signaling pathway by upregulating the phosphorylation of IκB-α and p65, and upregulated the MAPK signaling pathway by inducing phosphorylation of p38 [95]. Increased NO production in macrophages could be through the p38 MAPK and NF-κB signaling pathway [137]. A fractionated fucoidan (*Nizamuddinia zanardiinii*) named as F_3, could activate RAW264.7 macrophages by increasing the expression of cytokine mRNA (iNOS, NO, TNF-α, IIL-1β, and IL-6) and proteins that regulate the MAPK and NF-κB signaling pathway, such as p-NF-κB, p-JNK, p-ERK, and p-p38 proteins [128]. In summary, these results show that fucoidan activates RAW264.7 macrophages by upregulating the inflammatory cytokine, MAPK, and NF-κB signaling pathways.

Furthermore, fucoidan (*Laminaria japonica*) has been used to promote the differentiation of RAW264.7 macrophages from M0 to M1 phenotype macrophages [36]. Differentiation of RAW264.7n macrophages to M1 macrophages occurs via increasing the pro-inflammatory cytokines of IL-6, TNF-α, and NO [36]. Fucoidan compounds KCA (*Kjellmaniiella crassifolia, Astragalus polysaccharide*, and *Codonopsis pilosula*) and UCA (*Undaria pinnatifida, Astragalus polysaccharide*, and *Codonopsis pilosula*) may increase macrophage proliferation by increasing GM-CSF and TNF-α at concentrations below 200 μm/mL (KCA: 50–100 μm/mL; UCA: 25–200 μm/mL) [144]. However, when the concentrations of fucoidan compounds were above 200 μm/mL, fucoidan killed the RAW264.7 macrophages. Surprisingly, fucoidan from a few sources (for example, *Kjellmaniiella crassifolia* and *Undaria pinnatifida* fucoidan) showed different effects, such as inhibiting the growth of macrophages opposed to cell death [144].

3.5. Immunological Effect of Fucoidan on NK Cells

The NK cells are innate lymphoid cells that are essentially derived from common lymphoid progenitors [145]. The broad range of cytokines (e.g., IFN-γ, perforin, granzyme B) [127,130,145], and activating (e.g., NKp30, FasL) and inhibitory receptors (e.g., killer inhibitory receptor, KIR) located on the cell surface [145,146] allow them to interact with other immune cells or biomolecules which allow them to recognize tumor cells and then induce antitumor effects [145,147]. Furthermore, NK cells have also been described as DC promoters and T cell response regulators [147], suggesting that NK cells can enhance and maximize the antitumor effects of other immune cells in TME [145]. Ale et al. showed that intraperitoneally administered fucoidan (*Fucus vesiculosus*, 50 mg/kg) increased NK cell proliferation in C57BL/6 mice [129]. Fucoidan from *Fucus vesiculosus* and *Undaria pinnatifida* could significantly increase NK cells (NK1.1$^+$CD3$^-$) proliferation. Fucoidan from other sources (*Fucus vesiculosus, Undaria pinnatifida, Ascophyllum nodosum, Macrocystis pyrifera*) could activate NK cells (CD3$^-$NK1.1$^+$) via increasing killer cell lectin-like receptor and IFN-γ [127]. Furthermore, Zhang et al. (2019) further demonstrated that intraperitoneal administration of fucoidan (*Macrocystis pyrifera*, 50 mg/kg) in C57BL/6 mice could activate and increase NK cell proliferation of NK cells (NK1.1$^+$CD3$^-$) via increasing IFN-γ production and CD69 expression [148], suggesting that fucoidan activates NK cells through secreted cytokines (e.g., IFN-γ) and killer activating receptors (e.g., KLRG1). Exceptionally, CD3$^-$NK1.1$^+$ NK cells activated by all fucoidans from *Fucus vesiculosus*, *Undaria pinnatifida*, *Ascophyllum nodosum*, and *Macrocystis pyrifera* induced cytotoxic activity against YAC-1 cells [127]. Importantly, both Zhang et al. (2015) and Zhang et al. (2019) showed that fucoidan (*Macrocystis pyrifera*, 50 mg/kg)-activated CD3$^-$NK1.1$^+$ NK cells induced the highest cytotoxicity in mouse lymphoma YAC-1 cells [127,148], which suggest that fucoidan-activated CD3$^-$NK1.1$^+$ NK cells could induce antitumor effects, regardless of the fucoidan species. Consistent results were demonstrated in a recent study by Zhang et al. (2021); they showed that intraperitoneal administration of fucoidan (*Ecklonia cava*) in C57BL/6 mice induced the strongest CD3$^-$NK1.1$^+$ NK cell proliferation through increased CD69 expression and IFN-γ levels among the five fucoidans (*Fucus vesiculosus*, *Undaria pinnatifida*, *Ascophyllum nodosum*, *Macrocystis pyrifera*, and *Ecklonia cava*) at a concentration of 50 mg/kg [130]. Fucoidan (*Ecklonia cava*)-treated NK cells also induced strong antitumor effects in YAC-1 cells by significantly upregulating the expression of TRAIL, perforin, and granzyme B on the surface of fucoidan (*Ecklonia cava*)-treated NK cells [130]. Furthermore, an in vivo study by An et al. (2022) demonstrated that fucoidan (*Laminaria japonica*) could promote CD3$^-$NK1.1$^+$NK cells proliferation via increasing CD69 at a higher concentration of 100 mg/kg and killing targeted cells by secreting IFN-γ, perforin, and granzyme B at a lower concentration of 50 mg/kg [149]. Two other immunological mediators were also involved in the activation and cytotoxicity of fucoidan-mediated NK cells against other tumor cells in vitro, the death ligand FasL and the activating receptor NKp30 [146]. These data suggest that fucoidan would increase NK cells proliferation via increasing CD69 expression and IFN-γ levels and would induce cytotoxic effects of CD3$^-$NK1.1$^+$ NK cells in YAC-1 cells by upregulating surface markers, including perforin, granzyme B, NKp30, FasL, TRAIL, and KLRG1. Thus, cytotoxic mediators of IFN-γ, namely perforin and granzyme B, play a critical role for fucoidan in the promotion and activation of NK cells in mice.

Fucoidans could also induce cytotoxicity and the activation of NK cells in cyclophosphamide (CP)-treated immunosuppressed mice. It was reported that fucoidan (*Undaria pinnatifida*, 50 mg/kg, 100 mg/kg, 150 mg/kg) induced cytotoxicity against YAC-1 cells and increased NK1.1$^+$NK cells proliferation in CP-treated immunosuppressed mice [135], but it is unknown whether fucoidan secreted IFN-γ or promoted CD69 expression on the surface of NK1.1$^+$NK cells [135]. The HMWF (*Undaria pinnatifida*) markedly increased the proliferation of NK-92MI cells in the concentration range of 62.5 to 2000 μg/mL and induced a high cytotoxicity of NK-92MI cells against YAC-1 cells in CP-treated immunosuppressed mice by releasing granzyme B [49]. These results suggest that fucoidan could promote NK cell proliferation and activation by releasing granzyme B in CP-treated immunosuppressed mice. Oral administration of fucoidans (*Cladosiphon okamuranus*, HMWF: 110–138 kDa, LMWF: 6.5–40 kDa) has significantly increased the proliferation of NK cells in the spleen and reduced tumor weight in mice with tumors in the colon 26 [150], suggesting that fucoidan induces antitumor immunity effects by mediating NK cell activity [150].

It is noteworthy that it was previously suggested that "fucoidan-mediated NK cell activation depends on DC maturation" by showing that fucoidan (*Ecklonia cava*) was unable to increase CD69, IFN-γ, perforin, and granzyme B levels in NK cells after splenocytes depleted CD11c^{+}DCs [130,149]. However, uronic acid levels in fucoidans (*Fucus vesiculosus*, *Undaria pinnatifida*, *Ascophyllum nodosum*, *Macrocystis pyrifera*, and *Ecklonia cava*) have also been suggested to influence the immunological effects of fucoidan in NK cells [130]. Thus, further investigations are required to determine whether the depletion of DCs or the levels of uronic acid influence fucoidan to activate NK cells.

3.6. Factors Influencing Fucoidan-Activated Immune Cells

The dosage and molecular weight of fucoidan play a critical role in modulating the effect on macrophages. Indeed, LMWF fucoidan (*Undaria pinnatifida*) significantly enhances macrophage proliferation (CD11b +) and NK cells (CD3-CD19-CD49b+) by upregulating IL-6 secretion [35]. Furthermore, LMWF can restore cyclophosphamide (CTX)-induced immunosuppression without causing toxic effects. This natural multifunctional molecule is capable of alleviating CTX toxicity and acts as an immunomodulator in vivo [35]. These findings lay the basis for future studies to determine whether this optimal dose is appropriate for testing *Fucus vesiculosus* fucoidan using other immune cells, such as CD4+ and CD8+ T cells. Importantly, their findings establish the foundation for future researchers to select appropriate dose ranges that can be used in human clinical studies to examine their antitumor immunity in cancer patients and a suitable route of administration. However, it remains controversial whether the molecular weight of fucoidan influences its immune modulation effects on macrophages [144].

Furthermore, HMWF is also important in inducing immunomodulatory effects on macrophages. To determine whether molecular weight could be a factor that influences fucoidan to induce immunomodulatory effects on macrophages, Jiang et al. reported that HMWF-treated spleen cells, which include macrophages, enhanced the production of IFN-γ and NO production compared to LMWF treatment [138], suggesting that HMWF is more capable than LMWF of stimulating IFN-γ and NO production, increasing macrophage viability. However, increased NO production may be the result of contaminated HMWF used in the study; concern has been raised about endotoxin contamination in HMWF used in studies [95]. To overcome this concern, it is suggested that endotoxin-free LMWF is a better choice for future studies to investigate its immunomodulatory effects of fucoidan [35].

4. Relevance to Cancer Immunotherapy

Immunotherapy, i.e., immune checkpoint inhibitors and adoptive T cell transfer therapy (such as CAR-T cell therapy), has achieved an unprecedented clinical outcome in the treatment of homological malignancies. However, significant challenges remain ahead in the treatment of solid tumors. Effective treatment of solid tumor requires preferential activation of CTL-mediated cytotoxicity against cancer cells. To overcome these seemingly intractable obstacles, more 'powerful' immune cells or CAR-T cells with enhanced antitumor efficacy are required [20]. Fucoidan is a natural polysaccharide that has antitumor properties and immunopotentiating effects with low toxicity in both animal models and humans. This polysaccharide is a strong agonist of TLR4, which induces activation of DCs in humans. Therefore, fucoidan could be a desirable candidate for use in effective cancer immunotherapy. Figure 2 summarizes the immunopotentiation of fucoidan and its relevance to cancer immunotherapy.

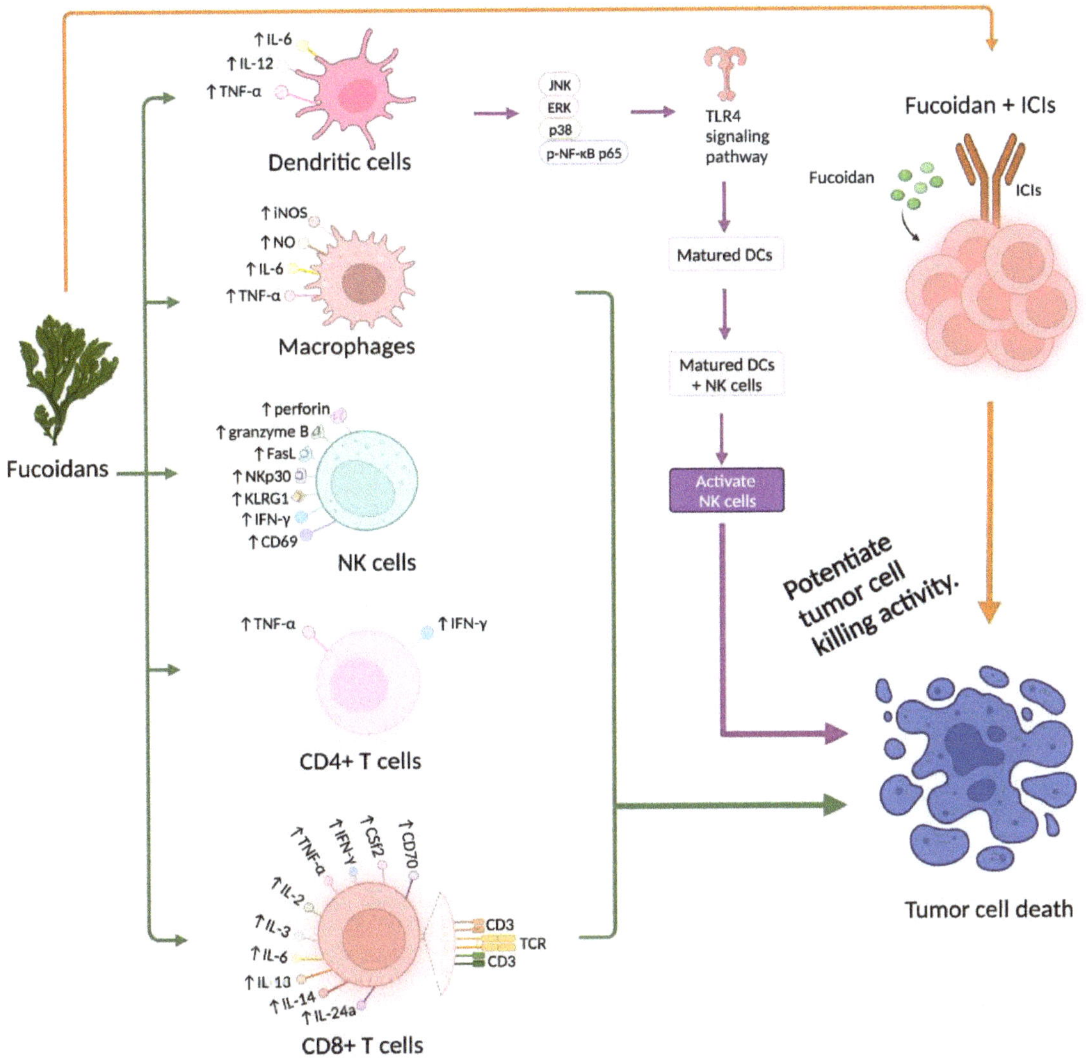

Figure 2. Immunopotentiation and antitumor immunity of fucoidan. Fucoidan activates DC maturation via secreting IL-6, IL-12, and TNF-α; matured DCs will then activate NK cells to induce antitumor immunity effects in tumor cells. Fucoidan can activate macrophages via increasing the production of iNOS, NO, IL-6, and TNF-α. Fucoidan increases NK cell proliferation by increasing CD69 expression and IFN-γ levels and activates NK cells by upregulating the cytotoxic mediators of perforin, granzyme B, activating the receptor NKp30, FasL, and KLRG1. Here, TNF-α and IFN-γ are the two common cytokines expressed on the surface of CD4+ and CD8+ T cells. Fucoidan activates these T cells via upregulating cytokines of TNF-α, IFN-γ, CD70, CSf2, IL-2, IL-3, IL-6, IL-13, IL-14, IL-24a, to induce tumor cell death. Fucoidan is co-administered with immune checkpoint inhibitors (ICIs) to enhance tumoricidal activity (this figure was created with BioRender.com, accessed on 5 February 2023).

4.1. Fucoidan Potentiates Cancer Immunotherapy

There is considerable evidence that fucoidan potentiates cancer immunotherapy when used in combination with immunotherapeutic products. A recent study has shown that fucoidan supplements significantly enhance the antitumor activities of PD-1 antibodies in vivo. Fucoidan consistently promotes the activation of tumor infiltrating CD8+ T cells. Therefore, fucoidan combined with ICB therapy could be a promising strategy to treat cancer. The underlying mechanism for this enhanced immunotherapy may be related to the activation of the JAK/STAT pathway to stimulate T cell activation [18]. Fucoidan (*Ecklonia cava*) combined with anti-PD-ligand 1 (anti-PD-L1) antibody treatment (administered intranasally) successfully prolonged survival for mice with metastatic lung cancer, and the body weight of the treated mice also increased. Furthermore, the combination treatment inhibits the infiltration of B16 tumor cells into the lung and prevents the growth of metastatic murine colon carcinoma CT-26 tumors in the lung [23]. When fucoidan was used together with Nivolumab, it increased the effects of Nivolumab on prostate cancer cells by enhancing the activity of human immune cells, and an additive effect was observed [136]. In a murine tumor model, a combination of fucoidan and anti-PD-L1 antibody inhibited CT-26 tumor growth more effectively than the anti-PD-L1 antibody. The study confirmed that the combination treatment with fucoidan enhanced anti-PD-L1 antibody-mediated anti-cancer immunity in the CT-26 carcinoma-bearing BALB/c mice, providing direct in vivo evidence [21].

4.2. Fucoidan Enhances the Efficacy of Immunotherapy via Novel Dosage Forms

Nanotechnology has emerged as a new approach to improve the efficiency of cancer immunotherapy by targeting the drug delivery system and the metabolism of immunotherapeutic agents [151]. Two preclinical studies have shown that fucoidans (*Fucus vesiculosus* and *Laminaria japonica*) have the potential to be used to improve the efficacy of immunotherapy in cancer treatments [152,153]. When fucoidan (*Fucus vesiculosus*) is packed as a therapeutic nanomedicine, it is capable of augmenting the therapeutic index of combination checkpoint immunotherapy and reducing toxicity: Chiang et al. reported the beneficial therapeutic effects of fucoidan–dextran-based magnetic nanomedicine (IO@FuDex3) conjugated with a checkpoint inhibitor (anti-PD-L1) and T cell activators (anti-CD3 and anti-CD28). The IO@FuDex3 medicine helped the repair of the immunosuppressive tumor microenvironment and potentiated the effect of the anti-PD-L1 antibody [126]. Fucoidan (*Fucus vesiculosus*)-based IL-2 delivery microcapsules, FPC2, loaded with IL-2 showed higher biological activity in ex vivo expansion of cytotoxic T cells than from Treg lymphocytes. A single intratumor administration of the FPC2/IL-2 complex with injectable gel had a favorable effect on the subpopulation ratio of tumor-infiltrating leukocytes as a result of the increased expansion of cytotoxic T lymphocytes and the decreased number of myeloid subpopulations, leading to increased activation of tumor-reactive T cells only at the tumor site. This represents a novel strategy in TCR-engineered T cell therapies for solid tumors [154].

More details on studies using fucoidans in novel dosage forms, such as nanoparticles and microcapsules, to improve immunotherapy efficacy, can be found in the following table (Table 3).

Table 3. Fucoidans in novel dosage form enhance immunotherapy efficacy.

Source of Fucoidan	Brief Description	Dosage Forms	Effects of Fucoidan	Ref.
Fucus vesiculosus	Combined fucoidan-based magnetic nanoparticles and immunomodulators enhance tumor-localized immunotherapy.	Nanoparticles (fucoidan-containing formulations: IO@FuDex1, IO@FuDex2, IO@FuDex3, M-IO@ FuDex1, M-IO@ FuDex3, and M-IO@ FuDex3)	IO@FuDex^2 -H: improved targeting efficiency; IO@FuDex^2 and IO@FuDex^3: increased the cell association via a slow elevation of median fluorescence index (MFI) in 4T1 cells; IO@FuDex^3-H: significantly increased the MFI in CD8$^+$T cells; targeted PD-L1 receptors and associated with 4T1 cells; inhibited lung metastasis in 4T1 cancer model; M-IOFuDex (magnetic navigation): enhanced tumor selectivity; increased T cell proliferation; decreased Tregs and TAMs in TME; IO@FuDex and IO@FuDex^3: inhibited the CT-26 tumor cell growth and extended the median survival to 62 days; reduced spleen Tregs; IO@FuDex^3 and M-IO@FuDex^3 increased TNF-α, VEGF, and TGF-β; IO@FuDex^1, IO@FuDex^2, IO@FuDex^3, and M-IO@Fu Dex^3 : ↑ antitumoral effects and median survival.	[126]
Fucus vesiculosus	Enhanced adoptive T cell therapy using fucoidan-based IL-2 delivery microcapsules.	Microcapsules (fucoidan-based coacervate-laden injectable hydrogel (FPC^2 − IG))	Acted as an IL-2 delivery vehicle for enhancing adoptive T cell therapy (ACT); increased tumor-infiltrating CD8$^+$ T cells in CT26-bearing mice with FPC^2 − IG − IL − 2 injection than FPC^2 − IG injection; Downregulated CD62L and enriched T$_{EM}$ and T$_{EFF}$ cell generation; promoted STAT5 phosphorylation in CD8$^+$ T cells; increased Treg, NK, DNT, NKT, B, CD8$^+$, and CD4$^+$ T cell populations; induced a higher Ki-67 expression in CT26-bearing mice; combination therapy (anti-PD-1 + FPC^2 − IG − IL − 2) reduced CT26 tumor cell growth and increased the IFN-γ levels in tumor-infiltrating CD8$^+$T cells; increased naïve OT-I T and NY-ESO-1 TCR- T cell proliferation; decreased the expression of PD-1, Tim-3, TIGIT, and LAG-3 in tumor-infiltrating NY-ESO-1 TCR T cells.	[154]
Fucus vesiculosus	Cytotoxicity and fabrication of fucoidan-cisplatin nanoparticles for macrophage and tumor cells.	Nanoparticles	Increased the cell viability of RAW264.7 macrophages; non-cytotoxic to RAW264.7 macrophages; reduced the cytotoxicity of cisplatin; inhibited HCT-8 cell growth.	[152]
Laminaria japonica	Fucoidan-based and tumor-activated nanoplatform overcame hypoxia and enhanced photodynamic therapy and antitumor immunity.	Nanoparticles	Significantly increased the VP fluorescent emission in FM@VP-treated MDA-MB-231 cells; MDA-MB-231 cells took up greater FM@VP nanoparticle clusters; inhibited MDA-MB-231 and MDA-MB-468 cell growth; decreased TNBC cell viability, upregulated P-selectin level; overcome tumor hypoxia; decreased pro-angiogenesis generated by hypoxic tumor-elicited pro-angiogenesis; inhibited YAP levels, CTGF, cyclin D1, and EGFR in MDA-MB-231 cells; attenuated the Hippo signaling; downregulated the protein levels of PD-L1; enhanced T cell-mediated cytotoxicity; suppressed orthotopic 4T1 tumor cells growth and metastatic colonization of lung tumor; downregulated Treg cell infiltration; increased the expressions of granzyme B and IFN-γ; increased CD4 and CD8 T cells but decreased TAMs.	[153]
Cladosiphon okamuranus	Immunomodulatory effects of fucoidan in mice.	Oral gavage	Increased the proliferation of splenocytes that activated by concanavalin A and LPS, and increased macrophage phagocytosis activity and the levels of IL-2, IFN-γ and serum IgM; decreased the levels of IL-4, IL-5 and serum IgE.	[2]
Fucus vesiculosus, Ascophyllu nodosum	Fucoidan-supplemented diet coordinated with ICBs to potentiate its antitumor immunity	Oral	Enhanced the therapeutic efficacy of PD-1 blockade; reduced B16 melanoma cell growth, volumes, and weights. Increased the proliferation of CD8$^+$T, NK, and tumor-infiltrating T cells; activated DC maturation; increased the proliferation of CD8$^+$T cells via increasing the production of IFN-γ and TNF-α; activated CD8$^+$T cells through the JAK/STAT pathway.	[18]

4.3. Fucoidan Enhances T Cell Activation via Increasing IL-2, IFN-γ, TNF-α

Several cytokines, including interleukin 2 (IL-2), interleukin 6 (IL-6), interleukin 12 (IL-12), TNF-α, and IFN-γ, have been shown to interact with fucoidan to enhance T cell activation. Here, IL-2 is a pro-inflammatory cytokine usually secreted by activated CD4+ and CD8+ T cells [155]. It is a known T cell growth factor responsible for T cell (CD4+, CD8+) expansion, and the production of TNF-α and IFN-γ [155]. Tomori et al. (2019) showed that the oral administration of fucoidan (*Cladosiphon okamuranus*) could significantly increase the secretion of IL-2 and IFN-γ in spleen cells (T and B cells) in mice, whilst reducing the secretion of IL-4, IL-5, and the serum antibody IgE [138]. They also showed that addition of concanavalin (Con A) in fucoidan-treated mice promotes T cell proliferation [2]. Increased production of pro-inflammatory cytokines (IL-2, IFN-γ) led to proliferation of T cells. Fucoidan administered with PD-1 antibodies induced synergistic effects in inhibiting B16 melanoma tumor cell proliferation, via increasing T cell infiltration to B16 tumor cells [18]. Fucoidan activated the JAK/STAT signaling pathway and augmented CD8+ T cell proliferation via interacting with the TCR/CD3 complex and increasing the production of TNF-α and IFN-γ [18].

These results suggest that fucoidan enhances antitumor immune responses in TME via regulating T cell activities. Another in vivo study by Lee et al. (2020) also demonstrated a similar trend; oral administration of fucoidan (*Undaria pinnatifida*) in cyclophosphamide (CP)-treated C57BL/6 mice significantly increases the proliferation of CD4+ and CD8+ T cells via increasing the production of TNF-α and IgM, at concentrations of 100 mg/kg and 150 mg/kg, respectively [135]. The results suggest that the production of TNF-α and IFN-γ plays a critical role in regulating fucoidan-mediated T cell activations.

More importantly, a very recent in vivo study conducted by Jeon et al. (2022) showed that a single intratumoral injection of fucoidan-based coacervate named as FPC^2– IG-IL-2 releases a higher level of IL-2 expression and increases the proliferation of CD4+ and CD8+ T cells [154]. They also showed that FPC^2– IG-IL-2 could enhance the antitumor effectiveness of a PD-1 blockade in both CT26-beraing mice and tumor-infiltrating CD8+ T cells [154]. These results confirmed that FPC^2– IG-IL-2 could enhance the activation of transferred tumor-reactive CD8+ T cells and antitumor immune responses. Thus, more preclinical studies are needed to investigate the effects of fucoidans on the production of IL-2 in T cells.

4.4. Fucoidan Enhance Immunotherapy through Regulating Cytokines Released by Macrophages and NK Cells

By producing various cytokines and interacting with other immune cells, such as DCs or natural killer (NK) cells, macrophages are involved in initiating, promoting, or, alternatively, inhibiting tumor development [156]. It has also been reported that macrophages can regulate the tumor microenvironment via producing iNOS, NO, or other pro-inflammatory cytokines (e.g., TNF-α and IL-6) [156]. Expression of iNOS in macrophages accelerates NO production, but excessive NO production can contribute to promoting tumor progression and metastasis [157]. Thus, inhibition of aberrant iNOS/NO production may improve the efficacy of cancer immunotherapy [157].

Anti-tumor immunity induced by fucoidan has been demonstrated in a study by Takeda et al. where they showed that fucoidan (*Cladosiphon okamuranus* Tokida)-treated RAW264.7 murine macrophages inhibited Sarcoma 180 (S-180) tumor cell growth in the S and G_2/M phase of the cell cycle. They also showed that the fucoidan activated RAW264.7 macrophages through increasing the iNOS level and NO production via activating NF-κB signaling pathway, respectively [158]. They also demonstrated that the inhibition of iNOS levels could suppress S-180 tumor cell growth [158].

Jiang et al. (2021) also demonstrated that fucoidan (sea cucumber *Stichopus chloronotus*) activates RAW264.7 macrophages via increasing the production of NO, TNF-α, IL-6, and IL-10, as well as being involved in the activation of the TLR4/2 and NF-κB signaling pathways [159]. These results suggest that fucoidan at low concentrations helps to avoid overexpression of iNOS and NO production in fucoidan-treated RAW264.7 macrophages. Thus, fucoidan is a critical regulator of iNOS expression and NO production in RAW264.7 macrophages.

Furthermore, Tabarsa et al. (2020) confirmed that crude fucoidan (*Nizamuddinia zanardinii*) could increase the proliferation of RAW264.7 macrophages at concentrations of 10–50 μg/mL without cytotoxicity and activate RAW264.7 macrophages by increasing NO production at 50 μg/mL [128]. However, they also showed that fucoidan fraction F_3 (*Nizamuddinia zanardinii*) upregulated the iNOS expression and NO production, accompanied with releasing several pro-inflammatory cytokines (e.g., TNF-α, IL-1β, IL-6) and IL-10 [128]. The IL-10 produced inhibited the overexpression of TNF-α, IL-1β, and IL-6, exhibiting immunological responses [159]. These results suggest that fucoidan could restrain the overactivation of RAW264.7 macrophages by secreting anti-inflammatory cytokines (e.g., IL-10), which helps to balance the ratio of pro- and anti-inflammatory cytokines in fucoidan activated RAW264.7 macrophages. Tabarsa et al. (2020) demonstrated fucoidan fraction F_3 (*Nizamuddinia zanardinii*) activated RAW264.7 macrophages increasing the amount of p-NF-κB, p-JNK, p-ERK, and p-p38 proteins [128], which suggests that the fucoidan fraction F_3 (*Nizamuddinia zanardinii*) activation of RAW264.7 macrophages involves the activation of the NF-κB and MAPK signaling pathways.

Fucoidan also activates NK cells by releasing cytokines (e.g., TNF-α, INF-γ) and activating the NF-B and MAPK signaling pathways [128]. For example, Tabarsa et al. (2020) demonstrated that fucoidan fraction F_3 (*Nizamuddinia zanardinii*) activates NK-92 cells via increasing the expressions of TNF-α, IFN-γ, granzyme-B, perforin, activating receptor NKG2D, and apoptosis-inducing ligand (FasL) [128]. They also demonstrated that fucoidan fraction F_3 (*Nizamuddinia zanardinii*) could increase the quantity of p-NF-κB, p-JNK, p-ERK, and p-p38 proteins [128]. Taken together, these results suggest that fucoidan fraction F_3 (*Nizamuddinia zanardinii*) in NK-92 cells activates NF-κB and MAPK signaling pathways.

Fucoidan is a natural and multifunctional agent that also has promising inhibitory effects on pro-inflammatory cytokines (TNF-α, IL-1β and IL-6) in LPS-treated RAW264.7 murine macrophages [96,97]. A previous in vitro study by Lee et al. (2012) found that three *Ecklonia cava* fucoidan fractions (F_1, F_2, F_3) were non-cytotoxic and reduced the expression of iNOS, NO, COX-2, and pro-inflammatory cytokines (TNF-α, IL-1β, and IL-6) in RAW 264.7 macrophages treated with LPS at a concentration of 12.5–100 μg/mL [99]. Notably, the F_3 fraction induced maximum inhibitory effects on these cytokines at a concentration of 100 μg/mL [99]. The in vitro study by Fernando et al. (2017) also showed that the fucoidan fraction (*Chnoospora minima*, MW = 95 kDa) fraction F2,4 was not cytotoxic and could decrease NO production and pro-inflammatory cytokine expression in pro-inflammatory cytokines (TNF-α, IL-1β, and IL-6) in RAW264.7 macrophages treated with LPS at a concentration of 50 μg/mL [100]. Similar results were also obtained by Ni et al. (2020) in an in vivo study and demonstrated that the fucoidan fraction LJSF4 (*Saccharina japonica*, fucoidan fraction: LJSF4) has no cytotoxicity and significantly inhibited the production of pro-inflammatory cytokines, including TNF-α, IL-1β, and IL-6 in LPS-treated RAW264.7 macrophages at 25 μg/mL [97]. These fucoidan fractions (e.g., F_1, F_2, F_3, F2,4, LJSF4) contained high level of fucose and sulfate content, suggesting that fucoidan fractions (e.g., F_1, F_2, F_3, F2,4, LJSF4) with the highest fucose and sulfate contents would have a greater ability to regulate and balance cytokine expressions in LPS-treated RAW264.7 macrophages. Therefore, the fucose and sulfate content in fucoidan could be one of the influential factors that affects its ability to induce inhibitory effects on pro-inflammatory cytokines in LPS-treated RAW264.7 macrophages. Jeong et al. also reported that fucoidan (*Fucus vesiculosus*) was not cytotoxic and only attenuated the production of pro-inflammatory cytokines of TNF-α and IL-1β in LPS-treated RAW264.7 murine macrophages at 100 μg/mL [96]. Ni et al. demonstrated that fucoidan fraction LJSF4 (*Saccharina japonica*, fucoidan fraction: LJSF4) has no cytotoxicity and significantly inhibits the production of pro-inflammatory cytokines, including TNF-α, IL-1β, and IL-6 in LPS-treated RAW264.7 macrophages at 25 μg/mL [97]. These results strongly suggest that fucoidan can inhibit the secretion and expression of pro-inflammatory cytokines (TNF-α, IL-1β, and Il-6) in RAW264.7 murine macrophages treated with LPS at a lower concentration ($\leq$100 μg/mL) [96], regardless of their species derivation.

Sanjeewa et al. (2018) reported that the fucoidan (*Sargassum horneri*) fraction f4 inhibited the production of iNOS, NO, and COX-2, and reduced the secretion of pro-inflammatory cytokines (TNF-α, IL-6) and the PEG_2 enzyme in LPS-treated RAW264.7 murine macrophages at concentrations of 25–100 μg/mL (the 50% inhibitory concentration (IC_{50}) = 87.12 μg/mL) without causing any toxicities [101], but it only slightly inhibited IL-6 production at the same concentration [101]. The f4 fraction also inhibited the phosphorylation of IκB-α and p-I κB-α [101]. In particular, the fucoidan fraction f4 (*Sargassum horneri*) contained lower fucose (36.86%) and sulfate (18.47%) contents [101]. Consistently, crude fucoidan (*Sargassum horneri*) was shown to be non-cytotoxic and could suppress NO production, the secretion of pro-inflammatory cytokines (TNF-α, IL-1β), and downregulate the expression levels of the iNOS and COX-2 proteins in macrophages [102]. They also demonstrated that crude fucoidan (*Sargassum horneri*) can inhibit the translocation of NF-κB p50 and p65 to the nucleus and downregulate the phosphorylation of p38 and ERK1/2 proteins in LPS-treated RAW264.7 macrophages at the same concentration [102]. These results suggest that fucoidan induced inhibitory effects on pro-inflammatory cytokines in LPS-treated RAW264.7 macrophages via NF-κB and MAPK signaling pathways.

All these results further strengthen the concept that fucoidan may induce its anti-inflammatory effects by inhibiting pro-inflammatory cytokine secretion and mRNA expression levels of pro-inflammatory cytokines (TNF-α, IL-1β, IL-6) in LPS-stimulated RAW264.7 murine macrophages [96,97,99,101,102,108]. More importantly, macrophages appear to play an essential role in the initial stage of the anti-inflammatory effects of fucoidan. However, the role and contributions of T cells (CD4+ and CD8+) are unknown. Therefore, further investigations are required to determine whether fucoidan-treated T cells (CD4+ and CD8+) are able to attenuate pro-inflammatory cytokines (TNF-α, IL-1β, IL-6).

4.5. Possible Combined Use of Fucoidan with Immunotherapeutic Products

Fucoidan extracts from three types of species (*Fucus vesiculosus*, *Undariia pinnatifidat*, *Macrocystis pyrifera*) are capable of independently promoting the activation and proliferation of human peripheral blood mononuclear cells (PBMC) in the presence of a T cell activator (anti-CD3) by increasing IFN-γ production. In these studies, fucoidan derived from *Fucus vesiculosus* was the optimal fucoidan based on the potency of these three different types of fucoidan [136]. Moreover, fucoidan induced antitumor effects by stimulating DC maturation and/or macrophage differentiation. Jin et al. (2014) found that when fucoidan was co-administered with ovalbumin antigen, it stimulated DC maturation and then promoted antigen-specific T cell immune responses [94,160].

Fucoidan (*Fucus vesiculosus*) has been developed as a therapeutic nanomedicine to enhance the efficacy of immune check inhibitors (anti-PD-L1) in immunosuppressive TME [126,161]. It has been shown that the fucoidan-based nanomedicine IO@FuDex^3 reduces adverse effects and extends patient survival in cancer treatments [5,126]. Although the development of fucoidan-based therapeutic nanoparticles is still in an early stage [152], it is important and promising to develop fucoidan as a nanotechnology-based cancer immunotherapy drug [162,163].

5. Relevant Clinical Trials-Anticancer and Immunomodulation Related Trials

In this section, we provide an overview of relevant clinical trials using fucoidan to treat cancer and modulate immune function that are listed on Clinicaltrials.gov and anzctr.org.au. A list of these trials is presented in Table 4.

Given the promising preclinical findings of experiments using fucoidan as an anti-cancer agent, some clinical trials have been conducted or are proposed to examine the therapeutic potential of fucoidan in the treatment of various human cancers, such as advanced lung cancer [85], breast cancer (ACTRN12615000673549) (Table 4) [24], metastatic colorectal cancer (NCT04066660) (Table 4) [164], and recurrent colorectal cancer [165]. These clinical trials demonstrate that fucoidan is a safe anticancer agent that can be combined with chemotherapeutic drugs to improve survival time and reduce the adverse effects of chemotherapy in cancer treatments. However, three clinical trials have no results published on the website (clinicaltrials.gov), including NCT04342949, NCT04597476, and NCT03130829 (as of 10 October 2022, Table 4). It is important to be aware that the focus of all registered clinical trials on these websites (clinicaltrials.gov, anzctr.org.au) has expanded their investigations from studying anticancer effects to immunomodulatory effects of fucoidan. For example, four clinical studies focused on investigating how fucoidan regulates biomarkers in the immune system (ACTRN12621000872831, ACTRN12605000021673, ACTRN12616000417482, and ACTRN12611000220965) (Table 4). Other clinical trials have not yet started to recruit participants for their study (Table 4). Therefore, a follow-up on the results of these clinical studies to evaluate the efficacy of fucoidan in cancer would provide more insight into the therapeutic potential of fucoidan.

A previous human clinical study conducted between April 2008 and June 2009 by Ikeguchi et al. [165], found that HMWF (*Cladosiphon okamuranus*) prolonged survival time in the HMWF treatment group and suppressed side effects (e.g., fatigue) of chemotherapy drugs in patients with unresectable and recurrent colorectal cancer [165]. They also demonstrated that HMWF (*Cladosiphon okamuranus*) did not exhibit side effects (e.g., allergic dermatitis) in these patients during the 6 months of fucoidan treatment, and no patient suffered severe toxicity [165]. All patients (n = 20) completed fucoidan treatment safely [165]. The results suggested that HMWF (*Cladosiphon okamuranus*) can protect patients from fatigue of grades 2 and 3 during chemotherapy [165]. In contrast, an open-label non-crossover study assessed the efficacy of co-administration of fucoidan with two hormonal therapies (letrozole and tamoxifen) in patients with breast cancer (ACTRN12615000673549) (Table 4) [24], they showed that the oral administration of fucoidan (*Undaria pinnatifida*) did not influence the plasma levels of the active metabolites of tamoxifen and did not cause significant changes in steady state plasma concentrations of hormonal therapies (letrozole, tamoxifen) in female patients with breast cancer (ACTRN12615000673549) [24]. Furthermore, there is no evidence to show that oral administration of fucoidan (*Undaria pinnatifida*) can cause liver metastases (ACTRN12615000673549) [24]. Tsai et al. (2017) conducted a prospective, randomized, double-blind, controlled human clinical trial in the southern city of Taiwan (NCT04066660) (Table 4) [164]. They found that LMWF (*Sargassum hemiphyllum*) significantly increased the disease control rate (DCR) by approximately 23.6% in the study group compared to the control group (NCT04066660) [164], indicating that fucoidan can manage the status of cancer progression. These results suggest that LMWF (*Sargassum hemiphyllum*) can act as a supplementary agent to induce auxiliary effects and there appears to be an improved overall survival trend in patients with metastatic colorectal cancer (NCT04066660) [164]. Furthermore, Hsu et al. (2018) demonstrated that combination therapy (fucoidan and cisplatin, $n = 50$) increased the survival rate by approximately 50% in the HiQ-fucoidan treatment group (*Laminaria japonica*) as compared to the control group [85]. The results suggest that HiQ-fucoidan (*Laminaria japonica*) can act as a supplementary agent in combination therapy to increase cisplatin absorption to prolong survival time in patients with advanced lung cancer [85]. However, the sample size of the control group was smaller than that of the HiQ-fucoidan group (*Laminaria japonica*) group [85]. Therefore, the precision of clinical results can be compromised. Furthermore, they did not monitor whether HiQ-fucoidan (*Laminaria japonica*) could reduce the side effects of cisplatin (e.g., fatigue) to improve quality of life [85]. Therefore, further human clinical studies are required to randomly select equal numbers of patients in each group and also to monitor whether fucoidan treatment can reduce the side effects of the chemotherapy drug (e.g., cisplatin) in patients with advanced lung cancer.

Table 4. List of all registered clinical trials using fucoidan to treat cancer and/or other immune dysfunctional diseases.

Clinical Trial Number	Starting Year (Status)	Description	Results
NCT04342949	2018 (unknown)	A double-blind, randomized, placebo-controlled, parallel study investigated fucoidan's auxiliary effects in patients with locally advanced rectal cancer who received a combined radio/chemotherapy before surgery. They aimed to observe whether fucoidan can improve the quality of life of these patients receiving the neoadjuvant CCRT.	No
NCT04066660	2019 (Recruiting)	A randomized, double-blind, controlled trial evaluated oligo-fucoidan's efficacy (500–800 Da) in patients with metastatic colorectal cancer. They have also observed whether fucoidan can improve the quality of life and prolong the overall survival rate of these patients.	Yes [164]
NCT04597476	2020 (Recruiting)	A randomized, double-blind phase II trial that evaluated fucoidan's clinical effect and safety in patients with stage III/IV head and neck squamous cell carcinoma.	No
NCT03130829	2019 (Withdrawn)	A pilot, randomized, double-blind, multicenter study evaluated whether orally administered oligo-fucoidan can improve the quality of life in patients receiving platinum-based chemotherapy with NSCLC.	No
NCT02875392	2016 (Completed)	A randomized, double-blind, parallel study demonstrated that fucoidan improves the metabolic profiles of patients with non-alcoholic fatty liver disease (NAFLD).	Yes [166]
NCT05437887	2022 (Not yet recruiting)	An open-label, prospective, single group study evaluated the effects of fucoidan on the gut microbiota in the patients of atopic dermatitis before and after fucoidan treatment.	No
NCT05461508	2023 (Recruiting)	An open-label, randomized, parallel study investigates the effects of the combination treatment (fucoidan and Vonoprazan) on Helicobacter Pylori eradication rate and gastrointestinal flora.	No
NCT03422055	2018 (Unknown)	An open-label, single-group phase I study that evaluated the tolerance, biodistribution, and dosimetry of fucoidan radiolabeled by Technetium-99 m in patients.	No
ACTRN126 16000417482	2016 (Completed recruitment)	A randomized, double-blind, placebo-controlled, cross-over phase I/II trial that investigated the measurement, modulation, and estimation of net endogenous non-carbonic acid production using the Australian food database following the administration of alkaline supplements in healthy adults.	N/A
ACTRN126 15000673549	2015 (Completed recruitment)	An open-label, non-randomized, single-group phase IV trial investigating the interaction between two systemic complementary and alternative medicines and standard therapy in patients with active breast cancer malignancy.	Yes [24]
ACTRN126 05000021673	2005 (Recruiting)	A non-randomized, double-blind, parallel phase I/II study that evaluated the effects of natural seaweed fucoidan (GFS) on the modulation of the immune system and the mobilization/release of hematopoietic progenitor stem cells from bone marrow to the peripheral blood.	No
ACTRN1262 1000872831	2021 (Not yet recruiting)	A randomized, double-blind, crossover trial determines whether daily fucoidan supplementation can upregulate immune biomarkers during three weeks of intensified exercise training in healthy, recreationally active adults.	No
ACTRN1260 5000021673	2005 (Recruiting)	A non-randomized, double-blind, parallel phase I/II study that evaluated the effects of natural seaweed fucoidan (GFS) on the modulation of the immune system and the mobilization/release of hematopoietic progenitor stem cells from bone marrow to the peripheral blood.	No

6. Concluding Remarks

Fucoidans have a range of immunomodulatory/immunopotentiating effects by acting through DCs, macrophages, NK cells, T cells, and B cells. However, very little is known about their effect on CAR-T cells and other engineered immune cells. Evidence is emerging concerning the benefits of combining fucoidans and immunotherapeutic agents, in particular ICIs and CAR-T cells, for the treatment of cancer. Rationally, fucoidan could play an important role in the new era of cancer immunotherapy through its immunopotentiating effects (Figure 2), anti-inflammatory effects, and antitumor properties. Human clinical studies are limited, and the results of clinical trials are not conclusive and inconsistent with preclinical data, indicating that more clinical studies on fucoidans are necessary. Furthermore, fucoidans may have great potential to be developed as a nanoparticle and used with other immunotherapeutic agents together as a novel strategy to treat cancer.

Despite many beneficial effects and promising future prospects for fucoidan, one of the challenges is the standardization of fucoidan, since not all fucoidans are equal in their pharmacological effects. The molecular structure, molecular weight, chemical composition, and bioactivity of fucoidans differ from species to species [16]. The extraction method is another major factor affecting the structural composition and bioactive properties of fucoidans. It is hoped that these problems will be gradually overcome as fucoidan moves forward toward more clinical applications.

Author Contributions: Conceptualization, Y.L. (Yiguang Lin) and Y.L. (Yani Li); software, Y.L. (Yani Li); resources, Y.L. (Yani Li), E.M., S.C., H.Y. and Y.L. (Yiguang Lin); writing—original draft preparation, Y.L. (Yani Li) and Y.L. (Yiguang Lin); writing—review and editing, E.M., S.C., H.Y. and Y.L. (Yiguang Lin); visualization, Y.L. (Yani Li); supervision, E.M., Y.L. (Yiguang Lin) and J.S. All authors have read and agreed to the published version of the manuscript.

Funding: This research is supported by an Australian Government Research Training Program Scholarship and a research grant from Natural Science Foundation of China (Grant number 32271225).

Institutional Review Board Statement: Not applicable.

Data Availability Statement: The data (figures and tables) used to support the findings of this study are included within the article.

Conflicts of Interest: The authors declare no conflict of interest.

References

1. Lin, Y.; Qi, X.; Liu, H.; Xue, K.; Xu, S.; Tian, Z. The anti-cancer effects of fucoidan: A review of both in vivo and in vitro investigations. *Cancer Cell Int.* **2020**, *20*, 154. [CrossRef] [PubMed]
2. Tomori, M.; Nagamine, T.; Miyamoto, T.; Iha, M. Evaluation of the Immunomodulatory Effects of Fucoidan Derived from Cladosiphon Okamuranus Tokida in Mice. *Mar. Drugs* **2019**, *17*, 547. [CrossRef] [PubMed]
3. Sanjeewa, K.K.A.; Herath, K.H.I.N.M.; Yang, H.-W.; Choi, C.S.; Jeon, Y.-J. Anti-Inflammatory Mechanisms of Fucoidans to Treat Inflammatory Diseases: A Review. *Mar. Drugs* **2021**, *19*, 678. [CrossRef] [PubMed]
4. Apostolova, E.; Lukova, P.; Baldzhieva, A.; Katsarov, P.; Nikolova, M.; Iliev, I.; Peychev, L.; Trica, B.; Oancea, F.; Delattre, C.; et al. Immunomodulatory and Anti-Inflammatory Effects of Fucoidan: A Review. *Polymers* **2020**, *12*, 2338. [CrossRef] [PubMed]
5. Kiselevskiy, M.V.; Anisimova, N.Y.; Ustyuzhanina, N.E.; Vinnitskiy, D.Z.; Tokatly, A.I.; Reshetnikova, V.V.; Chikileva, I.O.; Shubina, I.Z.; Kirgizov, K.I.; Nifantiev, N.E. Perspectives for the Use of Fucoidans in Clinical Oncology. *Int. J. Mol. Sci.* **2022**, *23*, 11821. [CrossRef]
6. Mak, W.; Hamid, N.; Liu, T.; Lu, J.; White, W.L. Fucoidan from New Zealand Undaria pinnatifida: Monthly variations and determination of antioxidant activities. *Carbohydr. Polym.* **2013**, *95*, 606–614. [CrossRef]
7. Wang, J.; Zhang, Q.; Zhang, Z.; Song, H.; Li, P. Potential antioxidant and anticoagulant capacity of low molecular weight fucoidan fractions extracted from Laminaria japonica. *Int. J. Biol. Macromol.* **2010**, *46*, 6–12. [CrossRef]
8. Li, B.; Lu, F.; Wei, X.; Zhao, R. Fucoidan: Structure and bioactivity. *Molecules* **2008**, *13*, 1671–1695. [CrossRef]
9. Priyanka, K.R.; Rajaram, R.; Sivakumar, S.R. A critical review on pharmacological properties of marine macroalgae. *Biomass Convers. Biorefinery* **2022**. [CrossRef]
10. Agency, E.M. *Assessment Report on Fucus vesiculosus L., thallus*; European Medicines Agency: London, UK, 2014.
11. Kylin, H. Zur Biochemie der Meeresalgen. 1913. Available online: https://www.degruyter.com/document/doi/10.1515/bchm2.1913.83.3.171/html (accessed on 15 December 2022).

12. Hsu, H.Y.; Hwang, P.A. Clinical applications of fucoidan in translational medicine for adjuvant cancer therapy. *Clin. Transl. Med.* **2019**, *8*, 15. [CrossRef]
13. Michel, G.; Tonon, T.; Scornet, D.; Cock, J.M.; Kloareg, B. The cell wall polysaccharide metabolism of the brown alga Ectocarpus siliculosus. Insights into the evolution of extracellular matrix polysaccharides in Eukaryotes. *New Phytol.* **2010**, *188*, 82–97. [CrossRef]
14. Berteau, O.; Mulloy, B. Sulfated fucans, fresh perspectives: Structures, functions, and biological properties of sulfated fucans and an overview of enzymes active toward this class of polysaccharide. *Glycobiology* **2003**, *13*, 29R–40R. [CrossRef]
15. Deniaud-Bouet, E.; Hardouin, K.; Potin, P.; Kloareg, B.; Herve, C. A review about brown algal cell walls and fucose-containing sulfated polysaccharides: Cell wall context, biomedical properties and key research challenges. *Carbohydr. Polym.* **2017**, *175*, 395–408. [CrossRef]
16. Ponce, N.M.A.; Stortz, C.A. A Comprehensive and Comparative Analysis of the Fucoidan Compositional Data Across the Phaeophyceae. *Front. Plant Sci.* **2020**, *11*, 556312. [CrossRef]
17. Obluchinskaya, E.D.; Pozharitskaya, O.N.; Shikov, A.N. In Vitro Anti-Inflammatory Activities of Fucoidans from Five Species of Brown Seaweeds. *Mar. Drugs* **2022**, *20*, 606. [CrossRef]
18. Yang, J.; Yang, X.; Pan, W.; Wang, M.; Lu, Y.; Zhang, J.; Fang, Z.; Zhang, X.; Ji, Y.; Bei, J.-X.; et al. Fucoidan-Supplemented Diet Potentiates Immune Checkpoint Blockage by Enhancing Antitumor Immunity. *Front. Cell Dev. Biol.* **2021**, *9*, 733246. [CrossRef]
19. Fucoidan, N.R.I.O. High-Molecular Weight Fucoidan & Low-Molecular Weight Fucoidan. Available online: https://www.fucoidan-life.com/en/info_fucoidan/fucoidan/ (accessed on 3 February 2023).
20. McGowan, E.; Lin, Q.; Ma, G.; Yin, H.; Chen, S.; Lin, Y. PD-1 disrupted CAR-T cells in the treatment of solid tumors: Promises and challenges. *Biomed. Pharmacother.* **2020**, *121*, 109625. [CrossRef]
21. Park, H.B.; Lim, S.M.; Hwang, J.; Zhang, W.; You, S.; Jin, J.O. Cancer immunotherapy using a polysaccharide from Codium fragile in a murine model. *Oncoimmunology* **2020**, *9*, 1772663. [CrossRef]
22. Park, H.B.; Hwang, J.; Lim, S.M.; Zhang, W.; Jin, J.O. Dendritic cell-mediated cancer immunotherapy with Ecklonia cava fucoidan. *Int. J. Biol. Macromol.* **2020**, *159*, 941–947. [CrossRef]
23. Zhang, W.; Hwang, J.; Yadav, D.; An, E.-K.; Kwak, M.; Lee, P.C.-W.; Jin, J.-O. Enhancement of Immune Checkpoint Inhibitor-Mediated Anti-Cancer Immunity by Intranasal Treatment of Ecklonia cava Fucoidan against Metastatic Lung Cancer. *Int. J. Mol. Sci.* **2021**, *22*, 9125. [CrossRef]
24. Tocaciu, S.; Oliver, L.J.; Lowenthal, R.M.; Peterson, G.M.; Patel, R.; Shastri, M.; McGuinness, G.; Olesen, I.; Fitton, J.H. The Effect of Undaria pinnatifida Fucoidan on the Pharmacokinetics of Letrozole and Tamoxifen in Patients With Breast Cancer. *Integr. Cancer Ther.* **2018**, *17*, 99–105. [CrossRef] [PubMed]
25. Zhao, Y.; Zheng, Y.; Wang, J.; Ma, S.; Yu, Y.; White, W.L.; Yang, S.; Yang, F.; Lu, J. Fucoidan Extracted from Undaria pinnatifida: Source for Nutraceuticals/Functional Foods. *Mar. Drugs* **2018**, *16*, 321. [CrossRef] [PubMed]
26. Phull, A.R.; Kim, S.J. Fucoidan from Undaria pinnatifida regulates type II collagen and COX-2 expression via MAPK and PI3K pathways in rabbit articular chondrocytes. *Biologia* **2017**, *72*, 1362–1369. [CrossRef]
27. Wang, J.; Zhang, Q.; Zhang, Z.; Zhang, H.; Niu, X. Structural studies on a novel fucogalactan sulfate extracted from the brown seaweed Laminaria japonica. *Int. J. Biol. Macromol.* **2010**, *47*, 126–131. [CrossRef] [PubMed]
28. Chen, A.; Lan, Y.; Liu, J.; Zhang, F.; Zhang, L.; Li, B.; Zhao, X. The structure property and endothelial protective activity of fucoidan from Laminaria japonica. *Int. J. Biol. Macromol.* **2017**, *105*, 1421–1429. [CrossRef]
29. Ale, M.T.; Mikkelsen, J.D.; Meyer, A.S. Important Determinants for Fucoidan Bioactivity: A Critical Review of Structure-Function Relations and Extraction Methods for Fucose-Containing Sulfated Polysaccharides from Brown Seaweeds. *Mar. Drugs* **2011**, *9*, 2106–2130. [CrossRef]
30. Holtkamp, A.D.; Kelly, S.; Ulber, R.; Lang, S. Fucoidans and fucoidanases—Focus on techniques for molecular structure elucidation and modification of marine polysaccharides. *Appl. Microbiol. Biotechnol.* **2009**, *82*, 1–11. [CrossRef]
31. Fletcher, H.R.; Biller, P.; Ross, A.B.; Adams, J.M.M. The seasonal variation of fucoidan within three species of brown macroalgae. *Algal Res.* **2017**, *22*, 79–86. [CrossRef]
32. Oliveira, C.; Ferreira, A.S.; Novoa-Carballal, R.; Nunes, C.; Pashkuleva, I.; Neves, N.M.; Coimbra, M.A.; Reis, R.L.; Martins, A.; Silva, T.H. The Key Role of Sulfation and Branching on Fucoidan Antitumor Activity. *Macromol. Biosci.* **2017**, *17*, 1600340. [CrossRef]
33. Zhang, Z.; Teruya, K.; Eto, H.; Shirahata, S. Induction of apoptosis by low-molecular-weight fucoidan through calcium- and caspase-dependent mitochondrial pathways in MDA-MB-231 breast cancer cells. *Biosci. Biotechnol. Biochem.* **2013**, *77*, 235–242. [CrossRef]
34. Cumashi, A.; Ushakova, N.A.; Preobrazhenskaya, M.E.; D'Incecco, A.; Piccoli, A.; Totani, L.; Tinari, N.; Morozevich, G.E.; Berman, A.E.; Bilan, M.I.; et al. A comparative study of the anti-inflammatory, anticoagulant, antiangiogenic, and antiadhesive activities of nine different fucoidans from brown seaweeds. *Glycobiology* **2007**, *17*, 541–552. [CrossRef]
35. Liu, L.; Yang, X.; Yuan, P.; Cai, S.; Bao, J.; Zhao, Y.; Aimaier, A.; Aipire, A.; Lu, J.; Li, J. In Vitro and In Vivo Dendritic Cell Immune Stimulation Effect of Low Molecular Weight Fucoidan from New Zealand Undaria pinnatifida. *Mar. Drugs* **2022**, *20*, 197. [CrossRef]

36. Deng, Z.; Wu, N.; Suo, Q.; Wang, J.; Yue, Y.; Geng, L.; Zhang, Q. Fucoidan, as an immunostimulator promotes M1 macrophage differentiation and enhances the chemotherapeutic sensitivity of capecitabine in colon cancer. *Int. J. Biol. Macromol.* **2022**, *222*, 562–572. [CrossRef]
37. Patankar, M.S.; Oehninger, S.; Barnett, T.; Williams, R.L.; Clark, G.F. A revised structure for fucoidan may explain some of its biological activities. *J. Biol. Chem.* **1993**, *268*, 21770–21776. [CrossRef]
38. Chollet, L.; Saboural, P.; Chauvierre, C.; Villemin, J.N.; Letourneur, D.; Chaubet, F. Fucoidans in Nanomedicine. *Mar. Drugs* **2016**, *14*, 145. [CrossRef]
39. Zayed, A.; El-Aasr, M.; Ibrahim, A.S.; Ulber, R. Fucoidan Characterization: Determination of Purity and Physicochemical and Chemical Properties. *Mar. Drugs* **2020**, *18*, 571. [CrossRef]
40. Chevolot, L.; Foucault, A.; Chaubet, F.; Kervarec, N.; Sinquin, C.; Fisher, A.-M.; Boisson-Vidal, C. Further data on the structure of brown seaweed fucans: Relationships with anticoagulant activity. *Carbohydr. Res.* **1999**, *319*, 154–165. [CrossRef]
41. Luthuli, S.; Wu, S.; Cheng, Y.; Zheng, X.; Wu, M.; Tong, H. Therapeutic Effects of Fucoidan: A Review on Recent Studies. *Mar. Drugs* **2019**, *17*, 487. [CrossRef]
42. Citkowska, A.; Szekalska, M.; Winnicka, K. Possibilities of Fucoidan Utilization in the Development of Pharmaceutical Dosage Forms. *Mar. Drugs* **2019**, *17*, 458. [CrossRef]
43. Shen, P.; Yin, Z.; Qu, G.; Wang, C. 11–Fucoidan and Its Health Benefits. In *Bioactive Seaweeds for Food Applications*; Qin, Y., Ed.; Academic Press: Cambridge, MA, USA, 2018; pp. 223–238. [CrossRef]
44. Nishino, T.; Nishioka, C.; Ura, H.; Nagumo, T. Isolation and partial characterization of a noval amino sugar-containing fucan sulfate from commercial Fucus vesiculosus fucoidan. *Carbohydr. Res.* **1994**, *255*, 213–224. [CrossRef]
45. Kopplin, G.; Rokstad, A.M.; Mélida, H.; Bulone, V.; Skjåk-Bræk, G.; Aachmann, F.L. Structural Characterization of Fucoidan from Laminaria hyperborea: Assessment of Coagulation and Inflammatory Properties and Their Structure–Function Relationship. *ACS Appl. Bio Mater.* **2018**, *1*, 1880–1892. [CrossRef]
46. Ustyuzhanina, N.E.; Bilan, M.I.; Ushakova, N.A.; Usov, A.I.; Kiselevskiy, M.V.; Nifantiev, N.E. Fucoidans: Pro- or antiangiogenic agents? *Glycobiology* **2014**, *24*, 1265–1274. [CrossRef]
47. Cabral, E.M.; Mondala, J.R.M.; Oliveira, M.; Przyborska, J.; Fitzpatrick, S.; Rai, D.K.; Sivagnanam, S.P.; Garcia-Vaquero, M.; O'Shea, D.; Devereux, M.; et al. Influence of molecular weight fractionation on the antimicrobial and anticancer properties of a fucoidan rich-extract from the macroalgae Fucus vesiculosus. *Int. J. Biol. Macromol.* **2021**, *186*, 994–1002. [CrossRef] [PubMed]
48. Yang, X.; Wang, S.; Trangle, S.S.; Li, Y.; White, W.L.; Li, J.; Ying, T.; Kong, Q.; Zhao, Y.; Lu, J. Investigation of Different Molecular Weight Fucoidan Fractions Derived from New Zealand Undaria pinnatifida in Combination with GroA Therapy in Prostate Cancer Cell Lines. *Mar. Drugs* **2018**, *16*, 454. [CrossRef]
49. Yoo, H.J.; You, D.J.; Lee, K.W. Characterization and Immunomodulatory Effects of High Molecular Weight Fucoidan Fraction from the Sporophyll of Undaria pinnatifida in Cyclophosphamide-Induced Immunosuppressed Mice. *Mar. Drugs* **2019**, *17*, 447. [CrossRef]
50. Chevolot, L.; Mulloy, B.; Ratiskol, J.; Foucault, A.; Colliec-Jouault, S. A disaccharide repeat unit is the major structure in fucoidans from two species of brown algae. *Carbohydr. Res.* **2001**, *330*, 529–535. [CrossRef]
51. Bilan, M.I.; Grachev, A.A.; Ustuzhanina, N.E.; Shashkov, A.S.; Nifantiev, N.E.; Usov, A.I. Structure of a fucoidan from the brown seaweed Fucus evanescens C.Ag. *Carbohydr. Res.* **2002**, *337*, 719–730. [CrossRef] [PubMed]
52. Lu, J.; Shi, K.K.; Chen, S.; Wang, J.; Hassouna, A.; White, L.N.; Merien, F.; Xie, M.; Kong, Q.; Li, J.; et al. Fucoidan Extracted from the New Zealand Undaria pinnatifida-Physicochemical Comparison against Five Other Fucoidans: Unique Low Molecular Weight Fraction Bioactivity in Breast Cancer Cell Lines. *Mar. Drugs* **2018**, *16*, 461. [CrossRef] [PubMed]
53. Mak, W.; Wang, S.K.; Liu, T.; Hamid, N.; Li, Y.; Lu, J.; White, W.L. Anti-Proliferation Potential and Content of Fucoidan Extracted from Sporophyll of New Zealand Undaria pinnatifida. *Front. Nutr.* **2014**, *1*, 9. [CrossRef]
54. van Weelden, G.; Bobinski, M.; Okla, K.; van Weelden, W.J.; Romano, A.; Pijnenborg, J.M.A. Fucoidan Structure and Activity in Relation to Anti-Cancer Mechanisms. *Mar. Drugs* **2019**, *17*, 32. [CrossRef]
55. Jin, J.O.; Chauhan, P.S.; Arukha, A.P.; Chavda, V.; Dubey, A.; Yadav, D. The Therapeutic Potential of the Anticancer Activity of Fucoidan: Current Advances and Hurdles. *Mar. Drugs* **2021**, *19*, 265. [CrossRef]
56. Jin, J.O.; Yadav, D.; Madhwani, K.; Puranik, N.; Chavda, V.; Song, M. Seaweeds in the Oncology Arena: Anti-Cancer Potential of Fucoidan as a Drug-A Review. *Molecules* **2022**, *27*, 6032. [CrossRef]
57. Guo, R.; Deng, M.; He, X.; Li, M.; Li, J.; He, P.; Liu, H.; Li, M.; Zhang, Z.; He, Q. Fucoidan-functionalized activated platelet-hitchhiking micelles simultaneously track tumor cells and remodel the immunosuppressive microenvironment for efficient metastatic cancer treatment. *Acta Pharm. Sin. B* **2022**, *12*, 467–482. [CrossRef]
58. do-Amaral, C.C.F.; Pacheco, B.S.; Seixas, F.K.; Pereira, C.M.P.; Collares, T. Antitumoral effects of fucoidan on bladder cancer. *Algal Res.* **2020**, *47*, 101884. [CrossRef]
59. Zhang, Z.; Till, S.; Jiang, C.; Knappe, S.; Reutterer, S.; Scheiflinger, F.; Szabo, C.M.; Dockal, M. Structure-activity relationship of the pro- and anticoagulant effects of Fucus vesiculosus fucoidan. *Thromb. Haemost.* **2014**, *111*, 429–437. [CrossRef]
60. Mansour, M.B.; Balti, R.; Yacoubi, L.; Ollivier, V.; Chaubet, F.; Maaroufi, R.M. Primary structure and anticoagulant activity of fucoidan from the sea cucumber Holothuria polii. *Int. J. Biol. Macromol.* **2019**, *121*, 1145–1153. [CrossRef]
61. Chandía, N.P.; Matsuhiro, B. Characterization of a fucoidan from Lessonia vadosa (Phaeophyta) and its anticoagulant and elicitor properties. *Int. J. Biol. Macromol.* **2008**, *42*, 235–240. [CrossRef]

62. Jin, W.; Zhang, Q.; Wang, J.; Zhang, W. A comparative study of the anticoagulant activities of eleven fucoidans. *Carbohydr. Polym.* **2013**, *91*, 1–6. [CrossRef]
63. Church, F.C.; Meade, J.B.; Treanor, R.E.; Whinna, H.C. Antithrombin Activity of Fucoidan: The interaction of fucoidan with heparin cofactor II, antithrombin III, and thrombin. *J. Biol. Chem.* **1989**, *264*, 3618–3623. [CrossRef]
64. Mauray, S.; de Raucourt, E.; Talbot, J.C.; Dachary-Prigent, J.; Jozefowicz, M.; Fischer, A.M. Mechanism of factor IXa inhibition by antithrombin in the presence of unfractionated and low molecular weight heparins and fucoidan. *Biochim. Biophys. Acta* **1998**, *1387*, 184–194. [CrossRef]
65. Kim, B.S.; Park, J.Y.; Kang, H.J.; Kim, H.J.; Lee, J. Fucoidan/FGF-2 induces angiogenesis through JNK- and p38-mediated activation of AKT/MMP-2 signalling. *Biochem. Biophys. Res. Commun.* **2014**, *450*, 1333–1338. [CrossRef] [PubMed]
66. Cong, Q.; Chen, H.; Liao, W.; Xiao, F.; Wang, P.; Qin, Y.; Dong, Q.; Ding, K. Structural characterization and effect on anti-angiogenic activity of a fucoidan from Sargassum fusiforme. *Carbohydr. Polym.* **2016**, *136*, 899–907. [CrossRef] [PubMed]
67. Matou, S.; Helley, D.; Chabut, D.; Bros, A.; Fischer, A.-M. Effect of fucoidan on fibroblast growth factor-2-induced angiogenesis in vitro. *Thromb. Res.* **2002**, *106*, 213–221. [CrossRef] [PubMed]
68. Chabut, D.; Fischer, A.M.; Helley, D.; Colliec, S. Low molecular weight fucoidan promotes FGF-2-induced vascular tube formation by human endothelial cells, with decreased PAI-1 release and ICAM-1 downregulation. *Thromb. Res.* **2004**, *113*, 93–95. [CrossRef] [PubMed]
69. Matsubara, K.; Xue, C.; Zhao, X.; Mori, M.; Sugawara, T.; Hirata, T. Effects of middle molecular weight fucoidans on in vitro and ex vivo angiogenesis of endothelial cells. *Int. J. Mol. Med.* **2005**, *15*, 695–699. [CrossRef]
70. Dinesh, S.; Menon, T.; Hanna, L.E.; Suresh, V.; Sathuvan, M.; Manikannan, M. In vitro anti-HIV-1 activity of fucoidan from Sargassum swartzii. *Int. J. Biol. Macromol.* **2016**, *82*, 83–88. [CrossRef]
71. Pomin, V.H.; Mourão, P.A. Structure, biology, evolution, and medical importance of sulfated fucans and galactans. *Glycobiology* **2008**, *18*, 1016–1027. [CrossRef]
72. Hayashi, K.; Nakano, T.; Hashimoto, M.; Kanekiyo, K.; Hayashi, T. Defensive effects of a fucoidan from brown alga Undaria pinnatifida against herpes simplex virus infection. *Int. Immunopharmacol.* **2008**, *8*, 109–116. [CrossRef]
73. Sun, T.; Zhang, X.; Miao, Y.; Zhou, Y.; Shi, J.; Yan, M.; Chen, A. Studies on Antiviral and Immuno-Regulation Activity of Low Molecular Weight Fucoidan from Laminaria japonica. *J. Ocean Univ. China* **2018**, *17*, 705–711. [CrossRef]
74. Song, S.; Peng, H.; Wang, Q.; Liu, Z.; Dong, X.; Wen, C.; Ai, C.; Zhang, Y.; Wang, Z.; Zhu, B. Inhibitory activities of marine sulfated polysaccharides against SARS-CoV-2. *Food Funct.* **2020**, *11*, 7415–7420. [CrossRef]
75. Lin, H.T.; Chen, C.C.; Chiao, D.J.; Chang, T.Y.; Chen, X.A.; Young, J.J.; Kuo, S.C. Nanoparticular CpG-adjuvanted SARS-CoV-2 S1 protein elicits broadly neutralizing and Th1-biased immunoreactivity in mice. *Int. J. Biol. Macromol.* **2021**, *193*, 1885–1897. [CrossRef]
76. Atashrazm, F.; Lowenthal, R.M.; Woods, G.M.; Holloway, A.F.; Dickinson, J.L. Fucoidan and cancer: A multifunctional molecule with anti-tumor potential. *Mar. Drugs* **2015**, *13*, 2327–2346. [CrossRef]
77. Kwak, J.-Y. Fucoidan as a Marine Anticancer Agent in Preclinical Development. *Mar. Drugs* **2014**, *12*, 851–870. [CrossRef]
78. Yamamoto, I.; Takahashi, M.; Suzuki, T.; Seino, H.; Mori, H. Antitumor effect of seaweeds. IV. Enhancement of antitumor activity by sulfation of a crude fucoidan fraction from Sargassum kjellmanianum. *Jpn. J. Exp. Med.* **1984**, *54*, 143–151.
79. Zhang, Z.; Teruya, K.; Eto, H.; Shirahata, S. Fucoidan Extract Induces Apoptosis in MCF-7 Cells via a Mechanism Involving the ROS-Dependent JNK Activation and Mitochondria-Mediated Pathways. *PLoS ONE* **2011**, *6*, e27441. [CrossRef]
80. Yamasaki-Miyamoto, Y.; Yamasaki, M.; Tachibana, H.; Yamada, K. Fucoidan induces apoptosis through activation of caspase-8 on human breast cancer MCF-7 cells. *J. Agric. Food Chem.* **2009**, *57*, 8677–8682. [CrossRef]
81. Abudabbus, A.; Badmus, A.J.; Shalaweh, S.; Bauer, R.; Hiss, D. Effects of Fucoidan and Chemotherapeutic Agent Combinations on Malignant and Non-malignant Breast Cell Lines. *Curr. Pharm. Biotechnol.* **2017**, *18*, 748–757. [CrossRef]
82. Yang, Y.; Liu, Q.; Shi, X.; Zheng, Q.; Chen, L.; Sun, Y. Advances in plant-derived natural products for antitumor immunotherapy. *Arch. Pharm. Res.* **2021**, *44*, 987–1011. [CrossRef]
83. Banafa, A.M.; Roshan, S.; Liu, Y.Y.; Chen, H.J.; Chen, M.J.; Yang, G.X.; He, G.Y. Fucoidan induces G1 phase arrest and apoptosis through caspases-dependent pathway and ROS induction in human breast cancer MCF-7 cells. *J. Huazhong Univ. Sci. Technol. Med. Sci.* **2013**, *33*, 717–724. [CrossRef]
84. Boo, H.J.; Hyun, J.H.; Kim, S.C.; Kang, J.I.; Kim, M.K.; Kim, S.Y.; Cho, H.; Yoo, E.S.; Kang, H.K. Fucoidan from Undaria pinnatifida induces apoptosis in A549 human lung carcinoma cells. *Phytother. Res.* **2011**, *25*, 1082–1086. [CrossRef]
85. Hsu, H.-Y.; Lin, T.-Y.; Hu, C.-H.; Shu, D.T.F.; Lu, M.-K. Fucoidan upregulates TLR4/CHOP-mediated caspase-3 and PARP activation to enhance cisplatin-induced cytotoxicity in human lung cancer cells. *Cancer Lett.* **2018**, *432*, 112–120. [CrossRef] [PubMed]
86. Hsu, H.Y.; Lin, T.Y.; Lu, M.K.; Leng, P.J.; Tsao, S.M.; Wu, Y.C. Fucoidan induces Toll-like receptor 4-regulated reactive oxygen species and promotes endoplasmic reticulum stress-mediated apoptosis in lung cancer. *Sci. Rep.* **2017**, *7*, 44990. [CrossRef] [PubMed]
87. Chen, X.; Sun, L.; Wei, X.; Lu, H.; Tan, Y.; Sun, Z.; Jiang, J. Antitumor effect and molecular mechanism of fucoidan in NSCLC. *BMC Complement Med.* **2021**, *21*, 25. [CrossRef]
88. Lee, H.; Kim, J.S.; Kim, E. Fucoidan from seaweed Fucus vesiculosus inhibits migration and invasion of human lung cancer cell via PI3K-Akt-mTOR pathways. *PLoS ONE* **2012**, *7*, e50624. [CrossRef] [PubMed]

89. Zhang, Z.; Teruya, K.; Yoshida, T.; Eto, H.; Shirahata, S. Fucoidan extract enhances the anti-cancer activity of chemotherapeutic agents in MDA-MB-231 and MCF-7 breast cancer cells. *Mar. Drugs* **2013**, *11*, 81–98. [CrossRef]
90. Chen, H.; Cong, Q.; Du, Z.; Liao, W.; Zhang, L.; Yao, Y.; Ding, K. Sulfated fucoidan FP08S2 inhibits lung cancer cell growth in vivo by disrupting angiogenesis via targeting VEGFR2/VEGF and blocking VEGFR2/Erk/VEGF signaling. *Cancer Lett.* **2016**, *382*, 44–52. [CrossRef]
91. Danforth, D.N. The Role of Chronic Inflammation in the Development of Breast Cancer. *Cancers* **2021**, *13*, 3918. [CrossRef]
92. Kundu, J.K.; Surh, Y.-J. Inflammation: Gearing the journey to cancer. *Mutat. Res./Rev. Mutat. Res.* **2008**, *659*, 15–30. [CrossRef]
93. Hu, Y.; Cheng, S.C.; Chan, K.T.; Ke, Y.; Xue, B.; Sin, F.W.; Zeng, C.; Xie, Y. Fucoidin enhances dendritic cell-mediated T-cell cytotoxicity against NY-ESO-1 expressing human cancer cells. *Biochem. Biophys. Res. Commun.* **2010**, *392*, 329–334. [CrossRef]
94. Jin, J.O.; Zhang, W.; Du, J.Y.; Wong, K.W.; Oda, T.; Yu, Q. Fucoidan can function as an adjuvant in vivo to enhance dendritic cell maturation and function and promote antigen-specific T cell immune responses. *PLoS ONE* **2014**, *9*, e99396. [CrossRef]
95. Bi, D.; Yu, B.; Han, Q.; Lu, J.; White, W.L.; Lai, Q.; Cai, N.; Luo, W.; Gu, L.; Li, S.; et al. Immune Activation of RAW264.7 Macrophages by Low Molecular Weight Fucoidan Extracted from New Zealand Undaria pinnatifida. *J. Agric. Food Chem.* **2018**, *66*, 10721–10728. [CrossRef]
96. Jeong, J.-W.; Hwang, S.J.; Han, M.H.; Lee, D.-S.; Yoo, J.S.; Choi, I.-W.; Cha, H.-J.; Kim, S.; Kim, H.-S.; Kim, G.-Y.; et al. Fucoidan inhibits lipopolysaccharide-induced inflammatory responses in RAW 264.7 macrophages and zebrafish larvae. *Mol. Cell. Toxicol.* **2017**, *13*, 405–417. [CrossRef]
97. Ni, L.; Wang, L.; Fu, X.; Duan, D.; Jeon, Y.J.; Xu, J.; Gao, X. In vitro and in vivo anti-inflammatory activities of a fucose-rich fucoidan isolated from Saccharina japonica. *Int. J. Biol. Macromol.* **2020**, *156*, 717–729. [CrossRef]
98. Multhoff, G.; Molls, M.; Radons, J. Chronic inflammation in cancer development. *Front. Immunol.* **2012**, *2*, 98. [CrossRef]
99. Lee, S.H.; Ko, C.I.; Ahn, G.; You, S.; Kim, J.S.; Heu, M.S.; Kim, J.; Jee, Y.; Jeon, Y.J. Molecular characteristics and anti-inflammatory activity of the fucoidan extracted from Ecklonia cava. *Carbohydr. Polym.* **2012**, *89*, 599–606. [CrossRef]
100. Fernando, I.P.S.; Sanjeewa, K.K.A.; Samarakoon, K.W.; Lee, W.W.; Kim, H.-S.; Kang, N.; Ranasinghe, P.; Lee, H.-S.; Jeon, Y.-J. A fucoidan fraction purified from Chnoospora minima; a potential inhibitor of LPS-induced inflammatory responses. *Int. J. Biol. Macromol.* **2017**, *104*, 1185–1193. [CrossRef]
101. Sanjeewa, K.K.A.; Fernando, I.P.S.; Kim, S.Y.; Kim, H.S.; Ahn, G.; Jee, Y.; Jeon, Y.J. In vitro and in vivo anti-inflammatory activities of high molecular weight sulfated polysaccharide; containing fucose separated from Sargassum horneri: Short communication. *Int. J. Biol. Macromol.* **2018**, *107*, 803–807. [CrossRef]
102. Sanjeewa, K.K.; Fernando, I.P.; Kim, E.A.; Ahn, G.; Jee, Y.; Jeon, Y.J. Anti-inflammatory activity of a sulfated polysaccharide isolated from an enzymatic digest of brown seaweed Sargassum horneri in RAW 264.7 cells. *Nutr. Res. Pract.* **2017**, *11*, 3–10. [CrossRef]
103. Lee, J.H.; Ryu, J.M.; Han, Y.-S.; Zia, M.F.; Kwon, H.Y.; Noh, H.; Han, H.J.; Lee, S.H. Fucoidan improves bioactivity and vasculogenic potential of mesenchymal stem cells in murine hind limb ischemia associated with chronic kidney disease. *J. Mol. Cell. Cardiol.* **2016**, *97*, 169–179. [CrossRef]
104. Barbosa, A.I.; Costa Lima, S.A.; Reis, S. Development of methotrexate loaded fucoidan/chitosan nanoparticles with anti-inflammatory potential and enhanced skin permeation. *Int. J. Biol. Macromol.* **2019**, *124*, 1115–1122. [CrossRef]
105. Ahmad, T.; Eapen, M.S.; Ishaq, M.; Park, A.Y.; Karpiniec, S.S.; Stringer, D.N.; Sohal, S.S.; Fitton, J.H.; Guven, N.; Caruso, V.; et al. Anti-Inflammatory Activity of Fucoidan Extracts In Vitro. *Mar. Drugs* **2021**, *19*, 702. [CrossRef] [PubMed]
106. Kim, H.-M.; Ahn, C.; Kang, B.-T.; Kang, J.-H.; Jeung, E.-B.; Yang, M.-P. Fucoidan suppresses excessive phagocytic capacity of porcine peripheral blood polymorphonuclear cells by modulating production of tumor necrosis factor alpha by lipopolysaccharide-stimulated peripheral blood mononuclear cells. *Res. Vet. Sci.* **2018**, *118*, 413–418. [CrossRef] [PubMed]
107. Hwang, P.A.; Phan, N.N.; Lu, W.J.; Ngoc Hieu, B.T.; Lin, Y.C. Low-molecular-weight fucoidan and high-stability fucoxanthin from brown seaweed exert prebiotics and anti-inflammatory activities in Caco-2 cells. *Food Nutr. Res.* **2016**, *60*, 32033. [CrossRef] [PubMed]
108. Fernando, I.P.S.; Sanjeewa, K.K.A.; Lee, H.G.; Kim, H.S.; Vaas, A.; De Silva, H.I.C.; Nanayakkara, C.M.; Abeytunga, D.T.U.; Lee, D.S.; Lee, J.S.; et al. Fucoidan Purified from Sargassum polycystum Induces Apoptosis through Mitochondria-Mediated Pathway in HL-60 and MCF-7 Cells. *Mar Drugs* **2020**, *18*, 196. [CrossRef] [PubMed]
109. Wang, Y.; Xing, M.; Cao, Q.; Ji, A.; Liang, H.; Song, S. Biological Activities of Fucoidan and the Factors Mediating Its Therapeutic Effects: A Review of Recent Studies. *Mar. Drugs* **2019**, *17*, 183. [CrossRef] [PubMed]
110. Koh, H.S.A.; Lu, J.; Zhou, W. Structure characterization and antioxidant activity of fucoidan isolated from Undaria pinnatifida grown in New Zealand. *Carbohydr. Polym.* **2019**, *212*, 178–185. [CrossRef] [PubMed]
111. Wang, X.; Yi, K.; Zhao, Y. Fucoidan inhibits amyloid-β-induced toxicity in transgenic Caenorhabditis elegans by reducing the accumulation of amyloid-β and decreasing the production of reactive oxygen species. *Food Funct.* **2018**, *9*, 552–560. [CrossRef]
112. Pozharitskaya, O.N.; Shikov, A.N.; Faustova, N.M.; Obluchinskaya, E.D.; Kosman, V.M.; Vuorela, H.; Makarov, V.G. Pharmacokinetic and Tissue Distribution of Fucoidan from Fucus vesiculosus after Oral Administration to Rats. *Mar. Drugs* **2018**, *16*, 132. [CrossRef]
113. Zhao, X.; Guo, F.; Hu, J.; Zhang, L.; Xue, C.; Zhang, Z.; Li, B. Antithrombotic activity of oral administered low molecular weight fucoidan from Laminaria Japonica. *Thromb. Res.* **2016**, *144*, 46–52. [CrossRef]

114. Zhan, E.; Chu, F.; Zhao, T.; Chai, Y.; Liang, H.; Song, S.; Ji, A. Determination of fucoidan in rat plasma by HPLC and its application in pharmacokinetics. *Pak. J. Pharm. Sci.* **2020**, *33*, 1–9.
115. Shikov, A.N.; Flisyuk, E.V.; Obluchinskaya, E.D.; Pozharitskaya, O.N. Pharmacokinetics of Marine-Derived Drugs. *Mar. Drugs* **2020**, *18*, 557. [CrossRef]
116. Tokita, Y.; Nakajima, K.; Mochida, H.; Iha, M.; Nagamine, T. Development of a fucoidan-specific antibody and measurement of fucoidan in serum and urine by sandwich ELISA. *Biosci. Biotechnol. Biochem.* **2010**, *74*, 350–357. [CrossRef]
117. Kadena, K.; Tomori, M.; Iha, M.; Nagamine, T. Absorption Study of Mozuku Fucoidan in Japanese Volunteers. *Mar. Drugs* **2018**, *16*, 254. [CrossRef]
118. Zhang, W.; Sun, D.; Zhao, X.; Jin, W.; Wang, J.; Zhang, Q. Microanalysis and preliminary pharmacokinetic studies of a sulfated polysaccharide from Laminaria japonica. *Chin. J. Oceanol. Limnol.* **2016**, *34*, 177–185. [CrossRef]
119. Imbs, T.I.; Zvyagintseva, T.N.; Ermakova, S.P. Is the transformation of fucoidans in human body possible? *Int. J. Biol. Macromol.* **2020**, *142*, 778–781. [CrossRef]
120. Bai, X.; Zhang, E.; Hu, B.; Liang, H.; Song, S.; Ji, A. Study on Absorption Mechanism and Tissue Distribution of Fucoidan. *Molecules* **2020**, *25*, 1087. [CrossRef]
121. Marinova Pty. Ltd. *Determination of the Generally Recognized as Safe (Gras) Status of Fucoidan from Fucus Vesiculosus as a Food Ingredient*; Food and Drug Administration: College Park, MD, USA, 2016.
122. Fitton, H.J.; Stringer, D.S.; Park, A.Y.; Karpiniec, S.N. Therapies from Fucoidan: New Developments. *Mar. Drugs* **2019**, *17*, 571. [CrossRef]
123. Sugawara, I.; Ishizaka, S. Polysaccharides with sulfate groups are human T-cell mitogens and murine polyclonal B-cell activators (PBAs). I. Fucoidan and heparin. *Cell. Immunol.* **1982**, *74*, 162–171. [CrossRef]
124. Zapopozhets, T.S.; Besednova, N.N.; Loenko Iu, N. [Antibacterial and immunomodulating activity of fucoidan]. *Antibiot. Khimioter.* **1995**, *40*, 9–13.
125. Liu, J.N.; Yoshida, Y.; Wang, M.Q.; Okai, Y.; Yamashita, U. B cell stimulating activity of seaweed extracts. *Int. J. Immunopharmacol.* **1997**, *19*, 135–142. [CrossRef]
126. Chiang, C.-S.; Lin, Y.-J.; Lee, R.; Lai, Y.-H.; Cheng, H.-W.; Hsieh, C.-H.; Shyu, W.-C.; Chen, S.-Y. Combination of fucoidan-based magnetic nanoparticles and immunomodulators enhances tumour-localized immunotherapy. *Nat. Nanotechnol.* **2018**, *13*, 746–754. [CrossRef] [PubMed]
127. Zhang, W.; Oda, T.; Yu, Q.; Jin, J.-O. Fucoidan from Macrocystis pyrifera Has Powerful Immune-Modulatory Effects Compared to Three Other Fucoidans. *Mar. Drugs* **2015**, *13*, 1084–1104. [CrossRef] [PubMed]
128. Tabarsa, M.; Dabaghian, E.H.; You, S.; Yelithao, K.; Cao, R.; Rezaei, M.; Alboofetileh, M.; Bita, S. The activation of NF-κB and MAPKs signaling pathways of RAW264.7 murine macrophages and natural killer cells by fucoidan from Nizamuddinia zanardinii. *Int. J. Biol. Macromol.* **2020**, *148*, 56–67. [CrossRef] [PubMed]
129. Ale, M.T.; Maruyama, H.; Tamauchi, H.; Mikkelsen, J.D.; Meyer, A.S. Fucoidan from Sargassum sp. and Fucus vesiculosus reduces cell viability of lung carcinoma and melanoma cells in vitro and activates natural killer cells in mice in vivo. *Int. J. Biol. Macromol.* **2011**, *49*, 331–336. [CrossRef]
130. Zhang, W.; An, E.K.; Park, H.B.; Hwang, J.; Dhananjay, Y.; Kim, S.J.; Eom, H.Y.; Oda, T.; Kwak, M.; Lee, P.C.; et al. Ecklonia cava fucoidan has potential to stimulate natural killer cells in vivo. *Int. J. Biol. Macromol.* **2021**, *185*, 111–121. [CrossRef]
131. Yang, M.; Ma, C.; Sun, J.; Shao, Q.; Gao, W.; Zhang, Y.; Li, Z.; Xie, Q.; Dong, Z.; Qu, X. Fucoidan stimulation induces a functional maturation of human monocyte-derived dendritic cells. *Int. Immunopharmacol.* **2008**, *8*, 1754–1760. [CrossRef]
132. Jin, J.O.; Park, H.Y.; Xu, Q.; Park, J.I.; Zvyagintseva, T.; Stonik, V.A.; Kwak, J.Y. Ligand of scavenger receptor class A indirectly induces maturation of human blood dendritic cells via production of tumor necrosis factor-alpha. *Blood* **2009**, *113*, 5839–5847. [CrossRef]
133. Sun, J.; Sun, J.; Song, B.; Zhang, L.; Shao, Q.; Liu, Y.; Yuan, D.; Zhang, Y.; Qu, X. Fucoidan inhibits CCL22 production through NF-κB pathway in M2 macrophages: A potential therapeutic strategy for cancer. *Sci. Rep.* **2016**, *6*, 35855. [CrossRef]
134. Makarenkova, I.D.; Logunov, D.Y.; Tukhvatulin, A.I.; Semenova, I.B.; Besednova, N.N.; Zvyagintseva, T.N. Interactions between sulfated polysaccharides from sea brown algae and Toll-like receptors on HEK293 eukaryotic cells in vitro. *Bull. Exp. Biol. Med.* **2012**, *154*, 241–244. [CrossRef]
135. Lee, H.H.; Cho, Y.; Kim, G.H.; Cho, H. Undaria pinnatifida Fucoidan-Rich Extract Recovers Immunity of Immunosuppressed Mice. *J. Microbiol. Biotechnol.* **2020**, *30*, 439–447. [CrossRef]
136. Park, A.Y.; Nafia, I.; Stringer, D.N.; Karpiniec, S.S.; Fitton, J.H. Fucoidan Independently Enhances Activity in Human Immune Cells and Has a Cytostatic Effect on Prostate Cancer Cells in the Presence of Nivolumab. *Mar. Drugs* **2022**, *20*, 12. [CrossRef]
137. Nakamura, T.; Suzuki, H.; Wada, Y.; Kodama, T.; Doi, T. Fucoidan induces nitric oxide production via p38 mitogen-activated protein kinase and NF-κB-dependent signaling pathways through macrophage scavenger receptors. *Biochem. Biophys. Res. Commun.* **2006**, *343*, 286–294. [CrossRef]
138. Jang, J.-Y.; Moon, S.-Y.; Joo, H.-G. Differential effects of fucoidans with low and high molecular weight on the viability and function of spleen cells. *Food Chem. Toxicol.* **2014**, *68*, 234–238. [CrossRef]
139. Reis e Sousa, C. Toll-like receptors and dendritic cells: For whom the bug tolls. *Semin. Immunol.* **2004**, *16*, 27–34. [CrossRef]
140. Gordon, S. Pattern recognition receptors: Doubling up for the innate immune response. *Cell* **2002**, *111*, 927–930. [CrossRef]

141. Kaliński, P.; Hilkens, C.M.U.; Wierenga, E.A.; Kapsenberg, M.L. T-cell priming by type-1and type-2 polarized dendritic cells: The concept of a third signal. *Immunol. Today* **1999**, *20*, 561–567. [CrossRef]
142. Yang, J.W.; Yoon, S.Y.; Oh, S.J.; Kim, S.K.; Kang, K.W. Bifunctional effects of fucoidan on the expression of inducible nitric oxide synthase. *Biochem. Biophys. Res. Commun.* **2006**, *346*, 345–350. [CrossRef]
143. Chen, L.M.; Tseng, H.Y.; Chen, Y.A.; Al Haq, A.T.; Hwang, P.A.; Hsu, H.L. Oligo-Fucoidan Prevents M2 Macrophage Differentiation and HCT116 Tumor Progression. *Cancers* **2020**, *12*, 421. [CrossRef]
144. Peng, Y.; Song, Y.; Wang, Q.; Hu, Y.; He, Y.; Ren, D.; Wu, L.; Liu, S.; Cong, H.; Zhou, H. In vitro and in vivo immunomodulatory effects of fucoidan compound agents. *Int. J. Biol. Macromol.* **2019**, *127*, 48–56. [CrossRef]
145. Chiossone, L.; Dumas, P.-Y.; Vienne, M.; Vivier, E. Natural killer cells and other innate lymphoid cells in cancer. *Nat. Rev. Immunol.* **2018**, *18*, 671–688. [CrossRef]
146. Surayot, U.; Lee, S.; You, S. Effects of sulfated fucan from the sea cucumber Stichopus japonicus on natural killer cell activation and cytotoxicity. *Int. J. Biol. Macromol.* **2018**, *108*, 177–184. [CrossRef] [PubMed]
147. Wang, M.; Zhou, Z.; Wang, X.; Zhang, C.; Jiang, X. Natural killer cell awakening: Unleash cancer-immunity cycle against glioblastoma. *Cell Death Dis.* **2022**, *13*, 588. [CrossRef] [PubMed]
148. Zhang, W.; Okimura, T.; Oda, T.; Jin, J.-O. Ascophyllan Induces Activation of Natural Killer Cells in Mice In Vivo and In Vitro. *Mar. Drugs* **2019**, *17*, 197. [CrossRef] [PubMed]
149. An, E.K.; Hwang, J.; Kim, S.J.; Park, H.B.; Zhang, W.; Ryu, J.H.; You, S.; Jin, J.O. Comparison of the immune activation capacities of fucoidan and laminarin extracted from Laminaria japonica. *Int. J. Biol. Macromol.* **2022**, *208*, 230–242. [CrossRef]
150. Azuma, K.; Ishihara, T.; Nakamoto, H.; Amaha, T.; Osaki, T.; Tsuka, T.; Imagawa, T.; Minami, S.; Takashima, O.; Ifuku, S.; et al. Effects of oral administration of fucoidan extracted from Cladosiphon okamuranus on tumor growth and survival time in a tumor-bearing mouse model. *Mar. Drugs* **2012**, *10*, 2337–2348. [CrossRef]
151. Shukla, S.; Steinmetz, N.F. Emerging nanotechnologies for cancer immunotherapy. *Exp. Biol. Med. (Maywood)* **2016**, *241*, 1116–1126. [CrossRef]
152. Hwang, P.A.; Lin, X.Z.; Kuo, K.L.; Hsu, F.Y. Fabrication and Cytotoxicity of Fucoidan-Cisplatin Nanoparticles for Macrophage and Tumor Cells. *Materials* **2017**, *10*, 291. [CrossRef]
153. Chung, C.H.; Lu, K.Y.; Lee, W.C.; Hsu, W.J.; Lee, W.F.; Dai, J.Z.; Shueng, P.W.; Lin, C.W.; Mi, F.L. Fucoidan-based, tumor-activated nanoplatform for overcoming hypoxia and enhancing photodynamic therapy and antitumor immunity. *Biomaterials* **2020**, *257*, 120227. [CrossRef]
154. Jeon, E.Y.; Choi, D.S.; Choi, S.; Won, J.Y.; Jo, Y.; Kim, H.B.; Jung, Y.; Shin, S.C.; Min, H.; Choi, H.W.; et al. Enhancing adoptive T-cell therapy with fucoidan-based IL-2 delivery microcapsules. *Bioeng. Transl. Med.* **2023**, *8*, e10362. [CrossRef]
155. Moghbeli, M.; Khedmatgozar, H.; Yadegari, M.; Avan, A.; Ferns, G.A.; Ghayour Mobarhan, M. Chapter Five—Cytokines and the immune response in obesity-related disorders. In *Advances in Clinical Chemistry*; Makowski, G.S., Ed.; Elsevier: Amsterdam, The Netherlands, 2021; Volume 101, pp. 135–168.
156. Duan, Z.; Luo, Y. Targeting macrophages in cancer immunotherapy. *Signal Transduct. Target. Ther.* **2021**, *6*, 127. [CrossRef]
157. Ekmekcioglu, S.; Grimm, E.A.; Roszik, J. Targeting iNOS to increase efficacy of immunotherapies. *Hum. Vaccin Immunother.* **2017**, *13*, 1105–1108. [CrossRef]
158. Takeda, K.; Tomimori, K.; Kimura, R.; Ishikawa, C.; Nowling, T.K.; Mori, N. Anti-tumor activity of fucoidan is mediated by nitric oxide released from macrophages. *Int. J. Oncol.* **2012**, *40*, 251–260. [CrossRef]
159. Jiang, S.; Yin, H.; Li, R.; Shi, W.; Mou, J.; Yang, J. The activation effects of fucoidan from sea cucumber Stichopus chloronotus on RAW264.7 cells via TLR2/4-NF-κB pathway and its structure-activity relationship. *Carbohydr. Polym.* **2021**, *270*, 118353. [CrossRef]
160. Yu, L.; Jin, Y.; Song, M.; Zhao, Y.; Zhang, H. When Natural Compounds Meet Nanotechnology: Nature-Inspired Nanomedicines for Cancer Immunotherapy. *Pharmaceutics* **2022**, *14*, 1589. [CrossRef]
161. Yadav, D.; Kwak, M.; Chauhan, P.S.; Puranik, N.; Lee, P.C.W.; Jin, J.-O. Cancer immunotherapy by immune checkpoint blockade and its advanced application using bio-nanomaterials. *Semin. Cancer Biol.* **2022**, *86*, 909–922. [CrossRef]
162. Sanaei, M.J.; Pourbagheri-Sigaroodi, A.; Kaveh, V.; Sheikholeslami, S.A.; Salari, S.; Bashash, D. The application of nano-medicine to overcome the challenges related to immune checkpoint blockades in cancer immunotherapy: Recent advances and opportunities. *Crit. Rev. Oncol. Hematol.* **2021**, *157*, 103160. [CrossRef]
163. Martin, J.D.; Cabral, H.; Stylianopoulos, T.; Jain, R.K. Improving cancer immunotherapy using nanomedicines: Progress, opportunities and challenges. *Nat. Rev. Clin. Oncol.* **2020**, *17*, 251–266. [CrossRef]
164. Tsai, H.L.; Tai, C.J.; Huang, C.W.; Chang, F.R.; Wang, J.Y. Efficacy of Low-Molecular-Weight Fucoidan as a Supplemental Therapy in Metastatic Colorectal Cancer Patients: A Double-Blind Randomized Controlled Trial. *Mar. Drugs* **2017**, *15*, 122. [CrossRef]
165. Ikeguchi, M.; Yamamoto, M.; Arai, Y.; Maeta, Y.; Ashida, K.; Katano, K.; Miki, Y.; Kimura, T. Fucoidan reduces the toxicities of chemotherapy for patients with unresectable advanced or recurrent colorectal cancer. *Oncol. Lett.* **2011**, *2*, 319–322. [CrossRef]
166. Yang, M.; Xuan, Z.; Wang, Q.; Yan, S.; Zhou, D.; Naman, C.B.; Zhang, J.; He, S.; Yan, X.; Cui, W. Fucoxanthin has potential for therapeutic efficacy in neurodegenerative disorders by acting on multiple targets. *Nutr. Neurosci.* **2022**, *25*, 2167–2180. [CrossRef]

Disclaimer/Publisher's Note: The statements, opinions and data contained in all publications are solely those of the individual author(s) and contributor(s) and not of MDPI and/or the editor(s). MDPI and/or the editor(s) disclaim responsibility for any injury to people or property resulting from any ideas, methods, instructions or products referred to in the content.

marine drugs MDPI

Review

Marine Migrastatics: A Comprehensive 2022 Update

Marzia Vasarri [1,*], Emanuela Barletta [1] and Donatella Degl'Innocenti [1,2]

1 Department of Experimental and Clinical Biomedical Sciences, University of Florence, Viale Morgagni 50, 50134 Florence, Italy; emanuela.barletta@unifi.it (E.B.); donatella.deglinnocenti@unifi.it (D.D.)
2 Interuniversity Center of Marine Biology and Applied Ecology "G. Bacci" (CIBM), Viale N. Sauro 4, 57128 Livorno, Italy
* Correspondence: marzia.vasarri@unifi.it

Abstract: Metastasis is responsible for the bad prognosis in cancer patients. Advances in research on metastasis prevention focus attention on the molecular mechanisms underlying cancer cell motility and invasion to improve therapies for long-term survival in cancer patients. The so-called "migrastatics" could help block cancer cell invasion and lead to the rapid development of antimetastatic therapies, improving conventional cancer therapies. In the relentless search for migrastatics, the marine environment represents an important source of natural compounds due to its enormous biodiversity. Thus, this review is a selection of scientific research that has pointed out in a broad spectrum of in vitro and in vivo models the anti-cancer power of marine-derived products against cancer cell migration and invasion over the past five years. Overall, this review might provide a useful up-to-date guide about marine-derived compounds with potential interest for pharmaceutical and scientific research on antimetastatic drug endpoints.

Keywords: marine compounds; migrastatics; cell migration; cell invasion; metastasis; anti-cancer

Citation: Vasarri, M.; Barletta, E.; Degl'Innocenti, D. Marine Migrastatics: A Comprehensive 2022 Update. *Mar. Drugs* **2022**, *20*, 273. https://doi.org/10.3390/md20050273

Academic Editors: Celso Alves and Marc Diederich

Received: 24 March 2022
Accepted: 15 April 2022
Published: 19 April 2022

Publisher's Note: MDPI stays neutral with regard to jurisdictional claims in published maps and institutional affiliations.

Copyright: © 2022 by the authors. Licensee MDPI, Basel, Switzerland. This article is an open access article distributed under the terms and conditions of the Creative Commons Attribution (CC BY) license (https://creativecommons.org/licenses/by/4.0/).

1. Introduction

Worldwide, cancer ranks among the leading causes of death. An estimated 19.3 million new cases occurred in 2020, with a mortality rate exceeding 50% [1]. Cancer develops due to complex biological processes such as uncontrolled cell proliferation, resistance to cell death, neo-angiogenesis, invasion, and metastasis [2].

The most common cause of cancer-related death is invasion and metastasis, in which cancer cells spread throughout the body, causing secondary sites of invasion and severe organ damage [3].

Significant progress has been made in treating malignant tumors thanks to the development of new technologies and combination therapies used as multiple approaches to affect several signaling pathways simultaneously [4]. However, traditional cytotoxic chemotherapeutic agents are still the most commonly used. Conventionally, the progression of solid cancers is defined by the increase in tumor size. Therefore, it is understandable that tumor shrinkage is considered one of the indices of therapeutic efficacy. However, tumor shrinkage is never absolute and is not predictive of antimetastatic effect and may divert attention from cancer metastasis, which is responsible for more than 90% of mortality [5].

Therefore, blocking cancer cell migration and the possibility of secondary tumor formation is crucial to significantly improve cancer treatment by eliminating the risk of systemic disease and reducing reliance on therapies with harmful side effects. Combining antimetastatic therapy with standard cytotoxic cancer therapies appears to be a promising approach for treating metastases [6,7].

In light of these considerations, Gandalovičová et al. (2017) coined the term "migrastatics" to define a new class of drugs capable of interfering with cancer cell migration and invasion, and thus with the ability to metastasize [5]. Migrastatic agents, which differ from conventional cytostatic compounds that primarily target cell proliferation, are important for treating cancer with a propensity for early metastasis. This new definition shifts the focus from primary cancer therapy to the treatment of metastasis development and from tumor shrinkage as a measure of treatment efficacy to metastasis-free survival as the most representative endpoint for antimetastatic drugs [5].

Despite the large arsenal of anti-cancer drugs available, inadequate selectivity toward cancer cells and developed resistance account for the serious side effects of therapy. This has made it more urgent than ever to find new drugs, and for this purpose, it has often proven useful to consider the pharmacological properties of natural compounds. To date, the majority (at least 60%) of anti-cancer drugs are derived from natural products of both terrestrial and marine origin. However, unlike the terrestrial environment, marine biodiversity represents a vast and largely unexplored source of bioactive compounds characterized by structural novelty, complexity, and diversity. The unique conditions of life in the marine environment require special mechanisms for organisms to adapt to growth in the ocean that are fundamentally different from those of terrestrial organisms. One important adaptation mechanism is the production of biologically active secondary metabolites. Secondary metabolites are not produced using biological or regular metabolic pathways and do not serve any primary function relevant to the development, growth, or propagation of a species. However, they provide a wealth of chemical diversity potentially useful for drug development because of their biological activities [8].

In addition, continued improvements in undersea life support systems have provided new opportunities for harvesting from unexplored regions and depths. The sea's treasures have made fundamental contributions to modern medicine, providing important scientific discoveries for human health [9]. Thus, marine bio-discovery has become a frontier pursuit for many scientists in academia and industry in recent decades. Continued exploration of the marine environment and characterization and screening of its inhabitants for unique bioactive chemicals has already proven fruitful in the search for new anti-cancer therapies [10,11]. Clinical trials are underway for a large number of marine-derived anti-cancer compounds [12], and the field is currently expanding rapidly.

It is conceivable that many marine species have yet to be discovered, which could lead to the identification of a myriad of marine natural products that could enhance and complement existing anti-cancer therapies. The literature is full of reviews on natural anti-cancer products and their various mechanisms of action, but what are the latest findings on marine anti-cancer agents with migrastatic potential? Here is a selection of marine anti-cancer compounds described in the last five years (coining of the term "migrastatics") for their ability to inhibit cancer cell migration and invasion. This review represents a useful tool for pharmaceutical industries and basic biomedical science to improve the knowledge of marine migrastatics as potential candidates for developing new anti-cancer strategies.

2. Biomechanisms Underlying Cancer Metastasis as Therapeutic Molecular Targets

Metastasis originates from the spread of tumor cells into tissues and organs beyond their primary site and their establishment at secondary sites with the formation of new tumors [13]. The first step in the metastatic process is the migration of cancer cells through the extracellular matrix (ECM) of the surrounding tissue and penetration into the lymphatic or vascular circulation. After the extravasation process through the basement membrane of the vessels, the invasive cells will attach to a new site and proliferate to produce the secondary tumor [3] (Figure 1).

The dynamics of this process depend on multiple biomechanisms and signaling pathways that promote the metastatic progression of cancer cells. Understanding these biomechanisms is essential to identifying molecular targets to reverse the pro-metastatic behavior of cancer cells.

Below we will briefly present the biomechanisms underlying metastasis described as potential druggable targets of marine migrastatics over the past five years (2017–2022).

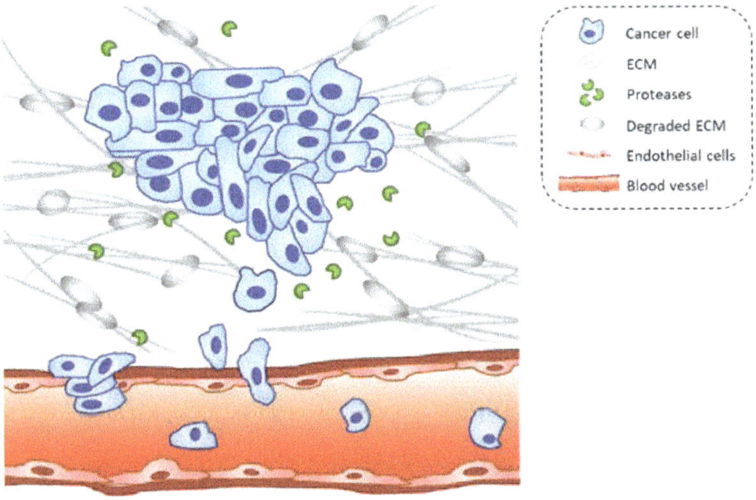

Figure 1. Schematic representation of the migration and invasion process of cancer cells. Cells penetrate the basement membrane and invade surrounding tissues; cancer cells invade blood vessels and give rise to metastasis.

2.1. Epithelial-Mesenchymal Transition (EMT) and EMT-Related Signaling Pathways

The invasiveness and metastatic potential of malignant epithelial tumors, which represent about 90% of all cancer cases, are supported by the so-called epithelial-mesenchymal transition (EMT). This is a process by which epithelial cells acquire fibroblastoid properties [14]. During EMT, there is loss of cell-cell adhesion, cytoskeletal remodeling, and alteration in cell-ECM adhesion. This process is triggered by complex regulatory networks involving transcriptional control within the affected epithelial cells, such as the suppression of E-cadherin (a known epithelial marker) expression by key regulators of EMT (such as Snail, Slug, and Twist) [15,16]. As a result, cells become more motile and adhesive to endothelial cells. Furthermore, the EMT process is regulated by many molecular events, including multiple signaling pathways in various cancers [14]. Among them, the Hedgehog (Hh) signaling pathway has been described to play a role in regulating EMT [17–20]. Aberrant activation of the Hh signaling pathway has been associated with cancer onset and metastasis formation [21]. Thus, EMT and related signaling pathways are meaningful targets for blocking the pro-metastatic behavior of cancer cells.

2.2. ECM Disassembly and the Role of Matrix Metalloproteinases (MMPs)

Cancer cell migration and invasion are also influenced by ECM disassembly. The ECM is a source of cell-binding proteins and growth factors important to tumor cell survival. ECM can be modified significantly by proteases generated by tumor cells or stromal cells. These ECM proteases affect the cell-cell and cell-ECM interactions. Among ECM proteases, matrix metalloproteinases (MMPs)—a family of zinc-dependent endoproteinases—play an important role as early markers in cancer progression. They facilitate invasion by degrading components of the ECM, such as collagen, laminin, and proteoglycans [22]. However, it has become clear that MMPs play a role in ECM modification and regulate numerous other biological events, including cell growth, inflammation, and angiogenesis, by cleaving cell surface proteins and adhesion molecules [23]. Among all members of the MMPs, it has been reported that MMP-2 and MMP-9 correlate with tumor metastasis [24]. Therefore, targeting the expression and/or activity of MMPs or other ECM proteases has long been considered promising targets for cancer therapy.

2.3. Anoikis Resistance

As part of normal development and tissue homeostasis, a cell death called anoikis (detachment-induced apoptosis) acts to prevent detached cells from reattaching to the wrong ECM and growing dysplastically. During the detachment of ECM-anchored cells, anoikis is triggered [25]. A tumor cell exhibiting pro-metastatic behavior develops altered cell adhesion mechanisms and anoikis resistance. A detached cell from a localized tumor can escape anoikis, resulting in uncontrolled growth. Cancer cells employ many mechanisms to abrogate anoikis, promoting invasion and metastasis [26]. By providing adequate structural support, ECM-based adhesion is crucial for cell survival. Several factors have been identified for modulating anoikis resistance, such as cell adhesion molecules, growth proteins, oxidative stress, stemness, autophagy, non-coding RNAs, and signaling pathways [26].

2.4. Cytoskeletal Remodeling and Cell Adhesion

The formation of membrane protrusions is essential for cancer cell migration in response to migratory and chemotactic stimuli. The polymerization of submembrane actin filaments is the driving force behind membrane protrusions that provide rigidity to cancer cells. Filiform structures, generated by the cytoskeletal remodeling of submembrane actin filaments, are critical factors for metastatic cancer cells to adhere to secondary tissues/organs. Through the filopodia, one of the filiform structures, metastatic tumor cells play an important role in signal sensing and cancer cell adhesion, as well as migration and invasion [27,28]. Promoting cell detachment from the ECM by limiting filopodia formation and thus inhibiting cell adhesion could improve cell anoikis and be a valuable target in anti-metastatic therapy.

Focal adhesions, i.e., clustering sites of integrins, are vital for cell survival. Connecting the actin cytoskeleton to the ECM provides a physical attachment of cells to the ECM. Thus, integrins, important cell adhesion receptors, are implicated in almost all stages of cancer progression from primary tumor development to metastasis. Numerous pieces of evidence draw attention to the function of focal adhesion kinase (FAK)—a non-receptor tyrosine kinase—in mediating inside-out signaling of focal adhesion to regulate cell proliferation, survival, and migration [29]. Therefore, targeting integrin and its downstream signaling could help antimetastatic treatment.

The coordination of dynamic reorganization between actin filaments and microtubules is critical for the transmigration of cancer cells through the vasculature and their metastasis. Microtubules exist as a component of the cytoskeleton, and they are important for maintaining the physical and plastic properties of migrating cells and random movement. Therefore, microtubule-interfering agents could serve as potential antimetastatic agents [30].

2.5. Hypoxia and Neo-Angiogenesis

Oxygen plays an important role in regulating developmental processes and tissue homeostasis. At the cellular level, oxygen is required for oxidative metabolism and cell survival. Therefore, hypoxia and hypoxic signaling are potent contributing factors to tumor progression to metastasis [31].

The rapid proliferation of cancer cells results in a high oxygen consumption in the tumor microenvironment. Oxygen deprivation in the tumor causes apoptosis and necrosis. Briefly, hypoxia triggers the response of hypoxia-inducible factors (HIFs), transcriptional factors that coordinate an adaptive cellular response to low oxygen levels. Additionally, hypoxia triggers the release of angiogenic growth factors to restore a functional vascular system. In particular, HIF-1α promotes the late phases of metastasis in the distant site by stimulating neo-angiogenesis through the up-regulation of vascular endothelial growth factor (VEGF) [31,32]. Thus, neo-angiogenesis-targeted therapy might strike cancer cells in addition to its effect on vasculature.

2.6. Apoptosis and Autophagy

Apoptosis and autophagy are physiological cell death processes that can counteract tumor progression. Apoptosis is programmed cell death that leads to the removal of damaged cells. Apoptosis can block metastatic dissemination by killing misplaced cells resulting in an important process for limiting metastasis formation [33,34]. Deregulation of apoptosis is recognized as a hallmark of cancer as it promotes tumor progression and resistance to therapy [35].

Autophagy is a process that involves the action of lysosomes to degrade damaged organelles and macromolecular substances. Although the role of autophagy in cancer remains controversial, autophagy has been reported to act in an antimetastatic role by limiting cancer necrosis and inflammatory responses in the early stages of cancer metastasis. In early metastasis, autophagy also reduces the migration and invasion of cancer cells from the sites of origin [36]. Therefore, the regulation of apoptosis and autophagy is a potential approach to cancer advancement.

2.7. Epigenetic Control

Metastatic traits are increasingly thought to derive from the epigenetically modified transcriptional output of oncogenic signals that initiate and drive tumor development. Evidence points to a broad role for epigenetic mechanisms in key steps of metastasis, including DNA methylation, histone modifications, nucleosome changes, and non-coding RNAs [37]. Unlike genetic abnormalities, epigenetic changes are reversible and thus potential druggable targets for anti-cancer strategies. Epigenetic therapies thus have great potential to reprogram cancer cells and thereby halt the advancement of cancer [38].

3. Marine Compounds as Migrastatics

Marine bioactive compounds have attracted a great deal of interest in human health. Human health research has long been concerned with exploring and identifying natural products that can be useful in designing and developing novel therapeutic approaches against cancer [39].

In light of growing evidence that cell migration is crucial to cancer development, scientific research seeks new molecules that could prevent cancer cells from spreading.

For years, researchers and experts have navigated the molecular treasures of the sea to search for and identify structurally novel and biologically active metabolites of natural products. The following sections review the last five years of research on new or known marine compounds for which a migrastatic role has been described and then proposed to the scientific community as potential agents for cancer therapy. As reported in Figure 2, the discussed bioactive marine compounds belong to several categories, namely polysaccharides, peptides and proteins, phenolic compounds, and alkaloids.

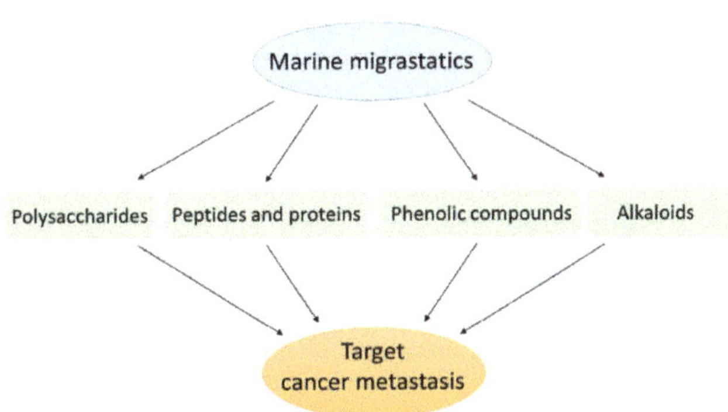

Figure 2. Bioactive compounds from marine entities as migrastatics for anti-cancer application.

3.1. Marine Polysaccharides

Sulfated polysaccharides such as carrageenan, fucoidan, and laminaran from various marine organisms and microorganisms have shown potent anti-migratory activity against several in vitro and vivo cancer models.

Exopolysaccharide 11 [EPS11] from the marine bacterium *Bacillus* sp. 11. was found to inhibit the migration of human lung cancer A549 cells by destroying filiform structures [40]. These structures are organelles widely found in cancer cells, which promote the invasion and migration of cancer cells. By the same mechanism, EPS11 was found to inhibit the migration of human hepatoma Huh7.5 [41], HepG2 and Bel-7402 cells [42] by acting on the cell membrane surface, i.e., destroying filiform structures and down-regulating the expression of CD99, an essential factor for cell adhesion, migration and cancer metastasis. Moreover, it has been revealed that EPS11 inhibits the metastatic process in vivo in animal models of metastatic melanoma [41].

Algae are an important source of polysaccharides with diverse biological activities among marine organisms. In this context, Ou et al. (2017) demonstrated the migrastatic potential of the water-soluble fucoidan-like polysaccharide STPC2 isolated from the brown alga *Sargassum thunbergii*. This polysaccharide was able to significantly inhibit the migration of lung cancer cells A549 via downregulation of MMP-2 activity—which is associated with cancer metastasis—and affect cell viability at a high concentration [43].

Laminaran sulfate isolated from the brown alga *Fucus evanescens* was shown to be a potent anti-migratory agent by inhibiting MMP-2 and MMP-9 activity in human colorectal adenocarcinoma (HCT116 cells), malignant melanoma (SK-MEL-5 cells), and breast adenocarcinoma (MDA-MB-231 cells) [44].

Malyarenko and colleagues (2019) also conducted a study that demonstrated for the first time the ability of sulfated laminaran from the brown alga *Dictyota dichotoma* to significantly increase the inhibitory effect of X-rays on SK-MEL-28 melanoma cell migration by regulating MMP-2 and MMP-9 activity. These results may provide a new combination strategy for radiation treatment in oncology [45].

Migrastatic properties have also been described for sulfated polysaccharides (SPUP) from the brown alga *Undaria Pinnatifida*. In particular, it could inhibit the migration of MCF7 breast cancer cells [46] and SKOV-3 and A2780 ovarian cancer cells by suppressing the Hedgehog signaling pathway [47].

Preventive effects against the migratory and invasive behavior of A2780 ovarian cancer cells were also attributed to a novel water-soluble polysaccharide (BFP-3) [48] isolated from the red alga *Bangia fuscopurpurea* by Wu et al. (2021). The migrastatic action of BFP-3 was likely due to mechanisms that promote apoptotic and autophagic cell death through the mitochondria-dependent pathway [49].

Fucoidan from the sea cucumber *Cucumaria frondosa* has been reported to inhibit in vitro migration of human osteosarcoma U2OS cells by impairing dynamic cytoskeletal remodeling through the suppression of the phosphorylation of FAK and paxillin and activation of the Rac1/PAK1/LIMK1/cofilin signaling axis [50].

The sulfated polysaccharide (SIP-SII) from *Sepiella maindroni* ink was shown to inhibit EGF-induced migration and invasion of human epidermoid carcinoma KB cells [51] and human ovarian carcinoma SKOV-3 cells [52] by suppressing the epidermal growth factor receptor (EGFR)-mediated Akt and p38 MAPK cascades and subsequently inhibiting MMP-2 expression.

Reduced phosphorylation of EGFR is linked to phosphorylation of ERK1/2, which is the downstream effector of FAK and E-cadherin. Up-regulation of FAK and down-regulation of E-cadherin are crucial in promoting cancer cell migration. In this context, sulfated galactan (SG) [53], from the red alga *Gracilaria fisheri*, suppresses HuCCA-1 cholangiocarcinoma cell migration by downregulating the EGFR-ERK signaling pathway. Specifically, SG inhibits ligand-induced EGFR dimerization by binding itself to the dimerization arms of unbound EGFR [54]. The up-regulation of FAK and down-regulation of E-cadherin are crucial to promoting cancer cell migration. Reduced phosphorylation of EGFR is related to the phosphorylation of ERK1/2, which is the downstream effector of FAK and E-cadherin [55].

Fractions rich in sulfated polysaccharides have also been attributed to migrastatic activity, such as those extracted from the green alga *Caulerpa cupressoides* var. *flabellata*, which inhibit the migration of B16-F10 melanoma cells [56]. Crude sulfated polysaccharides isolated and purified from the brown algae *Padina tetrastromatica* have been shown to block the migration of human cervical adenocarcinoma HeLa cells. They inhibit cell migration by lowering the expression of MMP-2 and MMP-9 and hinder angiogenesis through the downregulation of angiogenic mediators VEGF and HIF-1-α expression [57].

Table 1 summarizes all the above-mentioned marine polysaccharides as migrastatics.

Table 1. Marine polysaccharide as migrastatics.

Polysaccharides	Marine Source	Composition	In Vivo Animal Model	Target
Exopolysaccharide 11	*Bacillus* sp. 11	Mannose, glucosamine, galacturonic acid, glucose and xylose, in a ratio of 1:2.58:0.68:0.13:3.09:1.41	Melanoma (mice model)	Filiform structures; cytoskeleton; CD99 [41]
Polysaccharides	**Marine source**	**Composition**	**In vitro cell model**	**Target**
Exopolysaccharide 11	*Bacillus* sp. 11	Mannose, glucosamine, galacturonic acid, glucose and xylose, in a ratio of 1:2.58:0.68:0.13:3.09:1.41	Human lung cancer (A549 cells); human hepatoma (Huh7.5, HepG2, Bel-7402 cells)	Filiform structures; cytoskeleton; CD99 [40–42]
Fucoidan-like STPC2	*S. thunbergii*	Fucose, xylose, galactose and glucuronic acid, in a ratio of 8.1:3.8:2.1:1.0	Human lung cancer (A549 cells)	MMP-2 [43]
Laminaran sulfate	*F. evanescens*	β-(1→3)-linked D-glucopyranose and single β-(1→6)-linked D-glucose residues. Branches at C6 can be glucose or gentiobiose.	Human colorectal adenocarcinoma (HCT116 cells); human malignant melanoma (SK-MEL-5 cells); human breast adenocarcinoma (MDA-MB-231 cells)	MMP-2/9 [44]
Laminaran sulfate	*D. dichotoma*	(1→3)-linked glucopyranose residues with the branches of single glucose residues at C6 (ratio of bonds 1.3:1.6 = 3:1)	Human melanoma (SK-MEL-28 cells)	MMP-2/9 [45]
SPUP	*U. Pinnatifida*	Fucose, glucose, and galactose, in a ratio of 27.22:19.32:53.46	Human breast cancer (MCF-7 cells); human ovarian cancer (SKOV-3 and A2780 cells)	Apoptosis [46]; Hedgehog signaling pathway [47]
BFP-3	*B. fuscopurpurea*	Rhamnose, arabinose, mannose, glucose, and galactose	Human ovarian cancer (A2780 cells)	Apoptosis, autophagy [49]
Fucoidan	*C. frondosa*	L-fucose and a sulfate ester group. Total carbohydrate content 72.5%; sulfate content 26.1%. (98% purity).	Human osteosarcoma (U2OS cells)	Cytoskeleton; FAK [50]
SIP-SII	*S. maindroni*	Fucose, N-acetylgalactosamine and mannose, in a molar ratio of 2:2:1, with a single branch of glucuronic acid at the C-3 position of mannose.	Human epidermoid carcinoma (KB cells); human ovarian carcinoma (SKOV-3 cells)	EGF-mediated signaling pathway; MMP-2 [51,52]

Table 1. *Cont.*

Polysaccharides	Marine source	Composition	In vitro cell model	Target
Sulfated galactans	*G. fisheri*	3-linked β-d-galactopyranose and 4-linked 3,6-anhydro-α-l-galactopyranose or α-l-galactose-6-sulfate with partial methylation at 2-O-methylated-3,6-andydro-α-l-galactopyranose, 6-O-methylated-β-d-galactopyranose and 4-O-methyl-β-l-galactopyranose attached to C-6 of 3-linked-β-d-galactopyranose units, together with sulfation on C-4 and C-6 of d-galactopyranose units.	Human intrahepatic cholangiocarcinoma (HuCCA-1 cells)	EGFR-ERK signaling pathway; FAK; E-cadherin [54,55]
CCB-F0.5	*C. cupressoides* var. *flabellata*	Galactose and mannose in a molar ratio of 1.0:0.1 and traces of xylose. Low protein content 0.17%	Murine melanoma (B16-F10 cells)	*Not described* [56]
CCB-F1.0	*C. cupressoides* var. *flabellata*	Galactose, mannose, and xylose in a molar ratio of 1.0:0.1:0.6 and traces of glucose and rhamnose. Low protein content 0.19%	Murine melanoma (B16-F10 cells)	*Not described* [56]
Crude sulfate polysaccharide extract	*P. tetrastromatica*	-	Human cervical adenocarcinoma (HeLa cells)	MMP-2/9; angiogenesis [57]

3.2. Marine Peptides and Proteins

In recent decades, natural marine peptides have attracted much attention because of their specific characteristics, including a broad spectrum of bioactivity and low toxicity, making them very promising candidates against a wide spectrum of diseases, including cancer. Today, several anti-cancer peptides and their derivatives from marine organisms and microorganisms have been widely applied to clinical research [11,58–60].

Peptides are molecules that participate in all processes of life activities. They can have anti-tumor roles in diverse aspects in different ways, such as preventing cell migration.

Several depsipeptides (nonribosomal peptides cyclized via an ester bond and often containing nonprotein amino acids) have been approved to treat various cancers or are undergoing clinical trials for potential utility as anti-cancer drugs [61].

A recent study isolated a novel cyclic depsipeptide, nobilamide I, from the marine-derived bacterium *Saccharomonospora* sp., strain CNQ-490 (Figure 3A). This showed significant migrastatic properties in three different cancer cell lines, lung cancer A549 cells, gastric cancer AGS cells, and colorectal cancer Caco2 cells, by modulating the expression levels of MMP-2/9 [62].

Molassamide (Figure 3B), isolated from the marine cyanobacterium DRTO-73, showed a dual action on the migration of highly invasive MDA-MB-231 breast cancer cells by modulating both elastase-induced intercellular adhesion molecule (ICAM)-1 gene expression and ICAM-1 proteolytic processing by elastase [63].

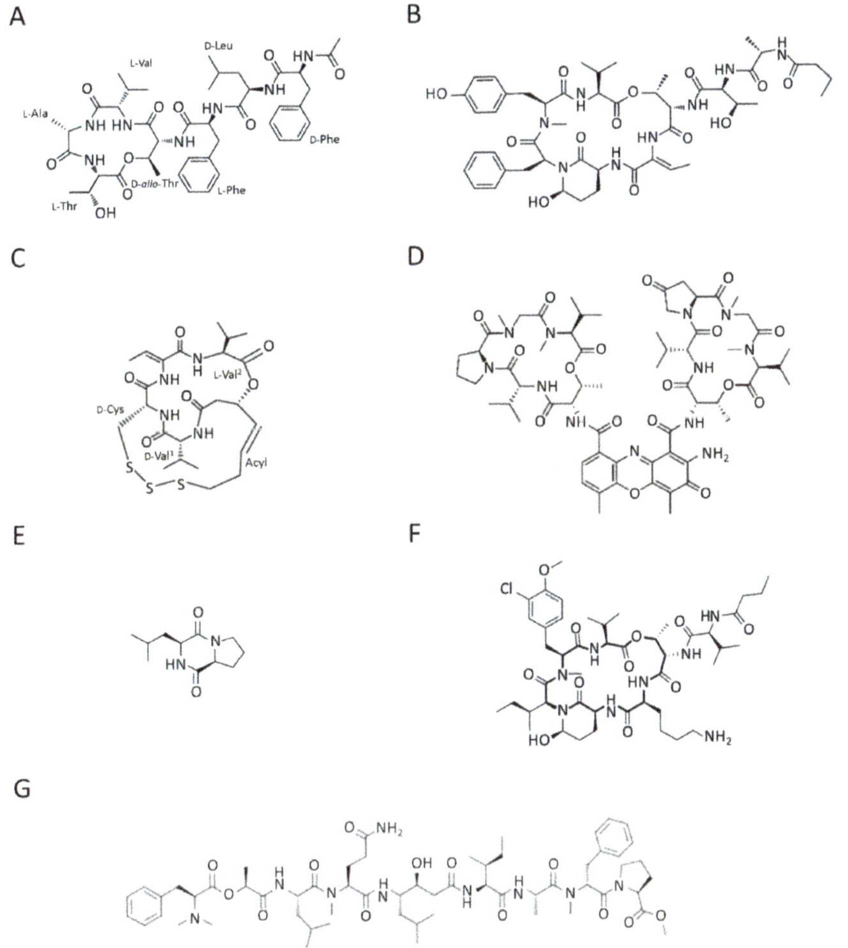

Figure 3. Chemical structure of (**A**) nobilamide I from the bacterium *Saccharomonospora* sp., strain CNQ-490; (**B**) molassamide from the Cyanobacterium DRTO-73; (**C**) chromopeptide A from the bacterium *Chromobacterium* sp. HS-13-94; (**D**) actinomycin V from *Streptomyces* sp.; (**E**) cyclo(L-leucyl-L-prolyl from marine microorganisms; (**F**) kempopeptin C from the cyanobacterium *Lyngbya* sp., (**G**) grassystatin F from the Cyanobacterium VPG 14-61.

Chromopeptide A (Figure 3C) is a depsipeptide isolated from the marine-derived bacterium *Chromobacterium* sp. HS-13-94 [64]. In in vitro and in vivo models of prostate cancer (PC3 cells), chromopeptide A showed effective anti-migratory and anti-metastatic properties by acting as an inhibitor of class I histone deacetylases (HDACs). It is well known that histone deacetylases are involved in posttranslational modification of gene expression [65]. Therefore, chromopeptide A, by affecting HDACs, can play a role in epigenetic mechanisms of regulation of several biological events. Notably, the peptide showed in vivo better body weight tolerance than FK228 (already FDA approved), implying controllable toxicity. These data capture attention for the potential applications of the marine-derived peptide in prostate cancer therapy [66]. HDACs play an important role in EMT regulation in a variety of cancers. It has been reported that treatment of cells with an HDAC inhibitor represses EMT and metastasis [67].

Actinomycin V (Figure 3D) is a cyclic chromopeptide produced by the marine actinomycete *Streptomyces* sp. Lin and colleagues reported a suppressive effect of actinomycin V on the migration and invasion of human breast cancer MDA-MB-231 cells. This effect may be explained by inhibiting EMT through the down-regulation of Snail and Slug protein expression [68].

The cyclic dipeptide cyclo(L-leucyl- L-prolyl) (CLP) from various marine microorganisms has a myriad of pharmaceutical significances (Figure 3E). Deepak Kgk and colleagues have demonstrated that CLP suppresses growth and migration by attenuating the cell cycle of MDA-MB-231 and MDA-MB-468 triple-negative breast cancer cells via CD151/EGFR signaling [69].

Kempopeptin C depsipeptide (Figure 3F), a protease inhibitor from the marine cyanobacterium *Lyngbya* sp., was also shown to suppress the migration of invasive MDA-MB-231 breast cancer cells [70].

Grassystatin F (Figure 3G), isolated from the marine cyanobacterium VPG 14-61, also acts as a protease inhibitor. This potent aspartic protease inhibitor can inhibit the migration of highly aggressive MDA-MD-231 triple-negative breast cancer cells [71].

Table 2 summarizes the specific information on the migrastatic marine depsipeptides described above.

Table 2. Marine depsipeptides as migrastatics.

Depsipeptides	Marine Source	In Vitro Cell Model	Target
Nobilamide I	*Saccharomonospora* sp., strain CNQ-490	Human lung cancer (A549 cells); human gastric cancer (AGS cells); human colorectal cancer (Caco2 cells)	MMP-2/9 [62]
Molassamide	Cyanobacterium DRTO-73, *Leptolyngbya* sp.	Human breast adenocarcinoma (MDA-MB-231 cells)	ICAM-1 [63]
Chromopeptide A	*Chromobacterium* sp., strain HS-13-94	Human prostate cancer (PC3 cells); mouse PC3 xenograft model	HDACs [66]
Actinomycin V	*Streptomyces* sp., strain N1510.2	Human breast adenocarcinoma (MDA-MB-231 cells)	EMT [68]
CLP	Marine microorganisms	Human breast adenocarcinoma (MDA-MB-231 and MDA-MB-468 cells)	CD151/EGFR signaling [69]
Kempopeptin C	*Lyngbya* sp.	Human breast adenocarcinoma (MDA-MB-231)	*Not described* [70]
Grassystatin F	Cyanobacterium VPG 14-61	Human breast adenocarcinoma (MDA-MB-231)	Protease inhibitor [71]

The marine abalone gastropod is a marine organism rich in vital elements, including proteins and peptides, and is known for its many biological properties [72]. Recent literature also describes a migrastatic role of some bioactive peptides obtained from boiled abalone (*Haliotis discus hannai*). In particular, BABP and AATP peptides inhibited the migration and invasion of human fibrosarcoma cells (HT1080) and human umbilical vein endothelial cells (HUVEC) by attenuating MMPs and VEGF [73,74].

An analysis of the activity of the αO-conotoxin GeXIVA from *Conus generalis* [75] in MDA-MB-157 breast cancer cells performed by Sun and colleagues revealed the inhibitory activity on cell migration of this conotoxin, probably downregulating α9-nAChR (α9 nicotinic acetylcholine receptor), essential for mediating tumor metastasis through EMT [76].

Enzyme proteins have also been described to have effects on cancer cell migration. This is the case of the N-V protease or Nereis active protease (NAP), which is a fibrinolytic active serine protease purified from the polychaeta *Nereis virens* [77]. An in vitro study conducted in 2019 demonstrated that NAP inhibited the migration of lung cancer H1299 cells probably by inducing apoptosis through the inhibition of the PI3K/AKT/mTOR pathway [78].

Adding to the list is the polypeptide PBN11-8, purified from the fermentation broth of *Bacillus* sp. N11-8. This, similar to the M84 peptidase from *Bacillus pumilus*, belonged to a type of zinc-dependent metalloprotease family. PBN11-8 was shown to suppress the invasion and migration of human hepatocellular carcinoma BEL-7402 cells by targeting the FAK pathways and MMP-2/9 [79].

Table 3 provides specific information about the peptides mentioned above and proteins with migrastatic action.

Table 3. The amino acid sequence and molecular mass of marine-derived migrastatic peptides and proteins.

Peptides and Proteins	Marine Source	Sequence	Molecular Mass	In Vitro Cell Model	Target
BABP	*H. discus hannai*	EMDEAQDPSEW	1234.41 Da	Human fibrosarcoma (HT1080 cells); human umbilical vein endothelial (HUVEC cells)	MMPs; VEGF [73]
AATP	*H. discus hannai*	KVEPQDPSEW	1214.30 Da	Fibrosarcoma (HT1080 cells); human umbilical vein endothelial (HUVEC cells)	MMPs; VEGF [74]
αO-conotoxin GeXIVA	*C. generalis*	TCRSSGRYCRSPYDR RRRYCRRITDACV [1]	3452 Da	Human breast cancer (MDA-MB-157 cells)	EMT [76]
N-V protease (or NAP)	*N. virens*	QAPNYSTASYNVVA VKINLFLSTNNKLYI HDTGVRAVYLAGM KVYLAANPTASSQT FNSDTLVYILDTGIN EPNYYINLY [2]	8888 Da	Human lung cancer (H1299 cells)	apoptosis [78]
PBN11-8	*B. pumilus*	ASTGSQKVTVYAVAD [3]	19,000 Da	Human hepatocellular carcinoma (BEL-7402 cells)	FAK; MMP-2/9 [79]

[1] C-terminal COOH sequence of αO-conotoxin GeXIVA. [2] N-V protease (No. P83433) in the Swiss-Prot protein sequence database. [3] N-terminal partial sequence of PBN11-8. The entire amino acid sequence of PBN11-8 shares 98.5% similarity with peptidase M84 of *Bacillus pumilus* (GenBank accession WP_025208148).

Not only single peptides or proteins but also crude protein extracts have demonstrated potent migrastatic bioactivity. This is the case of proteins extracted from sea cucumber (*Holothuria leucospilota*) that have shown a potential anti-cancer activity towards human hepatoma HepG2 cells, human lung carcinoma A549 cells, and human pancreatic cancer Panc02 cells, with a higher efficacy than a clinical anti-cancer drug [80].

3.3. Marine Phenolic Compounds

Polyphenols possess a variety of biological functions, making them one of the most important phytochemicals [81]. Several studies have shown natural polyphenols' protective effects against chronic diseases and an inverse correlation between polyphenol consumption and cancer development [82]. Various polyphenols have also been shown to inhibit cancer growth via pleiotropic mechanisms targeting multiple signaling pathways in charge of key cellular processes, including cancer cell migration [82].

Among phenolic compounds, phloroglucinol and its derivatives, which exist in brown algae, have attracted attention because of their good biological activity [83]. In particular, the phloroglucinol derivative 7-phloroeckol (7PE), derived from the brown alga *Ecklonia cava*, has recently shown migrastatic abilities in hepatoma cancer HepG2 cells and anti-angiogenic properties on human umbilical vein endothelial HUVEC cells. Furthermore, 7PE has been shown to act through PI3K/AKT/mTOR and Ras/ERK signaling pathways to inhibit HIF-1α protein expression from blocking VEGF protein production [84].

In addition, the phlorotannins dieckol and phlorofucofuroeckol obtained from *Ecklonia cava* were shown to be able to block LPS-induced migration and invasion of human breast cancer cells (MCF-7 and MDA-MB-231 cells) by reducing both MMP-2/9 or TLR-4 expression and NF-κB transcriptional activity, which was induced by LPS [85].

Many benzaldehyde derivatives produced as secondary metabolites by marine-derived fungi have also been described for their bioactive properties [86]. In this context, the marine fungus *Eurotium chevalieri*—an endophyte of the sponge *Grantia compressa*—was the source of the prenylated benzaldehyde derivative dihydroauroglaucin (DAG). DAG was found to inhibit the migration of human SH-SY5Y neuroblastoma cells by activating autophagy [87].

Cell migration is dependent on microtubule dynamics [30], and viriditoxin from the marine-derived fungus *Paecilomyces variotii* [88] was found to reduce the ability of human ovarian SKOV-3 cells to migrate by disrupting microtube dynamics [89].

Polyphenol-rich fractions have also proved to be valid biological tools against the migration of cancer cells, probably exploiting the synergistic action of several constituents [90]. This is the case of the polyphenolic fraction obtained from the brown seaweed *Padina boergeseni*, of which gallic acid, caffeic acid, rutin, quercetin ferulic acid were the main components; this was able to significantly inhibit the migration of renal cancer cells (A498 and ACHN cells) by involving cell cycle arrest and inducing apoptosis [91].

Additionally, phenolic phytoconstituents extracted from the red algae *Gelidiella acerosa* showed migrastatic properties in lung adenocarcinoma A549 cells by decreasing the expression level of MMP-2 [92].

In addition, the hydroalcoholic extract obtained from the marine plant *Posidonia oceanica* was found to be a rich reservoir of phenolic compounds, including catechin, epicatechin, gallic acid, ferulic acid, and chlorogenic acid. This has been shown to inhibit the migration of human fibrosarcoma HT1080 cells [93] and human neuroblastoma SH-SY5Y cells [94] by acting on MMPs and activating autophagy. Furthermore, the polyphenol-rich phytocomplex is suitable for use as a vehicle in nanoformulations that can improve bioavailability and its migrastatic bioactivity [95].

All polyphenols or polyphenol-rich fractions presented here (Table 4) share potential applicability in anti-cancer therapies.

Table 4. Marine phenolic compounds as migrastatics.

Phenolic Compound	Marine Source	Chemical Structure	In Vitro Cell Model	Target
7-phloroeckol	*E. cava*	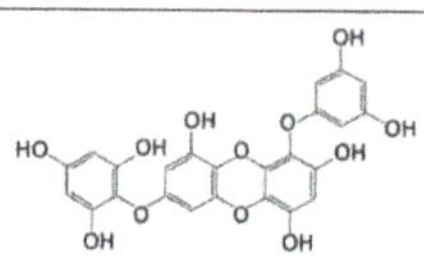	Human hepatoma cancer (HepG2 cells); human umbilical vein endothelial (HUVEC cells)	HIF-1α; angiogenesis [84]
Dieckol	*E. cava*	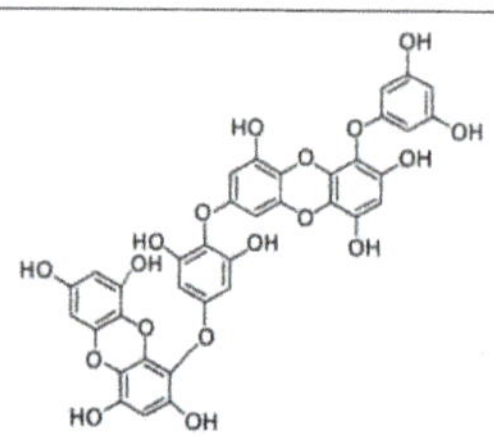	Human breast cancer (MCF-7, MDA-MB-231 cells)	MMP-2/9; TLR-4; NF-κB [85]

Table 4. *Cont.*

Phenolic Compound	Marine Source	Chemical Structure	In Vitro Cell Model	Target
Phlorofucofuroeckol	*E. cava*	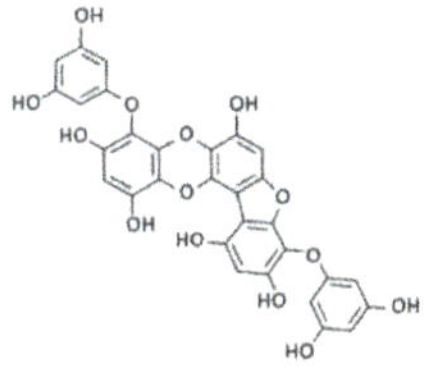	Human breast cancer (MCF-7, MDA-MB-231 cells)	MMP-2/9; TLR-4; NF-κB [85]
Dihydroauroglaucin	*E. chevalieri*	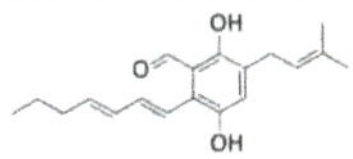	Human neuroblastoma (SH-SY5Y cells)	Autophagy [87]
Viriditoxin	*P. variotii*	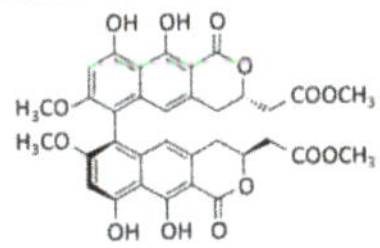	Human ovarian cancer (SKOV-3 cells)	Cytoskeleton [89]
Gallic acid	*P. boergeseni, P. oceanica*	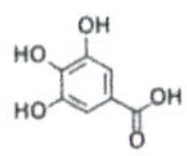	Human renal cancer (A498, ACHN cells); human fibrosarcoma (HT1080 cells); human neuroblastoma (SH-SY5Y cells)	Apoptosis [91]; autophagy [93]; autophagy, MMP-2 [94]
Caffeic acid	*P. boergeseni*	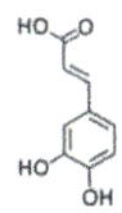	Human renal cancer (A498, ACHN cells)	Apoptosis [91]
Rutin	*P. boergeseni*	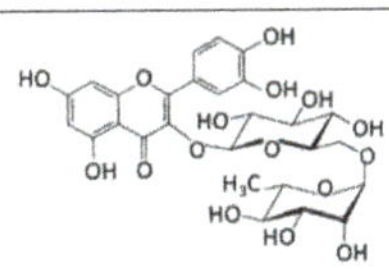	Human renal cancer (A498, ACHN cells)	Apoptosis [91]
Quercetin	*P. boergeseni*	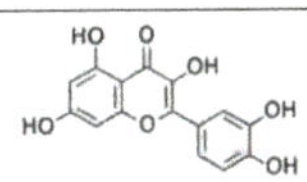	Human renal cancer (A498, ACHN cells)	Apoptosis [91]
Ferulic acid	*P. boergeseni, P. oceanica*	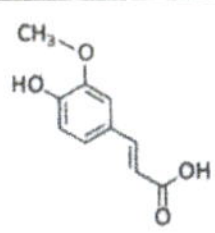	Human renal cancer (A498, ACHN cells); human fibrosarcoma (HT1080 cells); human neuroblastoma (SH-SY5Y cells)	Apoptosis [91]; autophagy [93]; autophagy, MMP-2 [94]
Catechin	*P. oceanica*	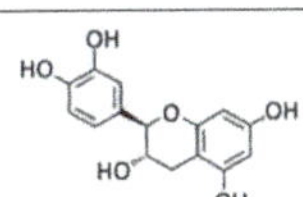	Human fibrosarcoma (HT1080 cells); human neuroblastoma (SH-SY5Y cells)	Autophagy [93]; autophagy, MMP-2 [94]
Epicatechin	*P. oceanica*	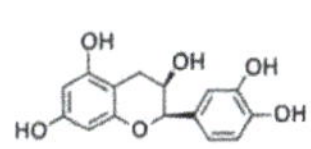	Human fibrosarcoma (HT1080 cells); human neuroblastoma (SH-SY5Y cells)	Autophagy [93]; autophagy, MMP-2 [94]
Chlorogenic acid	*P. oceanica*	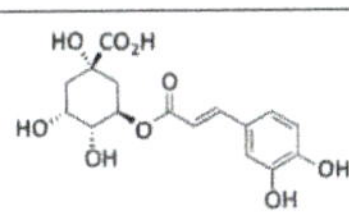	Human fibrosarcoma (HT1080 cells); human neuroblastoma (SH-SY5Y cells)	Autophagy [93]; autophagy, MMP-2 [94]

3.4. Marine Alkaloids

Marine organisms have been developed as a new source of naturally occurring alkaloids. Various alkaloids of marine origin have been reported to be potentially active against cancer metastasis [96].

A brominated alkaloid, aeroplysinin-1 (Figure 4A), isolated from the marine sponge *Aplysina aerophoba*, showed decreased migration and adhesion of mouse pheochromocytoma MTT cells in vitro by downregulating integrin β1 [97].

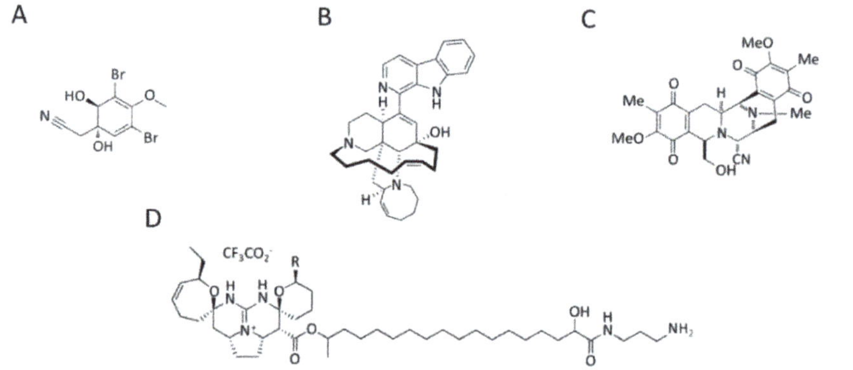

Figure 4. Chemical structure of (**A**) aeroplysinin-1 from the marine sponge *A. aerophoba;* (**B**) manzamine A from the sponge of the genera *Haliclona* sp., *Xestospongia* sp. and *Pellina* sp.; (**C**) jorunnamycin A from the sponge *Xestospongia* sp.; (**D**) normonanchocidines G (R=CH_3) and H (R=H) from the marine sponge *M. pulchra.*

In addition, manzamine A (Figure 4B), a pentacyclic β-carboline-fused alkaloid derived from a sponge of the genera *Haliclona* sp., *Xestospongia* sp. and *Pellina* sp., inactivates the EMT and the migratory capacity of human colorectal carcinoma HCT116 cells. This alkaloid suppresses several mesenchymal transcription factors (e.g., Snail, Slug and Twist) and simultaneously induces the epithelial marker E-cadherin leading to epithelial phenotype and migration suppression. This study showed that manzamine A is a potential migratory anti-cancer drug for colorectal cancer patients with tumors that undergo the EMT process and develop distal metastases [98].

In addition, the alkaloid jorunnamycin A (Figure 4C), a bistetrahydroisoquinolinequinone isolated from a Thai blue sponge *Xestospongia* sp. [99], showed the ability to inhibit EMT, sensitize anoikis, and suppress anchorage-independent survival in H460 human lung cancer cells. Since the loss of anchorage dependence is an important block to metastasis, jorunnamycin A could be an effective agent against lung cancer metastasis [100].

Two pentacyclic guanidine alkaloids, normonanchocidines G and H (Figure 4D), isolated from the marine sponge *Monanchora pulchra*, manifested a high impact on the capacity of human cervical epithelioid carcinoma HeLa [101].

Table 5 summarizes the specific information on the migrastatic marine alkaloids described above.

Table 5. Marine alkaloids as migrastatics.

Alkaloids	Marine Source	In Vitro Cell Model	Target
Aeroplysinin-1	*A. aerophoba*	Mouse pheocromocytoma cells (MTT cells)	Integrin β1 [97]
Manzamine A	*Haliclona* sp., *Xestospongia* sp. and *Pellina* sp.	Human colorectal carcinoma (HCT116 cells)	EMT [98]
Jorunnamycin A	*Xestospongia* sp.	Human lung cancer (H460 cells)	EMT; anoikis [100]
Normonanchocidines G and H	*M. pulchra*	Human cervical carcinoma (HeLa cells)	*Not described* [101]

4. Research Methodology

This review selected literature on marine migrastatics described since 2017, when the "migrastatics" term was coined.

Extensive searches were performed in PubMed, ScienceDirect, Web of Science, and Google Scholar databases using one or more of the following terms: "marine anti-cancer compounds", "marine anti-migratory compounds", "marine anti-invasive compounds", "marine compounds against metastasis", "marine migrastatics", and "migrastatics in cancer".

A total of 42 articles describing marine migrastatics in 2017–2022 were selected and included. Pre-2017 literature on marine anti-migratory and anti-invasive compounds were excluded. Chemical structures were adapted from PubChem, and figures were created using Microsoft PowerPoint per Microsoft 365 MSO (Version 2202 Build 16.0.14931.20128).

5. Summary and Future Perspectives

Although nearly two decades have passed since the six hallmarks of cancer were defined, anti-cancer therapeutic strategies have not focused enough on the mechanism responsible for the highest mortality in patients with solid tumors: metastasis.

Cancer cells undergo complex modifications in cancer progression and achieve an invasive phenotype to become metastatic.

Research is continually working to find new anti-cancer drugs to limit the pro-metastatic behavior of cancer cells. Hopes and expectations for more specific and less toxic therapies are ever-present.

However, not all available anti-cancer drugs can curb metastatic tumor aggressiveness. In 2017, the term "migrastatic" was coined to distinguish a category of anticancer agents capable of preventing cancer cell migration and invasion.

In the relentless search for migrastatics, the marine environment represents an untapped source of natural compounds due to its enormous biodiversity.

Data published in the past five years illustrate the migrastatic properties of compounds (e.g., polysaccharides, peptides and proteins, polyphenols, and alkaloids) obtained from microorganisms and marine organisms as a valuable tool to hit various molecular targets against cancer metastasis (Figures 5 and S1).

Considering the ever-growing market for marine biology, the plethora of naturally occurring migrastatic compounds has immense potential to provide numerous clinically relevant anti-migratory and anti-invasive compounds for cancer therapy in the near future. With this comprehensive 2022 update, we recommend the recent knowledge on marine migrastatic compounds to redirect pharmaceutical and scientific research efforts on antimetastatic drugs as endpoints of anti-cancer therapies.

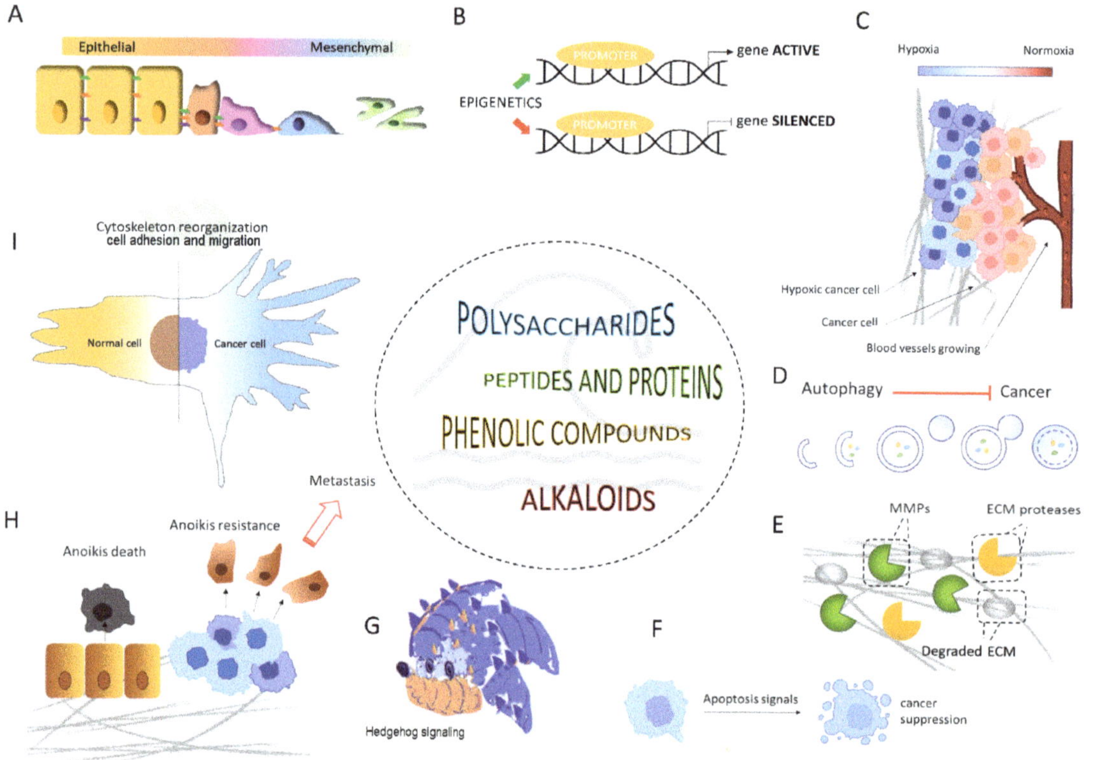

Figure 5. Schematic representation of potential molecular targets of marine migrastatics (2017–2022): (**A**) epithelial-mesenchymal transition; (**B**) epigenetic control; (**C**) neo-angiogenesis and hypoxia; (**D**) autophagy; (**E**) ECM degradation by MMPs and other proteases; (**F**) apoptosis; (**G**) Hedgehog signaling pathway; (**H**) resistance to anoikis; (**I**) cytoskeletal reorganization, cell adhesion and migration. In addition, as shown in Figure S1 of the Supplementary Materials, each of these pictorial representations of the molecular target for metastasis was linked to the migrastatic marine compounds described.

Supplementary Materials: The following supporting information can be downloaded at: https://www.mdpi.com/article/10.3390/md20050273/s1. Figure S1: Schematic representation of potential molecular targets of marine migrastatics (2017–2022).

Author Contributions: Conceptualization, M.V., E.B. and D.D.; writing—original draft preparation, M.V., E.B. and D.D.; writing—review and editing, M.V., E.B. and D.D. All authors have read and agreed to the published version of the manuscript.

Funding: This research received no external funding.

Conflicts of Interest: The authors declare no conflict of interest.

References

1. Sung, H.; Ferlay, J.; Siegel, R.L.; Laversanne, M.; Soerjomataram, I.; Jemal, A.; Bray, F. Global Cancer Statistics 2020: GLOBOCAN Estimates of Incidence and Mortality Worldwide for 36 Cancers in 185 Countries. *CA Cancer J. Clin.* **2021**, *71*, 209–249. [CrossRef]
2. Hanahan, D. Hallmarks of Cancer: New Dimensions. *Cancer Discov.* **2022**, *12*, 31–46. [CrossRef] [PubMed]
3. Lambert, A.W.; Pattabiraman, D.R.; Weinberg, R.A. Emerging Biological Principles of Metastasis. *Cell* **2017**, *168*, 670–691. [CrossRef] [PubMed]
4. El-Sayes, N.; Vito, A.; Mossman, K. Tumor Heterogeneity: A Great Barrier in the Age of Cancer Immunotherapy. *Cancers* **2021**, *13*, 806. [CrossRef] [PubMed]

5. Gandalovičová, A.; Rosel, D.; Fernandes, M.; Veselý, P.; Heneberg, P.; Čermák, V.; Petruželka, L.; Kumar, S.; Sanz-Moreno, V.; Brábek, J. Migrastatics-Anti-metastatic and Anti-invasion Drugs: Promises and Challenges. *Trends Cancer* **2017**, *3*, 391–406. [CrossRef] [PubMed]
6. Bayat Mokhtari, R.; Homayouni, T.S.; Baluch, N.; Morgatskaya, E.; Kumar, S.; Das, B.; Yeger, H. Combination therapy in combating cancer. *Oncotarget* **2017**, *8*, 38022–38043. [CrossRef] [PubMed]
7. Solomon, J.; Raškova, M.; Rösel, D.; Brábek, J.; Gil-Henn, H. Are We Ready for Migrastatics? *Cells* **2021**, *10*, 1845. [CrossRef] [PubMed]
8. Lindequist, U. Marine-Derived Pharmaceuticals–Challenges and Opportunities. *Biomol. Ther.* **2016**, *24*, 561–571. [CrossRef]
9. Lu, W.Y.; Li, H.J.; Li, Q.Y.; Wu, Y.C. Application of marine natural products in drug research. *Bioorg. Med. Chem.* **2021**, *35*, 116058. [CrossRef]
10. Dayanidhi, D.L.; Thomas, B.C.; Osterberg, J.S.; Vuong, M.; Vargas, G.; Kwartler, S.K.; Schmaltz, E.; Dunphy-Daly, M.M.; Schultz, T.F.; Rittschof, D.; et al. Exploring the Diversity of the Marine Environment for New Anti-cancer Compounds. *Front. Mar. Sci.* **2021**, *7*, 614766. [CrossRef]
11. Dyshlovoy, S.A.; Honecker, F. Marine Compounds and Cancer: Updates 2020. *Mar. Drugs* **2020**, *18*, 643. [CrossRef] [PubMed]
12. Marine Pharmacology. Available online: https://www.marinepharmacology.org/approved (accessed on 3 March 2022).
13. Fares, J.; Fares, M.Y.; Khachfe, H.H.; Salhab, H.A.; Fares, Y. Molecular principles of metastasis: A hallmark of cancer revisited. *Sig. Transduct. Target Ther.* **2020**, *5*, 28. [CrossRef] [PubMed]
14. Ribatti, D.; Tamma, R.; Annese, T. Epithelial-Mesenchymal Transition in Cancer: A Historical Overview. *Transl. Oncol.* **2020**, *13*, 100773. [CrossRef]
15. Garg, M. Epithelial-mesenchymal transition-activating transcription factors-multifunctional regulators in cancer. *World J. Stem Cells* **2013**, *5*, 188–195. [CrossRef] [PubMed]
16. Lamouille, S.; Xu, J.; Derynck, R. Molecular mechanisms of epithelial-mesenchymal transition. *Nat. Rev. Mol. Cell Biol.* **2014**, *15*, 178–196. [CrossRef] [PubMed]
17. Wang, F.; Ma, L.; Zhang, Z.; Liu, X.; Gao, H.; Zhuang, Y.; Yang, P.; Kornmann, M.; Tian, X.; Yang, Y. Hedgehog Signaling Regulates Epithelial-Mesenchymal Transition in Pancreatic Cancer Stem-Like Cells. *J. Cancer* **2016**, *7*, 408–417. [CrossRef]
18. Islam, S.S.; Mokhtari, R.B.; Noman, A.S.; Uddin, M.; Rahman, M.Z.; Azadi, M.A.; Zlotta, A.; van der Kwast, T.; Yeger, H.; Farhat, W.A. Sonic hedgehog (Shh) signaling promotes tumorigenicity and stemness via activation of epithelial-to-mesenchymal transition (EMT) in bladder cancer. *Mol. Carcinog.* **2016**, *55*, 537–551. [CrossRef]
19. Riaz, S.K.; Ke, Y.; Wang, F.; Kayani, M.A.; Malik, M.F.A. Influence of SHH/GLI1 axis on EMT mediated migration and invasion of breast cancer cells. *Sci. Rep.* **2019**, *9*, 6620. [CrossRef]
20. Yue, D.; Li, H.; Che, J.; Zhang, Y.; Tseng, H.H.; Jin, J.Q.; Luh, T.M.; Giroux-Leprieur, E.; Mo, M.; Zheng, Q.; et al. Hedgehog/Gli promotes epithelial-mesenchymal transition in lung squamous cell carcinomas. *J. Exp. Clin. Cancer Res.* **2014**, *33*, 34. [CrossRef]
21. Skoda, A.M.; Simovic, D.; Karin, V.; Kardum, V.; Vranic, S.; Serman, L. The role of the Hedgehog signaling pathway in cancer: A comprehensive review. *Bosn. J. Basic Med. Sci.* **2018**, *18*, 8–20. [CrossRef]
22. Kleiner, D.E.; Stetler-Stevenson, W.G. Matrix metalloproteinases and metastasis. *Cancer Chemother. Pharmacol.* **1999**, *43*, 42–51. [CrossRef] [PubMed]
23. Klein, T.; Bischoff, R. Physiology and pathophysiology of matrix metalloproteases. *Amino Acids* **2011**, *41*, 271–290. [CrossRef] [PubMed]
24. Egeblad, M.; Werb, Z. New functions for the matrix metalloproteinases in cancer progression. *Nat. Rev. Cancer* **2002**, *2*, 161–174. [CrossRef] [PubMed]
25. Gilmore, A. Anoikis. *Cell Death Differ.* **2005**, *12*, 1473–1477. [CrossRef]
26. Adeshakin, F.O.; Adeshakin, A.O.; Afolabi, L.O.; Yan, D.; Zhang, G.; Wan, X. Mechanisms for Modulating Anoikis Resistance in Cancer and the Relevance of Metabolic Reprogramming. *Front. Oncol.* **2021**, *11*, 626577. [CrossRef]
27. Jacquemet, G.; Hamidi, H.; Ivaska, J. Filopodia in cell adhesion, 3D migration and cancer cell invasion. *Curr. Opin. Cell Biol.* **2015**, *37*, 119. [CrossRef]
28. Arjonen, A.; Kaukonen, R.; Ivaska, J. Filopodia and adhesion in cancer cell motility. *Cell Adh. Migr.* **2011**, *5*, 421–430. [CrossRef]
29. Murphy, J.M.; Rodriguez, Y.A.R.; Jeong, K.; Ahn, E.E.; Lim, S.S. Targeting focal adhesion kinase in cancer cells and the tumor microenvironment. *Exp. Mol. Med.* **2020**, *52*, 877–886. [CrossRef]
30. Čermák, V.; Dostál, V.; Jelínek, M.; Libusová, L.; Kovář, J.; Rösel, D.; Brábek, J. Microtubule-targeting agents and their impact on cancer treatment. *Eur. J. Cell. Biol.* **2020**, *99*, 151075. [CrossRef]
31. Rankin, E.B.; Giaccia, A.J. Hypoxic control of metastasis. *Science* **2016**, *352*, 175–180. [CrossRef]
32. Rankin, E.B.; Nam, J.M.; Giaccia, A.J. Hypoxia: Signaling the Metastatic Cascade. *Trends Cancer* **2016**, *2*, 295–304. [CrossRef] [PubMed]
33. Pistritto, G.; Trisciuoglio, D.; Ceci, C.; Garufi, A.; D'Orazi, G. Apoptosis as anticancer mechanism: Function and dysfunction of its modulators and targeted therapeutic strategies. *Aging* **2016**, *8*, 603–619. [CrossRef] [PubMed]
34. Su, Z.; Yang, Z.; Xu, Y.; Chen, Y.; Yu, Q. Apoptosis, autophagy, necroptosis, and cancer metastasis. *Mol. Cancer* **2015**, *14*, 48. [CrossRef] [PubMed]
35. Neophytou, C.M.; Trougakos, I.P.; Erin, N.; Papageorgis, P. Apoptosis Deregulation and the Development of Cancer Multi-Drug Resistance. *Cancers* **2021**, *13*, 4363. [CrossRef] [PubMed]

36. Yun, C.W.; Lee, S.H. The Roles of Autophagy in Cancer. *Int. J. Mol. Sci.* **2018**, *19*, 3466. [CrossRef]
37. Fardi, M.; Solali, S.; Farshdousti Hagh, M. Epigenetic mechanisms as a new approach in cancer treatment: An updated review. *Genes Dis.* **2018**, *5*, 304–311. [CrossRef]
38. Ahuja, N.; Sharma, A.R.; Baylin, S.B. Epigenetic Therapeutics: A New Weapon in the War Against Cancer. *Annu. Rev. Med.* **2016**, *67*, 73–89. [CrossRef]
39. Karthikeyan, A.; Joseph, A.; Nair, B.G. Promising bioactive compounds from the marine environment and their potential effects on various diseases. *J. Genet. Eng. Biotechnol.* **2022**, *20*, 14. [CrossRef]
40. Cao, R.; Jin, W.; Shan, Y.; Wang, J.; Liu, G.; Kuang, S.; Sun, C. Marine Bacterial Polysaccharide EPS11 Inhibits Cancer Cell Growth via Blocking Cell Adhesion and Stimulating Anoikis. *Mar. Drugs* **2018**, *16*, 85. [CrossRef]
41. Wang, J.; Liu, G.; Ma, W.; Lu, Z.; Sun, C. Marine Bacterial Polysaccharide EPS11 Inhibits Cancer Cell Growth and Metastasis via Blocking Cell Adhesion and Attenuating Filiform Structure Formation. *Mar. Drugs* **2019**, *17*, 50. [CrossRef]
42. Liu, G.; Liu, R.; Shan, Y.; Sun, C. Marine bacterial exopolysaccharide EPS11 inhibits migration and invasion of liver cancer cells by directly targeting collagen I. *J. Biol. Chem.* **2021**, *297*, 101133. [CrossRef]
43. Ou, M.; Sun, X.; Liang, J.; Liu, F.; Wang, L.; Wu, X.; Tu, J. A polysaccharide from Sargassum thunbergii inhibits angiogenesis via downregulating MMP-2 activity and VEGF/HIF-1α signaling. *Int. J. Biol. Macromol.* **2017**, *94*, 451–458. [CrossRef]
44. Malyarenko, O.S.; Usoltseva, R.V.; Shevchenko, N.M.; Isakov, V.V.; Zvyagintseva, T.N.; Ermakova, S.P. In vitro anticancer activity of the laminarans from Far Eastern brown seaweeds and their sulfated derivatives. *J. Appl. Phycol.* **2017**, *29*, 543–553. [CrossRef]
45. Malyarenko, O.S.; Usoltseva, R.V.; Zvyagintseva, T.N.; Ermakova, S.P. Laminaran from brown alga *Dictyota dichotoma* and its sulfated derivative as radioprotectors and radiosensitizers in melanoma therapy. *Carbohydr. Polym.* **2019**, *206*, 539–547. [CrossRef] [PubMed]
46. Wu, J.; Li, H.; Wang, X.; Zhang, X.; Liu, W.; Wang, Y.; Zhang, Y.; Pan, H.; Wang, Q.; Han, Y. Effect of polysaccharide from *Undaria pinnatifida* on proliferation, migration and apoptosis of breast cancer cell MCF7. *Int. J. Biol. Macromol.* **2019**, *121*, 734–742. [CrossRef] [PubMed]
47. Yi, Y.; Qin, Z.; Yongping, X.; Gang, C.; Yukuan, Q. Sulfated Polysaccharide From *Undaria pinnatifida* Induces Apoptosis and Inhibits Proliferation, Migration, and Invasion in Ovarian Cancer via Suppressing the Hedgehog Signaling Pathway. *Front. Mater.* **2021**, *8*, 795061. [CrossRef]
48. Wu, J.; Chen, X.; Qiao, K.; Su, Y.; Liu, Z. Purification, structural elucidation, and in vitro antitumor effects of novel polysaccharides from *Bangia fuscopurpurea*. *Food Sci. Hum. Wellness.* **2021**, *10*, 63–71. [CrossRef]
49. Wu, J.; Lin, C.; Chen, X.; Pan, N.; Liu, Z. Polysaccharides isolated from *Bangia fuscopurpurea* induce apoptosis and autophagy in human ovarian cancer A2780 cells. *Food Sci. Nutr.* **2021**, *9*, 6707–6719. [CrossRef]
50. Zhang, M.; Chen, L.; Liu, Y.; Chen, M.; Zhang, S.; Kong, D. Sea cucumber *Cucumaria frondosa fucoidan* inhibits osteosarcoma adhesion and migration by regulating cytoskeleton remodeling. *Oncol. Rep.* **2020**, *44*, 469–476. [CrossRef]
51. Jiang, W.; Tian, W.; Ijaz, M.; Wang, F. Inhibition of EGF-induced migration and invasion by sulfated polysaccharide of *Sepiella maindroni* ink via the suppression of EGFR/Akt/p38 MAPK/MMP-2 signaling pathway in KB cells. *Biomed. Pharmacother.* **2017**, *95*, 95–102. [CrossRef]
52. Jiang, W.; Cheng, Y.; Zhao, N.; Li, L.; Shi, Y.; Zong, A.; Wang, F. Sulfated polysaccharide of *Sepiella Maindroni* ink inhibits the migration, invasion and matrix metalloproteinase-2 expression through suppressing EGFR-mediated p38/MAPK and PI3K/Akt/mTOR signaling pathways in SKOV-3 cells. *Int. J. Biol. Macromol.* **2018**, *107*, 349–362. [CrossRef] [PubMed]
53. Wongprasert, K.; Rudtanatip, T.; Praiboon, J. Immunostimulatory activity of sulfated *galactans* isolated from the red seaweed *Gracilaria fisheri* and development of resistance against white spot syndrome virus (WSSV) in shrimp. *Fish Shellfish. Immunol.* **2014**, *36*, 52–60. [CrossRef] [PubMed]
54. Boonsri, B.; Choowongkomon, K.; Kuaprasert, B.; Thitiphatphuvanon, T.; Supradit, K.; Sayinta, A.; Duangdara, J.; Rudtanatip, T.; Wongprasert, K. Probing the Anti-Cancer Potency of Sulfated *Galactans* on Cholangiocarcinoma Cells Using Synchrotron FTIR Microspectroscopy, Molecular Docking, and In Vitro Studies. *Mar. Drugs* **2021**, *19*, 258. [CrossRef] [PubMed]
55. Eke, I.; Cordes, N. Focal adhesion signaling and therapy resistance in cancer. *Semin. Cancer Biol.* **2015**, *31*, 65–75. [CrossRef]
56. da Silva Barbosa, J.; Palhares, L.C.G.F.; Silva, C.H.F.; Sabry, D.A.; Chavante, S.F.; Rocha, H.A.O. In Vitro Antitumor Potential of Sulfated Polysaccharides from Seaweed *Caulerpa cupressoides* var. flabellata. *Mar. Biotechnol.* **2021**, *23*, 77–89. [CrossRef]
57. Jose, G.M.; Kurup, G.M. Sulfated polysaccharides from *Padina tetrastromatica* arrest cell cycle, prevent metastasis and downregulate angiogenic mediators in HeLa cells. *Bioact. Carbohydr. Diet. Fibre.* **2017**, *12*, 7–13. [CrossRef]
58. Shakeel, E.; Arora, D.; Jamal, Q.M.S.; Akhtar, S.; Khan, M.K.A.; Kamal, M.A.; Siddiqui, M.H.; Lohani, M.; Arif, J.M. Marine Drugs: A Hidden Wealth and a New Epoch for Cancer Management. *Curr. Drug Metab.* **2018**, *19*, 523–543. [CrossRef]
59. Dyshlovoy, S.A.; Honecker, F. Marine Compounds and Cancer: The First Two Decades of XXI Century. *Mar. Drugs.* **2019**, *18*, 20. [CrossRef]
60. Lee, A.C.; Harris, J.L.; Khanna, K.K.; Hong, J.H. A Comprehensive Review on Current Advances in Peptide Drug Development and Design. *Int. J. Mol. Sci.* **2019**, *20*, 2383. [CrossRef]
61. Rangel, M.; de Santana, C.J.; Pinheiro, A.; Dos Anjos, L.; Barth, T.; Pires, O.R.; Fontes, W.; Castro, M.S. Marine Depsipeptides as Promising Pharmacotherapeutic Agents. *Curr. Protein Pept. Sci.* **2017**, *18*, 72–91. [CrossRef]

62. Le, T.C.; Pulat, S.; Lee, J.; Kim, G.J.; Kim, H.; Lee, E.Y.; Hillman, P.F.; Choi, H.; Yang, I.; Oh, D.C.; et al. Marine *Depsipeptide nobilamide* I Inhibits Cancer Cell Motility and Tumorigenicity via Suppressing Epithelial-Mesenchymal Transition and MMP2/9 Expression. *ACS Omega* **2022**, *7*, 1722–1732. [CrossRef] [PubMed]
63. Al-Awadhi, F.H.; Paul, V.J.; Luesch, H. Structural Diversity and Anticancer Activity of Marine-Derived Elastase Inhibitors: Key Features and Mechanisms Mediating the Antimetastatic Effects in Invasive Breast Cancer. *Chembiochem* **2018**, *19*, 815–825. [CrossRef] [PubMed]
64. Zhou, Z.; Wang, X.; Zhang, H.; Sun, J.; Zheng, L.; Liu, H.; Wang, J.; Shen, A.; Geng, M.; Guo, Y. Chromopeptide A, a highly cytotoxic depsipeptide from the marine sediment-derived bacterium *Chromobacterium* sp. HS-13-94. *Acta Pharm. Sin. B* **2015**, *5*, 62–66. [CrossRef] [PubMed]
65. Asfaha, Y.; Schrenk, C.; Alves Avelar, L.A.; Hamacher, A.; Pflieger, M.; Kassack, M.U.; Kurz, T. Recent advances in class IIa histone deacetylases research. *Bioorg. Med. Chem.* **2019**, *27*, 115087. [CrossRef] [PubMed]
66. Sun, J.Y.; Wang, J.D.; Wang, X.; Liu, H.C.; Zhang, M.M.; Liu, Y.C.; Zhang, C.H.; Su, Y.; Shen, Y.Y.; Guo, Y.W.; et al. Marine-derived chromopeptide A, a novel class I HDAC inhibitor, suppresses human prostate cancer cell proliferation and migration. *Acta Pharmacol. Sin.* **2017**, *38*, 551–560. [CrossRef]
67. Li, Y.; Seto, E. HDACs and HDAC Inhibitors in Cancer Development and Therapy. *Cold Spring Harb. Perspect. Med.* **2016**, *6*, a026831. [CrossRef]
68. Lin, S.; Zhang, C.; Liu, F.; Ma, J.; Jia, F.; Han, Z.; Xie, W.; Li, X. Actinomycin V Inhibits Migration and Invasion via Suppressing Snail/Slug-Mediated Epithelial-Mesenchymal Transition Progression in Human Breast Cancer MDA-MB-231 Cells In Vitro. *Mar. Drugs* **2019**, *17*, 305. [CrossRef]
69. Kgk, D.; Kumari, S.; Shailender, G.; Malla, R.R. Marine natural compound cyclo(L-leucyl-L-prolyl) peptide inhibits migration of triple negative breast cancer cells by disrupting interaction of CD151 and EGFR signaling. *Chem Biol. Interact.* **2020**, *315*, 108872. [CrossRef]
70. Al-Awadhi, F.H.; Salvador, L.A.; Law, B.K.; Paul, V.J.; Luesch, H. Kempopeptin C, a Novel Marine-Derived Serine Protease Inhibitor Targeting Invasive Breast Cancer. *Mar. Drugs* **2017**, *15*, 290. [CrossRef]
71. Al-Awadhi, F.H.; Law, B.K.; Paul, V.J.; Luesch, H. Grassystatins D-F, Potent Aspartic Protease Inhibitors from Marine *Cyanobacteria* as Potential Antimetastatic Agents Targeting Invasive Breast Cancer. *J. Nat. Prod.* **2017**, *80*, 2969–2986. [CrossRef]
72. Suleria, H.A.; Masci, P.P.; Gobe, G.C.; Osborne, S.A. Therapeutic potential of abalone and status of bioactive molecules: A comprehensive review. *Crit. Rev. Food Sci. Nutr.* **2017**, *57*, 1742–1748. [CrossRef] [PubMed]
73. Gong, F.; Chen, M.F.; Chen, J.; Li, C.; Zhou, C.; Hong, P.; Sun, S.; Qian, Z.J. Boiled Abalone Byproduct Peptide Exhibits Anti-Tumor Activity in HT1080 Cells and HUVECs by Suppressing the Metastasis and Angiogenesis In Vitro. *J. Agric. Food Chem.* **2019**, *67*, 8855–8867. [CrossRef] [PubMed]
74. Gong, F.; Chen, M.-F.; Zhang, Y.-Y.; Li, C.-Y.; Zhou, C.-X.; Hong, P.-Z.; Sun, S.-L.; Qian, Z.-J. A Novel Peptide from Abalone (*Haliotis discus hannai*) to Suppress Metastasis and Vasculogenic Mimicry of Tumor Cells and Enhance Anti-Tumor Effect In Vitro. *Mar. Drugs* **2019**, *17*, 244. [CrossRef] [PubMed]
75. Luo, S.; Zhangsun, D.; Harvey, P.J.; Kaas, Q.; Wu, Y.; Zhu, X.; Hu, Y.; Li, X.; Tsetlin, V.I.; Christensen, S.; et al. Cloning, synthesis, and characterization of αO-conotoxin GeXIVA, a potent α9α10 nicotinic acetylcholine receptor antagonist. *Proc. Natl. Acad. Sci USA* **2015**, *112*, E4026–E4035. [CrossRef]
76. Sun, Z.; Bao, J.; Zhangsun, M.; Dong, S.; Zhangsun, D.; Luo, S. αO-Conotoxin GeXIVA Inhibits the Growth of Breast Cancer Cells via Interaction with α9 Nicotine Acetylcholine Receptors. *Mar. Drugs* **2020**, *18*, 195. [CrossRef]
77. Zhang, Y.; Cui, J.; Zhang, R.; Wang, Y.; Hong, M. A novel fibrinolytic serine protease from the polychaete Nereis (*Neanthes*) virens (*Sars*): Purification and characterization. *Biochimie* **2007**, *89*, 93–103. [CrossRef]
78. Chen, Y.; Tang, Y.; Tang, Y.; Yang, Z.; Ding, G. Serine Protease from *Nereis virens* Inhibits H1299 Lung Cancer Cell Proliferation via the PI3K/AKT/mTOR Pathway. *Mar. Drugs* **2019**, *17*, 366. [CrossRef]
79. Zheng, L.; Zhu, X.; Yang, K.; Zhu, M.; Farooqi, A.A.; Kang, D.; Sun, M.; Xu, Y.; Lin, X.; Feng, Y.; et al. PBN11-8, a Cytotoxic Polypeptide Purified from *Marine bacillus*, Suppresses Invasion and Migration of Human Hepatocellular Carcinoma Cells by Targeting Focal Adhesion Kinase Pathways. *Polymers* **2018**, *10*, 1043. [CrossRef]
80. Ru, R.; Guo, Y.; Mao, J.; Yu, Z.; Huang, W.; Cao, X.; Hu, H.; Meng, M.; Yuan, L. Cancer Cell Inhibiting Sea Cucumber (*Holothuria leucospilota*) Protein as a Novel Anti-Cancer Drug. *Nutrients* **2022**, *14*, 786. [CrossRef]
81. Hussain, G.; Huang, J.; Rasul, A.; Anwar, H.; Imran, A.; Maqbool, J.; Razzaq, A.; Aziz, N.; Makhdoom, E.u.H.; Konuk, M.; et al. Putative Roles of Plant-Derived Tannins in Neurodegenerative and Neuropsychiatry Disorders: An Updated Review. *Molecules* **2019**, *24*, 2213. [CrossRef]
82. Briguglio, G.; Costa, C.; Pollicino, M.; Giambò, F.; Catania, S.; Fenga, C. Polyphenols in cancer prevention: New insights (Review). *Int. J. Funct. Nutr.* **2020**, *1*, 9. [CrossRef]
83. Montero, L.; Del Pilar Sánchez-Camargo, A.; Ibáñez, E.; Gilbert-López, B. Phenolic Compounds from Edible Algae: Bioactivity and Health Benefits. *Curr. Med. Chem.* **2018**, *25*, 4808–4826. [CrossRef] [PubMed]
84. Yang, S.; Liu, Y.; Xiao, Z.; Tang, Y.; Hong, P.; Sun, S.; Zhou, C.; Qian, Z.J. Inhibition effects of 7-phloro-eckol from *Ecklonia cava* on metastasis and angiogenesis induced by hypoxia through regulation of AKT/mTOR and ERK signaling pathways. *Arab. J. Chem.* **2021**, *14*, 103187. [CrossRef]

85. Lee, Y.J.; Park, J.H.; Park, S.A.; Joo, N.R.; Lee, B.H.; Lee, K.B.; Oh, S.M. *Dieckol* or *Phlorofucofuroeckol* extracted from *Ecklonia cava* suppresses lipopolysaccharide-mediated human breast cancer cell migration and invasion. *J. Appl. Phycol.* **2020**, *32*, 631–640. [CrossRef]
86. Vitale, G.A.; Coppola, D.; Palma Esposito, F.; Buonocore, C.; Ausuri, J.; Tortorella, E.; de Pascale, D. Antioxidant Molecules from Marine Fungi: Methodologies and Perspectives. *Antioxidants* **2020**, *9*, 1183. [CrossRef] [PubMed]
87. Vasarri, M.; Vitale, G.A.; Varese, G.C.; Barletta, E.; D'Auria, M.V.; de Pascale, D.; Degl'Innocenti, D. Dihydroauroglaucin Isolated from the Mediterranean Sponge *Grantia compressa* Endophyte Marine Fungus *Eurotium chevalieri* Inhibits Migration of Human Neuroblastoma Cells. *Pharmaceutics* **2022**, *14*, 616. [CrossRef]
88. Liu, J.; Li, F.M.; La Kim, E.; Hong, J.K.; Jung, J.H. Viriditoxin, from a Jellyfish-derived Fungus, is Antibiotic to Fish Pathogens. *Nat. Prod. Sci.* **2013**, *19*, 61–65.
89. Su, M.; Zhao, C.; Li, D.; Cao, J.; Ju, Z.; Kim, E.L.; Jung, Y.-S.; Jung, J.H. Viriditoxin Stabilizes Microtubule Polymers in SK-OV-3 Cells and Exhibits Antimitotic and Antimetastatic Potential. *Mar. Drugs* **2020**, *18*, 445. [CrossRef]
90. Chojnacka, K.; Lewandowska, U. Chemopreventive effects of polyphenol-rich extracts against cancer invasiveness and metastasis by inhibition of type IV collagenases expression and activity. *J. Funct. Foods* **2018**, *46*, 295–311. [CrossRef]
91. Rajamani, K.; Thirugnanasambandan, S.S. Polyphenols from brown alga, *Padina boergesenii* (Allendar & Kraft) decelerates renal cancer growth involving cell cycle arrest and induction of apoptosis in renal carcinoma cells. *Environ. Toxicol.* **2018**, *33*, 1135–1142. [CrossRef]
92. Begum, S.M.F.M.; Chitra, K.; Joseph, B.; Sundararajan, R.; Hemalatha, S. *Gelidiella acerosa* inhibits lung cancer proliferation. *BMC Complement Altern. Med.* **2018**, *18*, 104. [CrossRef]
93. Leri, M.; Ramazzotti, M.; Vasarri, M.; Peri, S.; Barletta, E.; Pretti, C.; Degl'Innocenti, D. Bioactive Compounds from *Posidonia oceanica* (L.) Delile Impair Malignant Cell Migration through Autophagy Modulation. *Mar. Drugs* **2018**, *16*, 137. [CrossRef] [PubMed]
94. Vasarri, M.; Leri, M.; Barletta, E.; Pretti, C.; Degl'Innocenti, D. *Posidonia oceanica* (L.) Delile Dampens Cell Migration of Human Neuroblastoma Cells. *Mar. Drugs* **2021**, *19*, 579. [CrossRef] [PubMed]
95. Piazzini, V.; Vasarri, M.; Degl'Innocenti, D.; Guastini, A.; Barletta, E.; Salvatici, M.C.; Bergonzi, M.C. Comparison of Chitosan Nanoparticles and Soluplus Micelles to Optimize the Bioactivity of *Posidonia oceanica* Extract on Human Neuroblastoma Cell Migration. *Pharmaceutics* **2019**, *11*, 655. [CrossRef]
96. Tohme, R.; Darwiche, N.; Gali-Muhtasib, H. A journey under the sea: The quest for marine anti-cancer alkaloids. *Molecules* **2011**, *16*, 9665–9696. [CrossRef]
97. Bechmann, N.; Ehrlich, H.; Eisenhofer, G.; Ehrlich, A.; Meschke, S.; Ziegler, C.G.; Bornstein, S.R. Anti-Tumorigenic and Anti-Metastatic Activity of the Sponge-Derived Marine Drugs Aeroplysinin-1 and Isofistularin-3 against Pheochromocytoma In Vitro. *Mar. Drugs* **2018**, *16*, 172. [CrossRef]
98. Lin, L.-C.; Kuo, T.-T.; Chang, H.-Y.; Liu, W.-S.; Hsia, S.-M.; Huang, T.-C. Manzamine A Exerts Anticancer Activity against Human Colorectal Cancer Cells. *Mar. Drugs* **2018**, *16*, 252. [CrossRef]
99. Charupant, K.; Suwanborirux, K.; Amnuoypol, S.; Saito, E.; Kubo, A.; Saito, N. Jorunnamycins A-C, new stabilized renieramycin-type bistetrahydroisoquinolines isolated from the Thai nudibranch *Jorunna funebris*. *Chem. Pharm. Bull.* **2007**, *55*, 81–86. [CrossRef]
100. Ecoy, G.A.U.; Chamni, S.; Suwanborirux, K.; Chanvorachote, P.; Chaotham, C. Jorunnamycin A from *Xestospongia* sp. Suppresses Epithelial to Mesenchymal Transition and Sensitizes Anoikis in Human Lung Cancer Cells. *J. Nat. Prod.* **2019**, *82*, 1861–1873. [CrossRef]
101. Tabakmakher, K.M.; Makarieva, T.N.; Denisenko, V.A.; Popov, R.S.; Kuzmich, A.S.; Shubina, L.K.; Lee, H.-S.; Lee, Y.-J.; Fedorov, S.N. Normonanchocidins G and H, New Pentacyclic Guanidine Alkaloids from the Far-Eastern Marine Sponge Monanchora pulchra. *Nat. Prod. Commun.* **2017**, *12*, 7. [CrossRef]

marine drugs

MDPI

Article

Type-I Hemins and Free Porphyrins from a Western Australian Sponge *Isabela* sp.

Samuele Sala [1,2,*], Stephen A. Moggach [1], Gareth L. Nealon [1,3], Jane Fromont [4], Oliver Gomez [4], Daniel Vuong [5], Ernest Lacey [5] and Gavin R. Flematti [1,*]

1 School of Molecular Sciences, The University of Western Australia, Crawley, WA 6009, Australia
2 Australian National Phenome Centre and Centre for Computational and Systems Medicine, Health Futures Institute, Murdoch University, Harry Perkins Building, Perth, WA 6150, Australia
3 Centre for Microscopy, Characterisation and Analysis, The University of Western Australia, Crawley, WA 6009, Australia
4 Collection and Research, Western Australian Museum, Welshpool, WA 6106, Australia
5 Microbial Screening Technologies Pty. Ltd., Smithfield, NSW 2164, Australia
* Correspondence: samuele.sala@murdoch.edu.au (S.S.), gavin.flematti@uwa.edu.au (G.R.F.); Tel.: +61-4-0116-9864 (S.S.); +61-8-64884461 (G.R.F.)

Abstract: Two novel free porphyrins, isabellins A and B, as well as the known compounds corallistin D and deuteroporphyrin IX were isolated from a marine sponge *Isabela* sp. LC-MS analysis of the crude extract revealed that the natural products were present both as free porphyrins and iron(III) coordinated hemins, designated isabellihemin A, isabellihemin B, corallistihemin D and deuterohemin IX, respectively. Structures were determined via high-resolution mass spectrometry, UV-Vis spectroscopy and extensive NOESY NMR spectroscopic experiments. The type-I alkyl substitution pattern of isabellin A and isabellihemin A was assigned unambiguously by single crystal X-ray diffraction. Biological evaluation of the metabolites revealed potent cytotoxicity for isabellin A against the NS-1 murine myeloma cell line.

Keywords: porphyrin; *Isabela*; hemin; X-ray diffraction; NOESY NMR; cytotoxic

check for updates

Citation: Sala, S.; Moggach, S.A.; Nealon, G.L.; Fromont, J.; Gomez, O.; Vuong, D.; Lacey, E.; Flematti, G.R. Type-I Hemins and Free Porphyrins from a Western Australian Sponge *Isabela* sp.. *Mar. Drugs* **2023**, *21*, 41. https://doi.org/10.3390/md21010041

Academic Editors: Marc Diederich and Celso Alves

Received: 12 December 2022
Revised: 29 December 2022
Accepted: 29 December 2022
Published: 3 January 2023

Copyright: © 2023 by the authors. Licensee MDPI, Basel, Switzerland. This article is an open access article distributed under the terms and conditions of the Creative Commons Attribution (CC BY) license (https://creativecommons.org/licenses/by/4.0/).

1. Introduction

Tetractinellid sponges of the *Corallistes* genus (Order: Tetractinellida; Family: Corallistes) have been reported to yield the microtubule stabilising macrolactone dictyostatin [1], and the poly-nitrogen compound corallistine [2], as well as the free porphyrins corallistins A-E and deuteroporphirin IX [3,4]. The assigned structures of corallistins A, B, C and E have been confirmed via total synthesis [5,6]. Recently, taxonomic re-identification of the sponges reported to produce corallistins A-E has suggested that the sponges are in fact members of the genus *Isabela* [7].

Metallated porphyrins and related macrocycles are expressed in most living organisms while synthetic porphyrins have been applied broadly in the area of photodynamic therapy [8]. They are however rarely encountered as functionalised secondary metabolites constituting a significant proportion of an organism's metabolic extract [4]. Given the biological importance of porphyrins as by-products of heme biosynthesis, their biosynthetic pathway has been well studied [9,10]. Beginning with glycine and succinyl-CoA, the enzymes ALA-synthase and ALA-dehydratase yield porphobilinogen in animals, fungi and α-proteobacteria. In plants, Archea and most other Bacteria, porphobilinogen is biosynthesised from two tRNA bound glutamyl starter units [10]. The enzyme PBG-deaminase then leads to the linear hydroxymethylbilane. From here, cyclisation can either occur chemically to afford the D_{4h} symmetrical uroporphyrinogen-I, or enzymatically with D-ring inversion via the UPG-III synthase, PBG-deaminase complex to afford uroporphirinogen-III [9,11]. In the case of uroporphirinogen-III, stepwise decarboxylation via the UPG-III decarboxylase enzyme affords coproporphyrinogen-III [11], which then loses a further two CO_2 groups via the CPG-oxidase enzyme leading to the formation of protoporphyrinogen IX [11]. From here, PPG-oxidase removes six hydrogens to give protoporphyrin IX, whereby two protons are substituted for one unit of Fe^{2+} via a ferrochelatase enzyme to afford heme B [10,11].

Our ongoing investigations [12,13] into the marine sponges of the Western Australian Marine Bio-resources Library (WAMBL) [14] yielded two novel free porphyrins from an *Isabela* marine sponge, herein named isabellins A and B (**1a**, **2a**, Figure 1). LC-MS analysis of the crude extract revealed that the compounds were present as both free porphyrins and as ferric hemin compounds (**1b, 2b**). Further analysis of the mixture revealed the presence of the known compounds corralistin D (**3a**) and deuteroporphyrin IX (**4a**) [4] as well as their corresponding hemin counterparts (**3b, 4b**). Nuclear magnetic resonance experiments of the compounds were complicated by intense signal suppression of the nuclei present on the aromatic scaffolds, as well as the difficulty in replication of experiments, presumably due to the effects of aromatic ring current on the rapidly aggregating/de-aggregating porphyrins in solution, as has been noted in prior literature [3–5]. To this end, the structures of the compounds were assigned unambiguously via detailed interpretation of 2D-NOESY experiments and single crystal X-ray crystallography of **1a/b**. The paramagnetic iron(III) hemin complexes **2b**, **3b** and **4b** were provisionally assigned via HR-ESI-MS. Biological evaluation of the isolated metabolites revealed compound **1a** as a potent inhibitor of the NS-1 murine myeloma cell line with strong selectivity for mammalian cell lines over bacterial pathogens and other Eukaryotes.

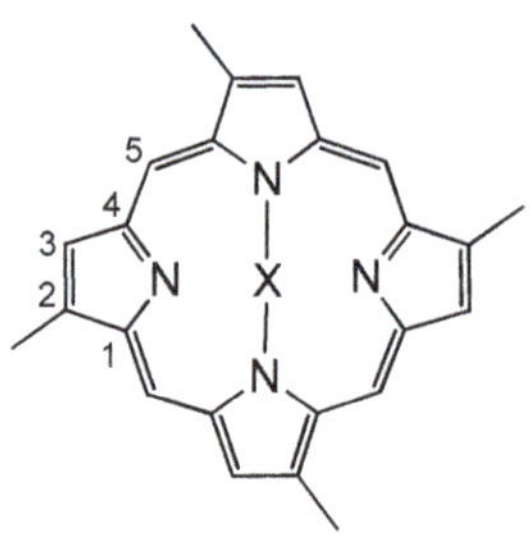

1a X = 2H
1b X = Fe(III)

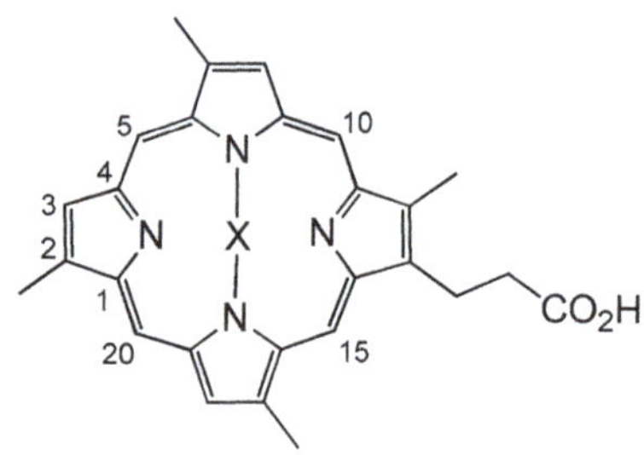

2a X = 2H
2b X = Fe(III)

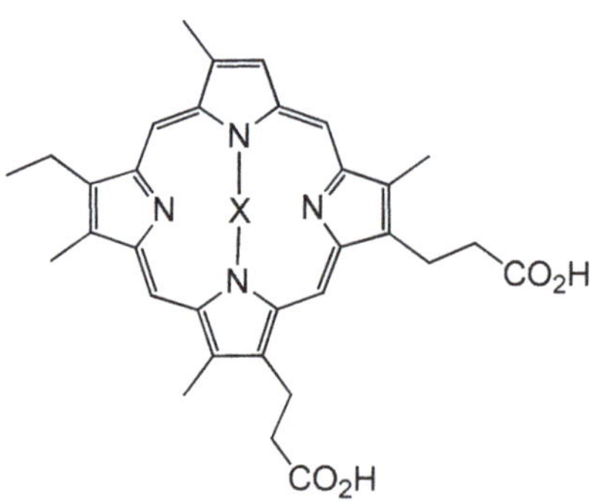

3a X = 2H
3b X = Fe(III)

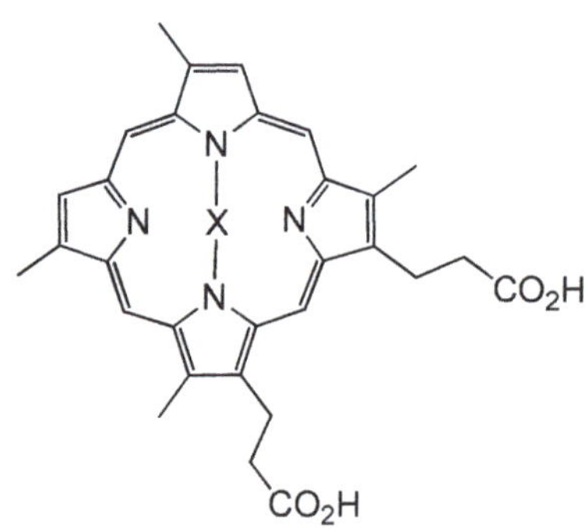

4a X = 2H
4b X = Fe(III)

Figure 1. Structures **1a/b** to **4a/b**.

2. Results

HPLC-photo diode array detector analysis of the crude solvent extract of the Isabela sponge revealed a series of etio-type porphyrins with a characteristic Soret band at approximately 390 nm and Q-bands with intensities in the order of IV > III > II > I [15]. Large scale isolation of the compounds was achieved using a combination of normal phase chromatography and reversed phase HPLC under acidic conditions.

Compound **1a** was isolated as a dark red crystalline solid. HR-ESIMS gave a protonated molecular ion $[M + H]^+$ at m/z 367.1924 consistent with the molecular formula $C_{24}H_{23}N_4$ (requires 367.1923). To our surprise, ^1H NMR of the compound in $CDCl_3$ (600 MHz) revealed the presence of a compound with four-fold rotational symmetry as revealed by three unique electronic environments (δ_H 10.12; CH-5, 9.14; CH-3, 3.76; C-2-CH_3). We note that appropriate ^1H NMR integration was achieved by applying a 10 second relaxation time to the pulse sequence. All attempts to obtain reliable ^{13}C NMR data for compound **1a** were hampered by significant signal suppression, presumably caused by the significant aromatic ring current present in the system. The difficulty in obtaining reliable ^{13}C NMR spectra for free base porphyrins has been documented elsewhere [5]. The structure of compound **1a** was subsequently assigned unambiguously via single crystal X-ray diffraction (Figure 2) and assigned the trivial name isabellin A. The extremely reduced state of compound **1a** is a biosynthetically anomaly, and to the best of our knowledge is the first report of a highly reduced geo-porphyrinoid [16] isolated from a living organism.

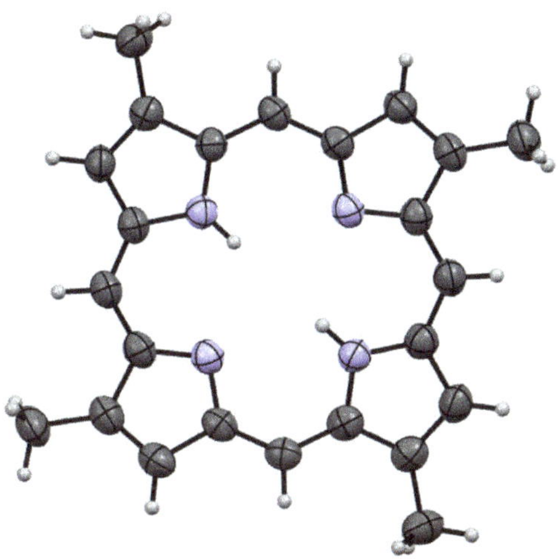

Figure 2. Single crystal X-ray structure of **1a**.

Compound **1b** was isolated as a brown solid which recrystallised in chloroform to give dark brown needles. HR-ESIMS of the compound gave a molecular ion cluster $[M - 2H + Fe(III)]^+$ with an isotopic distribution characteristic of an iron atom at m/z 420.1032, consistent with the molecular formula $C_{24}H_{20}N_4{}^{56}Fe^+$ (requires 420.1037), as well as a prominent acetonitrile adduct at m/z 461.1302 consistent with the molecular formula $C_{26}H_{23}N_5{}^{56}Fe^+$ (requires 461.1303), allowing us to conclude that we had isolated the ferric hemin counterpart to compound **1a**. The ^1H and ^{13}C NMR analysis of the paramagnetic Fe(III) complex proved unproductive. Ultimately, the structure of compound **1b** was assigned via single crystal X-ray diffraction as the trifluoroacetate (TFA) salt (Figure 3).

Compound **2a** was isolated as dark brown amorphous solid. HR-ESIMS gave a protonated molecular ion $[M + H]^+$ at m/z 439.2133 consistent with the molecular formula $C_{27}H_{27}N_4O_2$ (requires 439.2134). The ^1H NMR analysis of the compound in acidified DMSO-d_6 revealed the presence of four meso-proton environments (δ_H 10.37–10.34), three pyrrolic protons (δ_H 9.39–9.34), four methyl groups (δ_H 3.77, 3.75, 3.73 and 3.66) and a single propionate group as evidenced by two broad spin coupled triplets at δ_H 4.40 and δ_H 3.21. As with compound **1a**, extensive ^{13}C NMR experiments failed to resolve the majority of the ^{13}C nuclei attributable to a compound of this size. A range of NMR solvents and experimental parameters were trialled.

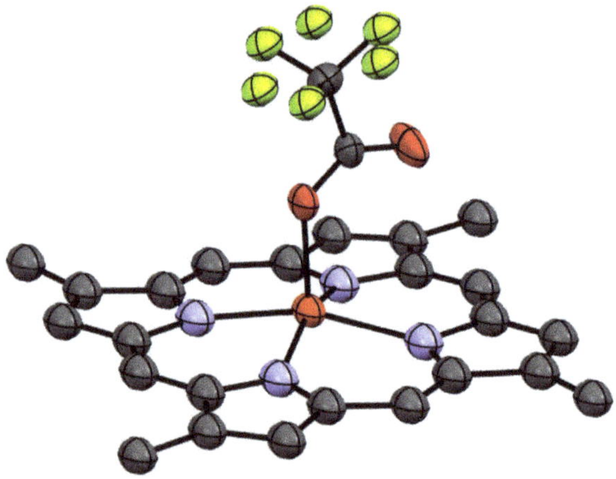

Figure 3. Single crystal X-ray structure of **1b** TFA salt. Hydrogen atoms have been omitted for clarity.

Given the capacity of the organism in question to produce porphyrins with both type-I (derived from a symmetrical APAPAPAP bearing uroporphirinogen precursor, with A = Acetyl and P = Propionyl) and type-III (derived from an asymmetrical APAPAPPA bearing uroporphirinogen precursor, featuring D-ring inversion) topology, configurational assignment of the alkyl substituents present on compound **2a** became a non-trivial exercise, with one potential type-I isomer and four potential type-III isomers possible. After some consideration it became clear that a simple experiment would be able to distinguish between naturally occurring type-I and type-III configurational isomers with four methyl groups present. The method can be summarised with the conditional statement: If every meso-proton of the porphyrin macrocycle shows a 2D-NOE correlation to a corresponding methyl group, then the porphyrin must be a type-I derived porphyrin. Extending the rationale, if one meso-proton does not show a correlation to a methyl group, then the porphyrin is either a natural type-III derived porphyrin, or a type-IV porphyrin, of which there are no naturally occurring derivatives.

Porphyrin **2a** showed clear correlations from each meso-proton to each methyl group, and was therefore assigned the type-I structure depicted (Figure 4). The compound was given the trivial name isabellin B (The authors here suggest that the new trivial name Isabellin be used to designate type-I porphyrins within the lithistid family of compounds, whereas the trivial name Corallistin be retained for porphirins with a type-III alkyl substitution pattern.). In similar fashion to **2a**, the type-III alkyl substitution patterns of the known metabolites corallistin D (**3a**) and deuteroporphyrin IX (**4a**) were confirmed using the methodology described above.

Reanalysis of the sponge crude extract by LC-HRMS revealed a series of ferric metabolites consistent in accurate mass measurements to be the hemin counterparts of **2a**, **3a** and **4a**, in similar relationship to that between **1a** and **1b** (Table 1). Given our previous difficulty in obtaining ^{1}H and ^{13}C NMR data for the paramagnetic **1b**, isolation of the compounds was not pursued. In support of their identity as the ferric counterparts to **2a**, **3a** and **4a**, treatment of the crude extract with concentrated H_2SO_4 led to the disappearance of the ferric metabolites when analysed by LC-MS. No new peaks (aside from those ascribed to **2a**, **3a** and **4a**) were seen in the chromatogram allowing for the provisional assignment of **2b**, **3b** and **4b** as illustrated.

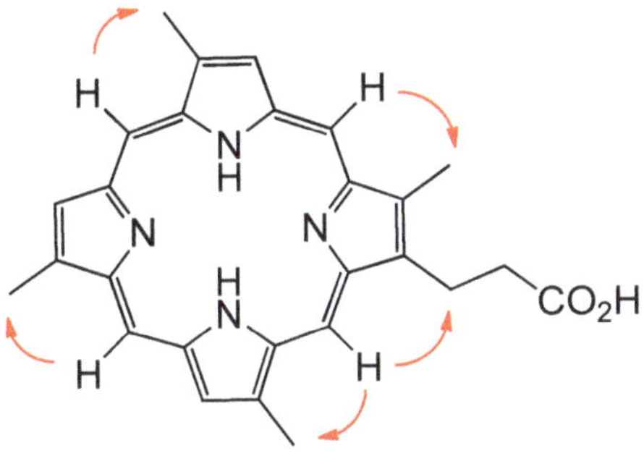

2a

Figure 4. Isabellin B (**2a**) with key NOE correlations indicated in red.

Table 1. Porphyrin-hemin mass correlation table for compounds **1a/b–4a/b**.

Compound Pair	[M + 2H + H]+	Molecular Formula (a)	[M + Fe + ACN]+	[M + Fe]+	Molecular Formula (b)
1a/b	367.1924	$C_{24}H_{22}N_4$	461.1302	420.1032	$C_{24}H_{20}N_4{}^{56}Fe^+$
2a/b	439.2133	$C_{27}H_{26}N_4O_2$	533.1522	492.1248	$C_{27}H_{24}N_4O_2{}^{56}Fe^+$
3a/b	539.2653	$C_{32}H_{34}N_4O_4$	633.2038	592.1772	$C_{32}H_{32}N_4O_4{}^{56}Fe^+$
4a/b	511.2345	$C_{30}H_{30}N_4O_4$	605.1718	564.1474	$C_{30}H_{28}N_4O_4{}^{56}Fe^+$

Biosynthetically, compounds **1a/b** and **2a/b** are presumably derived from uroporphyrinogen-I, whereas compounds **3a/b** and **4a/b** are divergent uroporphyrinogen-III derivatives. Given the degree of elaboration observed on the respective type-I and type-III derived compounds, it seems that **1a/b**, **2a/b** act as more efficient substrates for the UPG-decarboxylase, CPG-oxidase and PPG oxidase enzymes, as well as the subsequent reducing and devinylating enzymes active on the scaffolds. Whether the iron was chelated in its ferric state as isolated or in the ferrous state as has been reported for ferrochelatase enzymes [10,11] remains unknown, however LC-MS analysis of the sponge crude extract failed to detect any iron(II) metabolites.

Testing of the metabolites against a panel of micro-organisms and cell lines (Tables 2 and 3) revealed potent cytotoxicity of compound **1a** against the NS-1 myeloma cell line, with an MIC of 0.4 μg/mL at the 72-h time-point and 0.8 μg/mL at the 96-h time-point, comparable to the sparsomycin positive control. Testing against the neonatal foreskin fibroblast (NFF) cell line revealed marginal selectivity for the tumorigenic cell line with an MIC of 1.6 μg/mL at both time-points tested. In addition to this the compound was found to be moderately bacteriostatic towards the Gram-positive pathogens *Bacillus subtilis* and Staphylococcus aureus with an MIC of 25 μg/mL at the 24-h time-point, and inhibited the growth of *Giardia duodenalis* (MIC = 6.3 μg/mL). In stark contrast, metabolites **1b**, **2a**, **3a** and **4a** failed to display significant activity against any of the organisms and cell-lines tested, with the exception of mild activity towards NS-1 displayed by compound **3a** (MIC = 50 μg/mL at the 72-h time-point), and mild anti-bacterial activity displayed by compound **4a** towards *Staphylococcus aureus* (MIC = 50 μg/mL at the 72-h time-point). The cytotoxicity displayed by compound **1a** is in line with other porphyrin macrocycles [8]. We postulate that the discrepancy in activity between metabolite **1a** and other metabolites tested may be in part due to an increase in membrane permeability afforded to **1a** by its lipophilic structure, over that of the Fe(III) salt **1b** and the carboxylate bearing **2a**, **3a** and **4a**.

Table 2. Bioactivity profile of isabellins A and B (**1a** and **2a**), isabellihemin A (**1b**), corallistin D (**3a**) and deuteroporphyrin IX (**4a**) against select Bacteria and Fungi, MIC reported in μg/mL. [a].

Compound	*Bs 24 h*	*Bs 48 h*	*Sa 24 h*	*Sa 48 h*	*Ca 24 h*	*Ca 48 h*	*Sc 24 h*	*Sc 48 h*
1a	25	>100	25	>100	>200	>200	>200	>200
1b	>100	>100	>100	>100	>200	>200	>200	>200
2a	>100	>100	>100	>100	>200	>200	>200	>200
3a	>100	>100	>100	>100	>200	>200	>200	>200
4a	100	100	50	100	>200	>200	>200	>200
Control [b]	1.6	6.3	3.1	12.5	0.8	>200	1.6	3.1

[a] *Bs* = *Bacillus subtilis* (ATCC 6633); *Sa* = *Staphylococcus aureus* (ATCC 25923); *Ca* = *Candida albicans* (ATCC 10231); *Saccharomyces cerevisiae* (ATCC 9763); [b] Controls: *Bs*, *Sa* = tetracycline; *Ca*, *Sc* = blasticidin S HCl.

Table 3. Bioactivity profile of isabellins A and B (**1a** and **2a**), isabellihemin A (**1b**), corallistin D (**3a**) and deuteroporphyrin IX (**4a**) against select cell lines and protozoal parasites, MIC reported in μg/mL [a].

Compound	NS-1 *72 h*	NS-1 *96 h*	NFF *72 h*	NFF *96 h*	*Tf 48 h*	*Tf 72 h*	*Gi 96 h*
1a	0.4	0.8	1.6	1.6	>100	>100	6.3
1b	>100	>100	>100	>100	>100	>100	100
2a	>100	>100	>100	>100	>100	>100	>100
3a	50	100	>100	>100	>100	>100	100
4a	>100	>100	>100	>100	>100	>100	100
Control [b]	0.6	0.6	0.6	0.6	0.2	0.2	0.3

[a] NS-1 = Murine myeloma NS-1 (ATCC TIB-18); NFF = Neonatal foreskin fibroblast (ATCC PCS-201); *Tf* = *Tritrichomonas* foetus KV-1; *Gi* = *Giardia duodenalis* WB-1B. [b] Controls: NS-1, NFF = sparsomycin; Tf, Gi = metronidazole.

3. Discussion

Two new free porphyrins, isabellins A (**1a**) and B (**2a**), an iron (III) coordinated porphyrin, isabellihemin A (**1b**), and the known compounds corallistin D (**3a**) and deuteroporphyrin IX (**4a**) were isolated from a marine sponge *Isabela* sp. The type-I alkyl substitution pattern of **1a**, **1b** and **2a** was assigned unambiguously by NOESY NMR spectroscopic experiments and single crystal X-ray diffraction (Supplementary Materials). Testing of the isolated metabolites against a panel of micro-organisms and cell lines revealed potent cytotoxicity for **1a** against the NS-1 and NFF cell lines that was comparable to that of the sparsomycin positive control.

4. Materials and Methods

4.1. General Experimental

UV/Vis spectra were acquired on an Agilent Cary 60 UV/Vis spectrometer. Nuclear magnetic resonance (NMR) spectra were recorded on a Bruker Avance IIIHD 500 MHz spectrometer (500.1 MHz for ^{1}H and 125.8 MHz for ^{13}C) and a Bruker Avance IIIHD 600 MHz spectrometer (600.1 MHz for ^{1}H and 150 MHz for ^{13}C). Chemical shifts were calibrated against the residual solvent present: in $CDCl_3$ (^{1}H, δ 7.26 and ^{13}C, δ 77.16 ppm), in CD_3OD (^{1}H, δ 3.31 and ^{13}C, δ 49.00 ppm), in $(CD_3)_2SO$ (^{1}H, δ 3.50 and ^{13}C, δ 39.52 ppm), in $(CD_3)_2CO$ (^{1}H, δ 2.05 and ^{13}C, δ 29.84 ppm) and expressed relative to TMS [17]. NMR spectra measured in neat TFA were measured at 273 K. Deuterium lock was maintained via insertion of a $(CD_3)_2CO$ standard capillary tube insert. H_2O was suppressed via selective presaturation at 11.5 ppm. HPLC-mass spectrometry and HRMS were conducted using a Waters Alliance e2695 HPLC connected to a Waters 2998 diode array detector and Waters LCT Premier XE time-of-flight mass spectrometer using either an atmospheric pressure chemical ionization (APCI) source or an electrospray ionisation (ESI) source in either positive or negative mode. HRMS was conducted with either APCI or ESI in W-mode, using leucine enkephalin (200 pg/μL) as internal lock mass. For LC-MS separation an Altima C_{18} column (150 mm × 2.1 mm, 5 μm, Grace Discovery Sciences, Columbia, MD, USA) was used with a flow rate of 0.3 mL/min. Rapid silica filtration (RSF) under reduced pressure was conducted on a sintered glass column using chromatographic silica (Davisil LC60A 40-63 micron, Grace Discovery Sciences, Columbia, MD, USA). Flash silica chromatography was conducted using the Reveleris X2 flash chromatography system equipped with a cartridge containing silica gel as the stationary phase (120 g, 40 μm, p/n 145). Semi-preparative and analytical HPLC were performed using either an Agilent 1200 HPLC system with a diode array detector (DAD) and fraction collector or using a Hewlett Packard 1050 equipped with a DAD and Pharmacia Biotech RediFrac fraction collector. Analytical work was conducted using an Apollo C_{18} reversed phase column (250 mm × 4.6 mm, 5 μm, Grace Discovery Sciences) utilising 20 μL injections, and with a flow rate of 1.0 mL/min, and semi-preparative HPLC was undertaken with an Apollo C_{18} reversed-phase column (250 mm × 10 mm, 5 μm, Grace Discovery Sciences) with 300 μL injections at a flow rate of 4.0 mL/min.

4.2. Characterisation

A specimen of *Isabela* sp. (WAM Z35787) was collected at 97 m depth on hard substrate off Zuytdorp, WA (27°03′06″ S, 113°06′03″ E) by Sherman sled on 5 December 2005 aboard the CSIRO research vessel Southern Surveyor, and was stored frozen at −18 °C at the Western Australian Museum. The ethanol preserved portion of the sponge is a thick, erect plate 900 mm tall, 500 mm wide and 300 mm thick. It has a stony, incompressible texture and a smooth surface; it was dark purple alive and black-brown in ethanol, and it stains the ethanol dark brown. The spicules are desmas, blunt-ended oxeas 115 × 5 μm, blunt-ended dichotriaenes 1130 μm long, microrhabds 40 μm long and thin spirasters 20 μm long.

4.3. Extraction and Isolation

A portion of the *Isabela* sp. sponge (14.9 g, frozen weight) was sheared with scissors and extracted overnight, three times in MeOH:DCM (1:1, *v*/*v*) solution (3 × 500 mL) to which was added TFA (3 × 0.5 mL). The crude dark brown extract was filtered (Whatman No. 1, 18.5 cm) and reduced *in vacuo* to give a dark brown gum. The sample was reconstituted in acidified CH_2Cl_2 (1.0% TFA) and absorbed on celite (1 g) before separating with a Reveleris automated flash chromatography module. The column was eluted with an isocratic solvent system consisting of 100% EtOAc for 20 min. The mobile phase was then increased from EtOAc to 100% MeOH over a further 5 min and held for 10 min. The flow rate was set at 25 mL/min and fractions were collected in 25 mL aliquots throughout the run. The fraction eluting at six minutes was separated using semi-preparative reversed phase HPLC, eluting with an isocratic solvent system of 95% ACN/H_2O with 0.1% TFA to yield **1a** (3.5 mg). The fraction eluting at seven minutes was separated using semi-preparative reversed phase HPLC at a flow rate of 4 mL/min, eluting with an isocratic solvent system of 75% ACN/H_2O with 0.1% TFA over 40 min to yield **1b** (2.2 mg) eluting at 5 min and **2a** (3.2 mg) eluting between 15–20 min. The fraction eluting at twelve minutes was separated using semi-preparative reversed phase HPLC at a flow rate of 4 mL/min, eluting with an isocratic solvent system of 55% ACN/H_2O with 0.1% TFA over 40 min to yield **3a** (5.0 mg) and **4a** (4.2 mg).

4.4. Compound Characterization

Isabellin A **(1a)** dark red plate crystals, green in solution, pink when observed through a transmitted source of white light, bright red in acidified solution; UV/Vis (MeOH) λ_{max} (log ε) 390 (2.23), 495 (0.14), 530 (0.10), 565 (0.08), 615 (0.05) nm; ^{1}H NMR ($CDCl_3$, 600 MHz) δ [ppm] 10.12 (s, 1H), 9.14 (s, 1H), 3.76 (s, 3H); HRMS (ESI): *m/z* 367.1924 $[M + H]^+$ (calcd for $C_{24}H_{23}N_4$, 367.1923)

Isabellihemin A **(1b)** dark brown needles, brown in solution, UV/Vis (MeOH) λ_{max} (log ε) 385 (2.40), 490 (0.15), 605 (0.07) nm; HRMS (ESI): *m/z* 420.1032 $[M - 2H + Fe(III)]^+$ (calcd for $C_{24}H_{20}N_4{}^{56}Fe$, 420.1037), *m/z* 461.1302 $[M - 2H + ACN + Fe(III)]^+$ (calcd for $C_{26}H_{23}N_5{}^{56}Fe$, 461.1303)

Isabellin B **(2a)** Maroon solid, bright red in acidified solution; UV/Vis (MeOH) λ_{max} (log ε) 390 (0.74), 495 (0.06), 527 (0.04), 565 (0.03), 613 (0.02) nm; ^{1}H NMR (DMSO-d$_6$, 600 MHz) δ [ppm] 10.37 (s, 1H), 10.36 (s, 1H), 10.35 (s, 1H), 10.34 (s, 1H), 9.39 (s, 1H), 9.36 (s, 1H), 9.34 (s, 1H), 4.40 (bt, 2H), 3.77 (s, 3H), 3.76 (s, 3H), 3.73 (s, 3H), 3.66 (s, 3H), 3.20 (bt, 2H); HRMS (ESI): *m/z* 439.2133 [M + H]$^+$ (calcd for $C_{27}H_{27}N_4O_2$, 439.2134)

Isabellihemin B **(2b)** HRMS (ESI): *m/z* 492.1248 [M − 2H + Fe(III)]$^+$ (calcd for $C_{27}H_{24}N_4O_2{}^{56}Fe$, 492.1249), *m/z* 533.1522 [M − 2H + ACN + Fe(III)]$^+$ (calcd for $C_{29}H_{27}N_5O_2{}^{56}Fe$, 533.1514) *Corallistin D* **(3a)** Dark brown solid, bright pink in acidified solution: UV/Vis (MeOH) λ_{max} (log ε) 385 (3.55), 425 (0.21), 560 (0.26) nm; ^{1}H NMR (CDCl$_3$, 600 MHz) δ [ppm] 11.07 (bs, 1H) 10.69 (s, 1H), 10.66 (s, 1H), 10.65 (s, 1H) 9.40 (s, 1H), 4.46 (bt, 4H), 4.16 (q, 2H), 3.79 (s, 3H), 3.69 (s, 3H), 3.682 (s, 3H), 3.680 (s, 3H), 3.32 (bt, 4H), 2.41 (t, 3H); HRMS (ESI): *m/z* 539.2653 [M + H]$^+$ (calcd for $C_{32}H_{35}N_4O_4$, 539.2658)

Corallistihemin D **(3b)** HRMS (ESI): *m/z* 592.1772 [M − 2H + Fe(III)]$^+$ (calcd for $C_{32}H_{32}N_4O_4{}^{56}Fe$, 592.1773), *m/z* 633.2034 [M − 2H + ACN + Fe(III)]$^+$ (calcd for $C_{34}H_{35}N_5O_4{}^{56}Fe$, 633.2038) *Deuteroporphyrin IX* **(4a)** Dark brown solid, bright pink in acidified solution; UV/Vis (MeOH) λ_{max} (log ε) 390 (2.63), 500 (0.15), 525 (0.15), 560 (0.14), 600 (0.08) nm; ^{1}H NMR (CDCl$_3$, 600 MHz) δ [ppm] 11.10 (bs, 1H), 10.72 (s, 1H), 10.69 (s, 1H), 10.67 (s, 1H), 9.42 (s, 1H), 9.41 (s, 1H), 4.48 (bt, 4H), 3.80 (s, 3H), 3.79 (s, 3H), 3.71 (s, 3H), 3.68 (s, 3H), 3.22 (bt, 2H), 3.20 (bt, 2H); HRMS (ESI): *m/z* 511.2345 [M + H]$^+$ (calcd for $C_{30}H_{31}N_4O_4$, 511.2345)

Deuterohemin IX **(4b)** HRMS (ESI): *m/z* 564.1474 [M − 2H + Fe(III)]$^+$ (calcd for $C_{30}H_{28}N_4O_4{}^{56}Fe$, 564.1460), *m/z* 605.1718 [M − 2H + ACN + Fe(III)]$^+$ (calcd for $C_{32}H_{31}N_5O_4{}^{56}Fe$, 605.1725)

4.5. X-ray Crystallographic Analysis of **1a**

From a solution of MeOH:DCM (3:1) blood red plates were obtained, A suitable crystal with dimensions 0.08 × 0.05 × 0.04 mm^3 was selected and mounted on a XtaLAB Synergy, Single source at home/near, HyPix diffractometer. The crystal was kept at a steady T = 150.00(10) K during data collection. The structure was solved with the **ShelXT** 2018/2 [18] solution program using dual methods and by using **Olex2** 1.5 [19] as the graphical interface. The model was refined with **XL** [20] using full matrix least squares minimisation on F^2.

$C_{24}H_{22}N_4$, M_r = 366.45, monoclinic, $P2_1/c$ (No. 14), a = 11.7999(5) Å, b = 10.7615(5) Å, c = 14.9068(6) Å, b = 96.745(4)°, $a = g$ = 90°, V = 1879.83(14) Å^3, T = 150.00(10) K, Z = 4, Z' = 1, m(Cu K_a) = 0.609, 18158 reflections measured, 3906 unique (R_{int} = 0.0539) which were used in all calculations. The final wR_2 was 0.2031 (all data) and R_1 was 0.0621 (I ≥ 2 s(I)).

4.6. X-ray Crystallographic Analysis of 1b

From a solution of CHCl$_3$ dark brown needles were obtained. A suitable crystal with dimensions 0.10 × 0.05 × 0.03 mm^3 was selected and mounted on a XtaLAB Synergy, Single source at home/near, HyPix diffractometer. The crystal was kept at a steady T = 120.00(14) K during data collection. The structure was solved with the **ShelXT** 2018/2 [18] solution program using dual methods and by using **Olex2** 1.5 [19] as the graphical interface. The model was refined with **XL** [20] using full matrix least squares minimisation on F^2.

$C_{25}H_{20}F_{1.5}FeN_4O_{1.5}$, M_r = 484.80, monoclinic, $P2_1/c$ (No. 14), a = 9.6505(10) Å, b = 15.664(2) Å, c = 17.1896(19) Å, b = 100.170(10)°, $a = g$ = 90°, V = 2557.7(5) Å^3, T = 120.00(14) K, Z = 4, Z' = 1, m(Cu K_a) = 5.029, 13005 reflections measured, 1627 unique (R_{int} = 0.1153) which were used in all calculations. The final wR_2 was 0.3316 (all data) and R_1 was 0.1147 (I ≥ 2 s(I)).

4.7. Bioassays

Test compounds were dissolved in DMSO to provide 10 mg/mL stock solutions. An aliquot of each stock solution was transferred to the first lane of rows B to G in a 96-well microtiter plate and 2-fold serially diluted across the 12 lanes of the plate to provide a 2048-fold concentration gradient. Bioassay medium was added to an aliquot of each test solution to provide a 100-fold dilution into the final bioassay, thus yielding a test range of 100 to 0.05 μg/mL in 1% DMSO. Row A was used as the negative control (no inhibition), and Row H was used as the positive control (uninoculated).

CyTOX is an indicative bioassay platform for discovery of antitumor actives. NS-1 (ATCC TIB-18) mouse myeloma cells and NFF (ATCC PCS-201) human neonatal foreskin fibroblast cells were each inoculated in 96-well microtiter plates (190 μL) at 50,000 cells/mL in DMEM (Dulbecco's modified Eagle's medium + 10% fetal bovine serum (FBS) + 1% penicillin/streptomycin (10,000 U/mL/10,000 μg/mL, Life Technologies Cat. No. 15140122), together with resazurin (250 μg/mL; 10 μL) and incubated in a 37 °C (5% CO_2) incubator. The plates were incubated for 96 h during which time the positive control wells change colour from a blue to pink colour. MIC end points were determined visually.

ProTOX is a generic bioassay platform for antibiotic discovery. *Bacillus subtilis* (ATCC 6633) and *Staphylococcus aureus* (ATCC 25923) were used as indicative species for antibacterial activity. A bacterial suspension (50 mL in a 250 mL flask) was prepared in nutrient broth by cultivation for 24 h at 100–250 rpm, 28 °C. The suspension was diluted to an absorbance of 0.01 absorbance unit per mL, and 10 μL aliquots were added to the wells of a 96-well microtiter plate, which contained the test compounds dispersed in nutrient agar (Amyl) with resazurin (12.5 μg/mL). The plates were incubated at 28 °C for 48 h, during which time the negative control wells change from a blue to light pink color. MIC end points were determined visually.

EuTOX is a generic bioassay platform for antifungal discovery. The yeast *Candida albicans* (ATCC 10231) and *Saccharomyces cerevisiae* (ATCC 9763) wereused as indicative species for antifungal activity. A yeast suspension (50 mL in a 250 mL flask) was prepared in 1% malt extract broth by cultivation for 24 h at 250 rpm, 24 °C. The suspension was diluted to an absorbance of 0.005 and 0.03 absorbance units per mL for *C. albicans* and *S. cerevisiae*, respectively. Aliquots (20 μL and 30 μL) of *C. albicans* and *S. cerevisiae*, respectively, were applied to the wells of a 96-well microtiter plate, which contained the test compounds dispersed in malt extract agar containing bromocresol green (50 μg/mL). The plates were incubated at 24 °C for 48 h, during which time the negative control wells change from a blue to yellow color. MIC end points were determined visually.

GiTOX is a bioassay focused on the discovery of inhibitors of the parasite, *G. duodenalis*. In the present bioassay *G. duodenalis* (strain WB-1B) was inoculated in 96-well microtitre plates (200 μL) at 4 × 105 cells/mL in Giardia medium (0.2% tryptone, Oxoid; 0.1% yeast extract, Difco; 0.5% glucose; 0.106% L-arginine; 0.1% L-cysteine; 0.2% NaCl; 0.1% K_2HPO_4; 0.06% KH_2PO_4; 0.02% ascorbic acid; 0.0023% ferric ammonium citrate; 0.01% Bile (Sigma, Burlington, MA, USA); 1% penicillin/streptomycin (10,000 U/mL/10,000 μg/mL, Life Technologies Cat. No. 15140122), 10% newborn calf serum (NBCS), Life Technologies, Waltham, MA, USA). The plates were incubated in anaerobic jars (Oxoid AG25) containing an Anaerogen satchel (Oxoid AN25) in a 37 °C (5% CO_2) incubator. At 96 h, *G. duodenalis* proliferation was counted and % inhibition graphed to determine the MIC values.

TriTOX is a bioassay focused on the discovery of inhibitors of the animal protozoan pathogen *Tritrichomonas fetus* (strain KV-1). *T. fetus* were inoculated in 96-well microtiter plates (200 μL) at 4 × 10^4 cells/mL in *T. fetus* medium (0.2% tryptone, Oxoid; 0.1% yeast extract, Difco; 0.25% glucose; 0.1% l-cysteine; 0.1% K_2HPO_4; 0.1% KH_2PO_4; 0.1% ascorbic acid; 0.01% $FeSO_4 \cdot 7H_2O$; 1% penicillin/streptomycin (10 mL/L), 10% new born calf serum, Life Technologies, Waltham, MA, USA). The plates were incubated in anaerobic jars (Oxoid AG25) containing an Anaerogen satchel (Oxoid AN25) in a 37 °C (5% CO_2) incubator. At 48 h and 72 h, MIC end points were determined visually and absorbance was measured using Spectromax plate reader (Molecular Devices, Sunnyvale, CA, USA) at 570 nm [21].

Supplementary Materials: The following supporting information can be downloaded at: https://www.mdpi.com/article/10.3390/md21010041/s1, NMR (^{1}H, ^{13}C, ^{1}H-^{1}H-COSY, HSQC, HMBC, NOESY), Single crystal X-ray diffraction data of **1a** (CIF), Single crystal X-ray diffraction data of **1b** (CIF).

Author Contributions: Methodology, S.S., D.V. and G.R.F.; Software, S.A.M. and G.L.N.; Formal analysis, S.S., S.A.M., G.L.N., J.F. and E.L.; Investigation, S.S., O.G. and D.V.; Resources, S.A.M., J.F. and E.L.; Data curation, S.A.M., J.F. and O.G.; Writing—original draft, S.S.; Writing—review and editing, G.R.F.; Supervision, G.R.F.; Funding acquisition, S.A.M., Ernest Lacey and G.R.F. All authors have read and agreed to the published version of the manuscript.

Funding: S.A.M. thanks the Australian Research Council (ARC) for a Future Fellowship (FT200100243).

Data Availability Statement: Data available from zenodo: DOI:10.5281/zenodo.7425830. Link: https://zenodo.org/record/7425830#.Y5aOtJ5BxPY.

Acknowledgments: We thank J. Parthenay and M. Clarke from the Centre for Microscopy, Characterisation and Analysis for technical assistance with MS measurements. S.S. acknowledges F. Dhoro for the valuable discussions. S.S. also acknowledges financial support from an Australian Government Research Training Program scholarship.

Conflicts of Interest: The authors declare no conflict of interest.

References

1. Paterson, I.; Britton, R.; Delgado, O.; Wright, A.E. Stereochemical determination of dictyostatin, a novel microtubule-stabilising macrolide from the marine sponge *Corallistidae* sp. *Chem. Commun.* **2004**, 632–633. [CrossRef] [PubMed]
2. Debitus, C.; Cesario, M.; Guilhem, J.; Pascard, C.; Païs, M. Corallistine, a new polynitrogen compound from the sponge *Corallistes fulvodesmus* L. & L. *Tetrahedron Lett.* **1989**, *30*, 1534–1538.
3. D'Ambrosio, M.; Guerriero, A.; Debitus, C.; Ribes, O.; De Forges, B.R.; Pietra, F. Corallistin A, a second example of a free porphyrin from a living organism. Isolation from the demosponge *Corallistes* sp. of the coral see and inhibition of abnormal cells. *Helv. Chim. Acta* **1989**, *72*, 1451–1454. [CrossRef]
4. D'Ambrosio, M.; Guerriero, A.; Pietra, F.; Debitus, C.; Ribes, O. On the Novel Free Porphyrins Corallistin B, C, D, and E: Isolation from the demosponge *Corallistes* sp. of the Coral Sea and Reactivity of Their Nickel 55 (II) Complexes toward Formylating Reagents. *Helv. Chim. Acta* **1993**, *76*, 1489–1496. [CrossRef]
5. Pandey, R.K.; Leung, S.H.; Smith, K.M. Total synthesis of new porphyrins isolated from the coral sea demosponge *Corallistes* sp. *Tetrahedron Lett.* **1994**, *35*, 8093–8096. [CrossRef]
6. Yon-Hin, P.; Scott, A.I. Total synthesis of corallistin A. *Tetrahedron Lett.* **1991**, *32*, 4231–4234. [CrossRef]
7. Pisera, A.; Institute of Paleobiology, Polish Academy of Sciences, Warszawa, Poland. Personal communication, 2020.
8. Allison, R.R.; Downie, G.H.; Cuenca, R.; Hu, X.-H.; Childs, C.J.H.; Sibata, C.H. Photosensitizers in clinical PDT. *Photodiagnosis Photodyn. Ther.* **2004**, *1*, 27–42. [CrossRef] [PubMed]
9. Battersby, A.R.; Fookes, C.J.R.; Matcham, G.W.J.; McDonald, E. Biosynthesis of the pigments of life: Formation of the macrocycle. *Nature* **1980**, *285*, 17–21. [CrossRef] [PubMed]
10. Layer, G.; Reichelt, J.; Jahn, D.; Heinz, D.W. Structure and function of enzymes in heme biosynthesis. *Protein Sci.* **2010**, *19*, 1137–1161. [CrossRef] [PubMed]
11. Leeper, F.J. The biosynthesis of porphyrins, chlorophylls, and vitamin B12. *Nat. Prod. Rep.* **1985**, *2*, 19–47. [CrossRef] [PubMed]
12. Shrestha, S.; Sorolla, A.; Fromont, J.; Blancafort, P.; Flematti, G.R. Aurantoside C Targets and Induces Apoptosis in Triple Negative Breast Cancer Cells. *Mar Drugs* **2018**, *16*, 361. [CrossRef] [PubMed]
13. Shrestha, S.; Sorolla, A.; Fromont, J.; Blancafort, P.; Flematti, G.R. Crambescidin 800, Isolated from the Marine Sponge Monanchora viridis, Induces Cell Cycle Arrest and Apoptosis in Triple-Negative Breast Cancer Cells. *Mar Drugs* **2018**, *16*, 53. [CrossRef] [PubMed]
14. Fromont, J.; Althaus, F.; McEnnulty, F.R.; Williams, A.; Salotti, M.; Gomez, O.; Gowlett-Holmes, K. Living on the edge: The sponge fauna of Australia's southwestern and northwestern deep continental margin. *Hydrobiologia* **2012**, *687*, 127–142. [CrossRef]
15. Mandal, P.C.; Goto, M.; Sasaki, M. Removal of Nickel and Vanadium from Heavy Oils Using Supercritical Water. *J. Jpn. Pet. Inst.* **2014**, *57*, 18–28. [CrossRef]
16. William Louda, J. Porphyrins. In *Encyclopedia of Geochemistry: A Comprehensive Reference Source on the Chemistry of the Earth*; White, W.M., Ed.; Springer International Publishing: Cham, Switzerland, 2018; pp. 1247–1253.
17. Gottlieb, H.E.; Kotlyar, V.; Nudelman, A. NMR Chemical Shifts of Common Laboratory Solvents as Trace Impurities. *J. Org. Chem.* **1997**, *62*, 7512–7515. [CrossRef] [PubMed]
18. Sheldrick, G. Crystal structure refinement with SHELXL. *Acta Crystallogr. Sect. C* **2015**, *71*, 3–8. [CrossRef] [PubMed]
19. Dolomanov, O.V.; Bourhis, L.J.; Gildea, R.J.; Howard, J.A.K.; Puschmann, H. OLEX2: A complete structure solution, refinement and analysis program. *J. Appl. Crystallogr.* **2009**, *42*, 339–341. [CrossRef]

20. Sheldrick, G. A short history of SHELX. *Acta Crystallogr. Sect. A* **2008**, *64*, 112–122. [CrossRef] [PubMed]
21. Lam, A.Y.F.; Vuong, D.; Jex, A.R.; Piggott, A.M.; Lacey, E.; Emery-Corbin, S.J. TriTOX: A novel Trichomonas vaginalis assay platform for high-throughput screening of compound libraries. *Int. J. Parasitol. Drugs Drug Resist.* **2021**, *15*, 68–80. [CrossRef] [PubMed]

Disclaimer/Publisher's Note: The statements, opinions and data contained in all publications are solely those of the individual author(s) and contributor(s) and not of MDPI and/or the editor(s). MDPI and/or the editor(s) disclaim responsibility for any injury to people or property resulting from any ideas, methods, instructions or products referred to in the content.

marine drugs

MDPI

Article

Oxygenated Cembrene Diterpenes from *Sarcophyton convolutum:* Cytotoxic Sarcoconvolutum A–E

Tarik A. Mohamed [1], Abdelsamed I. Elshamy [2], Asmaa M. Abdel-Tawab [3], Mona M. AbdelMohsen [1], Shinji Ohta [4], Paul W. Pare [5,*] and Mohamed-Elamir F. Hegazy [1,6,*]

1 Chemistry of Medicinal Plants Department, National Research Centre, 33 El-Bohouth St., Dokki, Giza 12622, Egypt; ta.mourad@nrc.sci.eg (T.A.M.); monaamohsen@yahoo.com (M.M.A.)
2 Department of Natural Compounds Chemistry, National Research Centre, 33 El-Bohouth St., Dokki, Giza 12622, Egypt; ai.el-shamy@nrc.sci.eg
3 Marine Biotechnology and Natural Products Laboratory, National Institute of Oceanography and Fisheries, Cairo 11516, Egypt; am.eltawab@niof.sci.eg
4 Graduate School of Integrated Sciences for Life, Hiroshima University, 1-7-1 Kagamiyama, Higashi-Hiroshima 739-8521, Japan; ohta@hiroshima-u.ac.jp
5 Department of Chemistry & Biochemistry, Texas Tech University, Lubbock, TX 79409, USA
6 Department of Pharmaceutical Biology, Institute of Pharmaceutical and Biomedical Sciences, Johannes Gutenberg University, Staudinger Weg 5, 55128 Mainz, Germany
* Correspondence: paul.pare@ttu.edu (P.W.P.); mohegazy@uni-mainz.de (M.-E.F.H.); Tel.: +1-806-834-0461 (P.W.P.); +20-33-371-635 (M.-E.F.H.)

Abstract: The soft coral genus *Sarcophyton* contains the enzymatic machinery to synthesize a multitude of cembrene-type diterpenes. Herein, highly oxygenated cembrenoids, sarcoconvolutum A–E (**1–5**) were purified and characterized from an ethyl acetate extract of the red sea soft coral, *Sarcophyton convolutum*. Compounds were assemblies according to spectroscopic methods including FTIR, 1D- and 2D-NMR as well as HRMS. Metabolite cytotoxicity was tested against lung adenocarcinoma, cervical cancer, and oral-cavity carcinoma (A549, HeLa and HSC-2, respectively). The most cytotoxic compound, (**4**) was observed to be active against cell lines A549 and HSC-2 with IC_{50} values of 49.70 and 53.17 µM, respectively.

Keywords: *Sarcophyton convolutum*; sarcoconvolutum A–E; cembrenoids; cytotoxicity

Citation: Mohamed, T.A.; Elshamy, A.I.; Abdel-Tawab, A.M.; AbdelMohsen, M.M.; Ohta, S.; Pare, P.W.; Hegazy, M.-E.F. Oxygenated Cembrene Diterpenes from *Sarcophyton convolutum:* Cytotoxic Sarcoconvolutum A–E. *Mar. Drugs* **2021**, *19*, 519. https://doi.org/10.3390/md19090519

Academic Editors: Celso Alves and Marc Diederich

Received: 21 August 2021
Accepted: 11 September 2021
Published: 13 September 2021

Publisher's Note: MDPI stays neutral with regard to jurisdictional claims in published maps and institutional affiliations.

Copyright: © 2021 by the authors. Licensee MDPI, Basel, Switzerland. This article is an open access article distributed under the terms and conditions of the Creative Commons Attribution (CC BY) license (https://creativecommons.org/licenses/by/4.0/).

1. Introduction

Natural products and structural analogues are key for drug discovery, especially for pharmacotherapies for cancers and infectious diseases [1–5]. Such biologically active metabolites are characterized by scaffold diversity and structural complexity. For example, within *Sarcophyton* soft coral, isolated metabolites include cembrenoids [2,6–9], diterpene dimers [10,11], sesquiterpenes [12,13], ceramides [14], steroids [15,16], and prostaglandins [17,18]. Cembrenoids in particular exhibit a significant number of sp^3 carbon centers and oxygen atoms with no nitrogen or halogen atoms. Higher numbers of H-bond acceptors and donors confer hydrophilicity and ring structures provide significant molecular rigidity. Cembrenoids also exhibit promising biological activities including anticancer [6–8], anti-inflammatory [8], antifouling [19,20], ichthyotoxic [21], antifeedant [12], antiviral [22], and neuroprotective [23] properties.

In a pursuit of novel metabolites with biological activity, polyoxygenated cembrene-type diterpenoids (Figure 1) have been isolated from the Red Sea soft coral *S. convolutum*. Metabolite antiproliferative activity was assayed against a non-small-cell lung adenocarcinoma, a cervical cancer, and an oral-cavity squamous-cell carcinoma, A549, HeLa, and HSC-2, respectively.

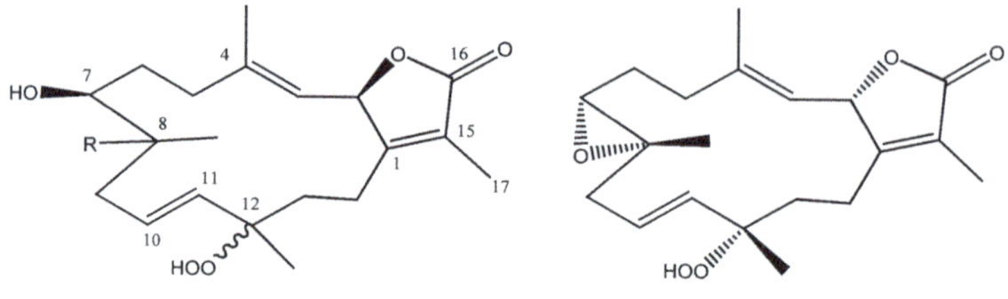

1 R= α-OH; α-OOH
2 R= β-OH; β-OOH
3 R= α-OMe; α-OOH

4

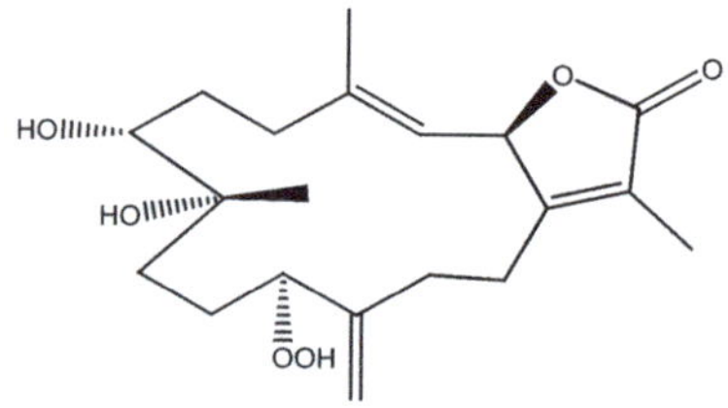

5

Figure 1. Sarcoconvolutum A–E (**1–5**) isolated from *S. convolutum*.

2. Results and Discussion

Sarcoconvolutum A (**1**) was isolated as yellow oil with a positive optical rotation (+10.6) in a MeOH solvent. The HRCIMS molecular ion peak at m/z 367.2122 $[M + H]^+$ was assigned predicting a molecular formula of $C_{20}H_{30}O_6$ (calcd. 367.2121, $[M + H]^+$) with six degrees of unsaturation suggesting a bicyclic skeleton. FTIR spectrum exhibited bands at 3465 cm^{-1} and 1765 cm^{-1} corresponding to hydroxyls and carbonyl groups. From ^1H NMR spectrum (Table 1), two oxygenated protons at δ_H 3.26 br d (J = 10.8 Hz) and 5.53 d (J = 10.4 Hz), three olefinic protons at δ_H 4.84 br d (J = 10.4 Hz), 5.48 br d (J = 16.3 Hz), and 5.50 m, in addition to four methyls were at δ_H 1.28 s, 1.37 s, 1.83 s, and 1.87 s were characterized. Twenty carbon resonances were predicted from ^{13}C NMR (Table 1) and categorized into 6 quaternary (including carbonyl at δ_C 175.3; three olefinics at δ_C 123.1, 143.9 and 162.3; alongside of two oxygenated carbons at δ_C 74.5 and 84.1), five methines (comprising two oxygenated carbons at δ_C 71.6 and 79.4; as well as three olefinic at δ_C 121.1, 127.8, and 134.8), five methylenes, four methyls (δ_C 8.8, 16.5, 20.3, and 24.2) depending upon DEPT and HSQC experiments. The above analyses of 1D NMR of **1** revealed the cembrene-based diterpenoid [6,7,24]. The 1D NMR of 1 was similar to 12-hydroperoxylsarcoph-10-ene isolated previously from *S. glaucum* [24]. Observed signal differences for the newly isolated compound included a down field shift of H-7 and C-7 by 0.73 and 12.1 ppm, respectively; a down field shift of 15.3 ppm for C-8; and a down field shift of 6 ppm for Me-19 consistent with the substitution of a hydroxyl group at C-7 instead of an epoxide ring coupling C-7 and C-8. The proposed structure was confirmed by ^1H ^1H COSY and HMBC spectral analysis. H-2 [δ_H 5.53 d (J = 10.4 Hz)]/C-4 (δ_C 143.9, J^3), and ^1H ^1H COSY of H-2/H-3 [δ_H 4.84 br d (J = 10.4 Hz)] indicated the location of $\Delta^{3(4)}$. The HMBC correlation of H_3-18 (δ_H 1.87 s) and C_{H2}-5 (δ_C 35.2, J^3) followed by ^1H ^1H COSY correlations of H_2-5 [δ_H 2.18 br d (J = 12.7 Hz)]/ H-6 (δ_H 1.77 br d (J = 13.4 Hz)], H-6/H-7 (δ_H 3.26 br d (J = 10.8 Hz) confirmed a hydroxyl group at C-7. HMBC correlation of H_3-19 (δ_H 1.28 s)/C-7 (δ_C 71.6, J^3), H_3-19/C-8 (δ_C 74.5, J^3), and H-7/C-8 (J^2) established hydroxylation of the C-8 quaternary carbon. Subsequently, HMBC correlation of H_3-19/C_{H2}-9 (δ_C 42.9, J^3), H_3-20 (δ_H 1.37 s)/C_{H2}-11 (δ_C 134.8, J^3), in addition to ^1H ^1H COSY of H_2-9 [δ_H 2.34 m]/H-10 (δ_H 5.50 m), H-10/H-11 [(δ_H 5.48 br d (J = 16.3 Hz)] established $\Delta^{10(11)}$. The down field shift of C-12 by ca. 7 ppm [24] as well as the HMBC correlation of H-11/C-12 (δ_C 84.1, J^3), H_3-20/C-12 (J^2), and H_3-20/C-13 (δ_C 34.4 J^3) indicated the presence of a hydroperoxide group at C-12. The C-1/C-2 included lactone ring was established via HMBC of H-2/C-16 (keto group, δ_C 175.3, J^3), H-2/C-15 (δ_C 123.1, J^3), H_3-17 (δ_H 1.83 s)/C-16 (J^3), H_3-17/C-1 (δ_C 162.3, J^3), and H_3-17/C-15 (Figure 2).

The relative configuration of 1 is based on coupling constants and NOESY data (Figure 3). From the coupling constant of H-2 (10.4 Hz) along with the vicinal coupling of H-3 (10.4 Hz), the *cis* orientation and α configuration of H-2 was established [7,24,25]. Starting from this point, the NOESY correlations of H-2α [δ_H 5.53 d (J = 10.4 Hz)]/ H_3-18 [δ_H 1.87 s], H_3-18/ H-5α [δ_H 2.18 br d (J = 12.7 Hz)], H_3-18/ H-6α [δ_H 1.77 br d (J = 13.4)], H-5α/ H-6α, and H-6α/ H-7 [δ_H 3.26 br d (J = 10.8 Hz)] established an α orientation for H-7. NOESY correlations of H-6β [δ_H 1.41 ddd (J = 13.7, 12.7, 10.9 Hz)]/ H_3-19 (δ_H 1.28 s), H-9β (δ_H 2.34 m)/ H_3-19, H-9β/ H-11 [δ_H 5.48 br d (J = 16.3 Hz)], H-11/ H-13β [δ_H 1.72 br t (J = 13.2 Hz)], H-13β/ H_3-20 [δ_H 1.37 s], H-11/ H_3-20 indicated β configurations for both Me-19 and Me-20. Based on the described spectral analysis, **1** was identified as 7β,8α-dihydroxy-12α-hydroperoxide-16-keto-cembra-1*E*,3*E*,10*E*-triene (sarcoconvolutum A).

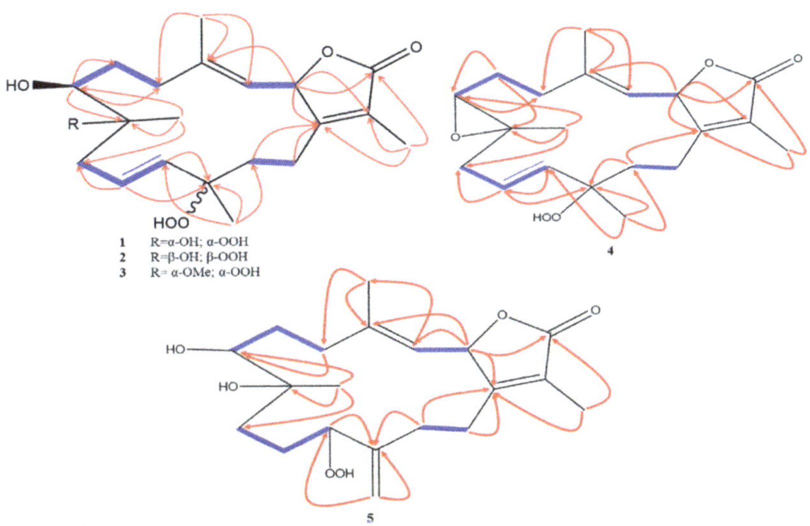

Figure 2. Key HMBC and $^1H\,^1H$ COSY of sarcoconvolutum A–E (**1–5**).

Sarcoconvolutum B (**2**) was isolated as yellow oil with a positive optical rotation (+43.1) in MeOH. From the HRCIMS molecular ion peak at *m/z* 367.2122 $[M + H]^+$, the molecular formula of $C_{20}H_{30}O_6$ (calcd. 367.2121, $[M + H]^+$) a bicylic skeleton with six degrees of unsaturation was predicted. The FTIR broad bands corresponding to hydroxyls and carbonyl groups were detected at 3462 cm^{-1} and 1768 cm^{-1}. The ^1H NMR spectrum (Table 1) displayed two oxygenated protons at δ_H 3.32 d (J = 10.9 Hz) and 5.45 d (J = 10.2 Hz), three olefinic protons at δ_H 4.88 d (J = 10.1 Hz), 5.50 d (J = 16.1 Hz), and 5.57 dt (J = 16.1, 7.2 Hz), along with four methyls were at δ_H 1.28 s, 1.42 s, 1.82 s, 1.85 s. From the observed twenty signals in the ^{13}C NMR spectrum (Table 1), 6 quartenary (including carbonyl at δ_C 174.8; three olefinics at δ_C 123.5, 143.5 and 161.9; alongside of two oxygenated carbons at δ_C 74.5 and 84.0), 5 methenes (comprising two oxygenated carbons at δ_C 78.7 and 71.1, as well as three olefinic signals at δ_C 121.6, 126.9, 134.6), 5 methylenes, 4 methyls (δ_C 8.9, 16.1, 23.6, and 24.1) were identified based on DEPT and HSQC signals. A down field shift of δ_C 84.0 by ca. 7 ppm suggested the presence of a hydroperoxyl unit at C-12 [24] which was consistent with mass spectral data. A ^{13}C NMR comparison of the two isolated compounds indicated a down field shift of Me-20 for **2**. The 2D NMR comparisons showed otherwise similar $^{1}H\,^{1}H$ COSY and HMBC signals (Figure 2). A ^{13}C NMR down field shift of 3.3 ppm for Me-20 indicated the opposite stereochemistry at C-12.

Relative stereochemistry was determined based on coupling constants and NOESY data (Figure 3). The coupling constant of H-2 (10.2 Hz) in addition to the vicinal coupling of H-3 (10.1 Hz) suggested a *cis* orientation and α configuration of H-2 [7,24,25]. The NOESY correlations of H-2α [δ_H 5.45 d (J = 10.2 Hz)]/ H_3-18 [δ_H 1.82 s], H-18/ H-5 [δ_H 2.37 td (J = 13.2t, 2.8 Hz)], H-18/ H-6 [δ_H 1.49 td (J = 13.7t, 3.6 Hz)], H-5α/ H-6, H-6/ H-7 [δ_H 3.32 br d (J = 10.9 Hz)], H-7/ H-19 [δ_H 1.28 s] and H-13β [δ_H 1.95 td (J = 13.1, 4.1 Hz)]/ H_3-19 indicated a H-7α Me-19 and Me-20orientation. Based upon these spectral data, **2** was identified as 7β,8α-dihydroxy-12β-hydroperoxide-16-keto-cembra-1*E*,3*E*,10*E*-triene (sarcoconvolutum B).

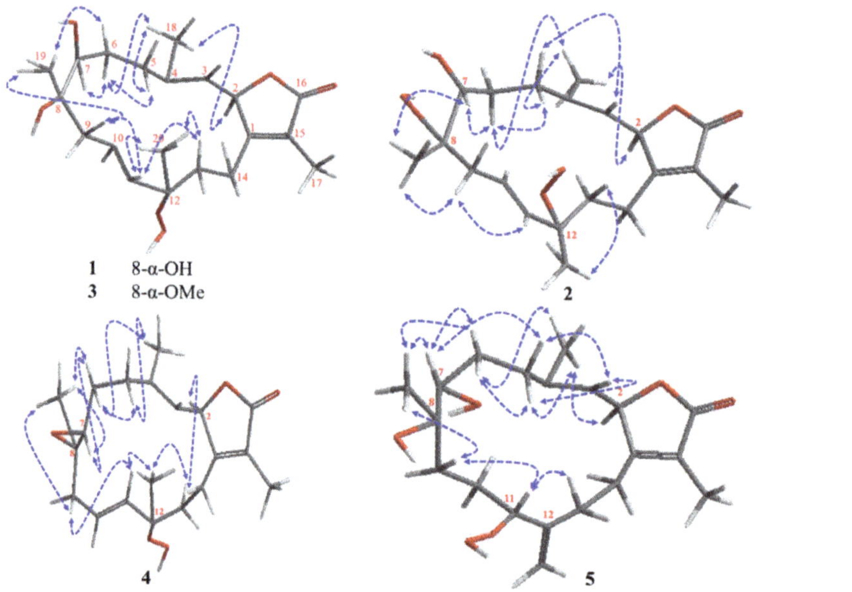

Figure 3. Significant NOESY of sarcoconvolutum A–E (**1**–**5**).

Sarcoconvolutum C (**3**) was isolated as yellow oil with a positive optical rotation (+33.1, *c* 0.003, CH_3OH). The molecular formula was deduced as $C_{21}H_{32}O_6$ (calcd. 364.2250, [M-OH + H]$^+$) based on a HREIMS molecular ion peak at m/z 364.2258 [M-OH + H]$^+$ indicating a bicylic skeleton with six degrees of unsaturation. FTIR broad bands corresponded to hydroxyls and carbonyl groups were detected at 3457 cm^{-1} and 1761 cm^{-1}. From ^{1}H NMR spectrum (Table 1), two oxygenated protons at δ_H 3.27 br d (J = 10.9 Hz) and δ_H 5.49 d (J= 9.9 Hz), three olefinic protons at δ_H 4.86 br d (J = 9.9 Hz), δ_H 5.44 br d (J = 16.1 Hz) and δ_H 5.56 dt (J = 15.6, 8.1t Hz), four methyls as well as one methyl of methoxy group at δ_H 3.23 s were assigned. Based on the ^{13}C NMR (Table 1), twenty-one carbon resonances were observed and were categorized by DEPT and HSQC analysis as 6 quaternary carbons (including carbonyl at δ_C 174.8; three olefinics at δ_C 123.3, 144.2 and 161.4; alongside of two oxygenated carbons at δ_C 78.3 and 84.4), 5 methines (comprising two oxygenated carbons at δ_C 78.3 and 71.9; as well as three olefinic at δ_C 121.2, 128.2, 134.0), 5 methylenes, 5 methyls (δ_C 9.0, 16.2, 18.2, 21.2, and 49.3). As with **1** and **2**, down field shift at δ_C 84.4 ppm of ca. 7 ppm along with a mass shift of [M-H_2O], suggested the addition of a hydroperoxy group [24]. The compound is similar to **1** and **2** except for a down field shift of δ_H 78.3 by 3.8 ppm associated with C-8 and a new methoxyl signal at δ_H 3.23 s and δ_C 49.3. HMBC correlations of a methyl proton at δ_H 3.23 and the C-12 at δ_H 78.3

confirm the localization of the methoxylation to C-12 (Figure 2). Thus, **3** was identified as 7-hydroxy-8-methoxy-12-hydroperoxide-16-keto-cembra-1*E*,3*E*,10*E*-triene.

Table 1. ^{1}H and ^{13}C NMR ($CDCl_3$, 500 Hz) of sarcoconvolutum A–E (**1**–**5**).

No	Sarcoconvolutum A (1)		Sarcoconvolutum B (2)		Sarcoconvolutum C (3)		Sarcoconvolutum D (4)		Sarcoconvolutum E (5)	
	^{1}H NMR (*J* Hz)	^{13}C	^{1}H NMR (*J* Hz)	^{13}C	^{1}H NMR (*J* Hz)	^{13}C	^{1}H NMR (*J* Hz)	^{13}C	^{1}H NMR (*J* Hz)	^{13}C
1	—	162.3	—	161.9	—	161.4	—	161.7	—	161.8
2	5.53 d (10.4)	79.4	5.45 d (10.2)	78.7	5.49 d (9.9)	79.0	5.45 d (9.4) *	78.8	5.47 d (10.1)	80.2
3	4.84 br d (10.4)	121.1	4.88 br d (10.1)	121.6	4.86 br d (9.9)	121.2	5.00 d (9.4)	121.1	4.92 br d (10.1)	119.2
4	—	143.9	—	143.5	—	144.2	—	144.4	—	145.9
5α	2.18 br d (12.7)	35.2	2.23 dt (13.2, 3.4t)	35.3	2.18 dt (13.4, 3.4t)	35.4	2.26 m *	36.6	2.35 dt (13.0, 7.6t)	37.9
5β	2.40 t (11.3)		2.37 td (13.2t, 2.8)		2.37 td (13.4, 7.4)		2.34 td (13.1t, 5.7)		2.10 td (13.0t, 5.1)	
6α	1.77 br d (13.4)	26.7	1.49 td (13.7t, 3.6)	26.3	1.87 td (13.4t, 3.6)	26.7	1.60 m	24.1	1.75 m *	30.5
6β	1.51 ddd (13.7, 12.7, 10.9)		1.83 m *		1.44 td (15.3t, 4.3)		1.82 m *		1.25 m *	
7	3.26 br d (10.8)	71.6	3.32 br d (10.9)	71.1	3.27 br d (10.9)	71.9	2.65 dd (6.8, 3.6)	57.0	3.45 br d (10.5)	75.0
8	—	74.5	—	74.5	—	78.3	—	60.0	—	73.9
9α	2.34 m *	42.9	2.44 dd (13.7, 7.8)	43.4	2.34 m *	37.2	2.41 dd (13.1, 5.7)	39.0	1.57 m	35.1
9β	2.34 m *		2.28 dd (13.4, 6.6)		2.34 m *		2.46 dd (13.3, 7.1)		1.51 m	
10α	5.50 m	127.8	5.57 dt (16.1, 7.2)	126.9	5.56 dt (15.6, 8.1t)	128.2	5.42 m *	125.8	1.57 m	25.2
10β									1.32 m	
11	5.48 br d (16.3)	134.8	5.50 br d (16.1)	134.6	5.44 br d (16.1)	134.0	5.47 m *	135.5	4.43 dd (9.0, 5.0)	89.3
12	—	84.1	—	84.0	—	84.4	—	84.6	—	146.0
13α	1.72 br t (13.2)	34.4	1.49 td (13.7, 3.6)	36.4	1.80 td (13.4t, 3.5)	35.1	1.58 m *	36.0	2.02 br t (15.1)	27.8
13β	1.68 td (13.2t, 5.6)		1.95 td (13.1, 4.1)		1.67 td (13.4t, 4.7)		1.89 m *		2.25 m	
14α	2.01 br t (13.2)	22.7	2.06 br t (13.7)	21.6	2.05 br t (13.4)	22.7	2.07 br t	22.0	2.13 m	24.5
14β	2.43 br t (13.2)		2.62 td (13.7, 4.0)		2.40 td (13.7, 4.3)		2.27 td * (13.2t, 5.5)		2.65 td (12.9, 4.9)	
15	—	123.1	—	123.5	—	123.3	—	123.6	—	124.3
16	—	175.3	—	174.8	—	174.8	—	174.8	—	174.9
17	1.83 s	8.8	1.85 s	8.9	1.85 s	9.0	1.86 s	9.1	1.86 s	8.9
18	1.87 s	16.5	1.82 s	16.1	1.83 s	16.2	1.87 s	15.8	1.86 s	16.4
19	1.28 s	24.2	1.28 s	24.1	1.19 s	18.2	1.31 s	22.2	1.26 s	24.8
20	1.37 s	20.3	1.42 s	23.6	1.41 s	21.2	1.41 s	18.8	5.07 s, 5.13 s	113.4
OMe					3.23 s	49.3				

* overlapped.

The relative configuration of **3** was deduced via the coupling constants and NOESY analysis (Figure 3). The coupling constant of H-2 (9.9 Hz) and the vicinal coupling of H-3 (9.9 Hz) identified an α and *cis* orientation for H-2 [7,24,25]. The NOESY experiments exhibited the same configuration of **1** that elucidated the α orientation of H-7 and β and both methyls, Me-19 and Me-20. Based on these spectral observations, **3** was identified as 7β-hydroxy-8α-methoxy-12α-hydroperoxide-16-keto-cembra-1*E*,3*E*,10*E*-triene (sarcoconvolutum C).

Sarcoconvolutum D (**4**) was obtained as dark yellow oil with a positive optical rotation (+37.2, *c* 0.003, CH_3OH). The HREIMS molecular ion peak at m/z 348.1939 $[M]^+$ that predicted a molecular formula of $C_{20}H_{28}O_5$ (calcd. 348.1937, $[M]^+$) with a bicylic skeleton and seven degrees of unsaturation. The corresponding FTIR broad bands to hydroxyls and carbonyl groups at 3456 cm^{-1} and 1763 cm^{-1} were assigned. The ^{1}H NMR (Table 1) revealed two oxygenated protons at δ_H 2.65 dd (J = 6.8, 3.6 Hz), and 5.45 d (J = 9.4 Hz), three olefineic protons at δ_H 5.00 d (J = 9.4 Hz), 5.42 m, and 5.47 m, in addition to four methyls at δ_H 1.31 s, 1.41 s, 1.86 s, and 1.87 s. From ^{13}C NMR, twenty carbon resonances were characterized and categorized to six quartenary (consisting of carbonyl at δ_C 174.8; three olefinics at δ_C 123.6, 144.4, and 161.7; and two oxygenated carbons at δ_C 60.0 and 84.6, five methenes (comprising two oxygenated carbons at δ_C 57.0, and 78.8; and two olefinic carbon (at δ_C 125.8 and 135.5), five methylenes, four methyls based on DEPT-135 and HSQC analysis. The compound is very similar to **1** except for an up-field shift of δ_H 2.65 dd (J = 6.8, 3.6 Hz) by 0.67 ppm and an up-field shift of δ_C 57.0 by 14.6 ppm both associated with C-7 and an up-field shift of δ_C 60 by 14.5 ppm associated with C-8. These chemical shift changes were deduced to be a result of a C-7/C-8 epoxide ring that was consistent with a molecular ion peak at m/z 348.1939 ($C_{20}H_{28}O_5$). The localization of this group was derived via the HMBC correlations of Me-19 (δ_H 1.31 s)/C-7 (J^3), Me-19/C-8 (J^2), H-6 (δ_H 1.60 m)/C-7 (J^2), and H-6/C-8 (J^3) (Figure 2).

The relative stereochemistry was identified via coupling constants [7,24,25] and NOESY analysis (Figure 3). Compound **4** exhibited almost same NOESY correlations as **1** except the correlations of Me-19/H-7, and H-6β/H-7 that elucidated the β orientation of H-7. These data confirmed **4** as 12α-hydroperoxide-16-keto-cembra-1*E*,3*E*,10*E*-triene-7α, 8α-epoxide (sarcoconvolutum D).

Sarcoconvolutum E (**5**) was obtained as yellow oil exhibiting a positive optical rotation (+61.7, *c* 0.003, CH_3OH). The mass spectroscopy exhibited a HREIMS molecular ion peak at m/z 367.2130 $[M + H]^+$ that was identified as $C_{20}H_{30}O_6$ (calcd. 367.2042, $[M + H]^+$) with a bicylic skeleton and six degrees of unsaturation. The FTIR broad bands corresponding to hydroxyls and carbonyl groups were detected at 3464 cm^{-1} and 1759 cm^{-1}. ^{1}H NMR (Table 1) displayed three oxygenated protons at δ_H 3.45 br d (J = 10.5 Hz), 4.43 dd (J = 9.0, 5.0 Hz), and 5.47 d (J = 10.1 Hz), one olefineic proton at δ_H 4.92 br d (J = 10.1 Hz), one exomethylene proton at δ_H 5.07 s, and 5.13 s, and three methyles at δ_H 1.26 s, 1.86 s (6H). The ^{13}C NMR showed twenty carbon resonances. Six quaternary (including carbonyl at δ_C 174.9; four olefinics at δ_C 124.3, 145.9, 146.0 and 161.8; and one oxygenated carbon at δ_C 73.9), four methenes (comprising two oxygenated carbons at δ_C 70.0 and 89.3; and one olefinic carbon (at δ_C 119.2), 7 methylenes (comprising exomethylene carbon at δ_C 113.4), three methyls (δ_C 8.9, 16.4, and 24.8) that were characterized via DEPT-135 and HSQC experiments. NMR spectral data of **5** were similar to **1** and **2** except for the following signals: (i) a down-field shift of δ_C 75.0, by ca. 3.5 ppm associated with C-7; (ii) an downfield shift of δ_H 3.45 brd (J = 10.5 Hz) by 0.2 ppm associated with H-7; and (iii) an up-field shift of δ_H 4.43 dd (J = 9.0, 5.0 Hz) by 1 ppm and a shift of ca. 45 ppm of δ_C 134.0 to 89.0 associated with C-11 indicating the oxygenation of this carbon; (iv) the appearance of δ_H 1.32 (m, 1.57) associated with H-10 and C-10 (at δ_C 25.0) indicating a disappearance of $\Delta^{10(11)}$; and (v) the presence of δ_C 146.0 associated with C-12 and signals δ_H 5.07 s, 5.13 s and δ_C 113.4 associated with an exomethylene carbon at C-20 indicating the presence of $\Delta^{12(20)}$. These new functional group assignments based on spectral data were consistent with 2D HMBC spectral signals including H_3-19 [δ_H 1.26 s]/C-7 [δ_C 75.0, J^3], H_3-19/C-7 [δ_C 73.9, J^2] confirmed the hydroxylation of both C-7 and C-8. The HMBC correlations of H_2-20 [at δ_H 5.07 s, 5.13 s]/C-12 [at δ_C 146.0, J^2], H_2-20/C-11 [at δ_C 89.0, J^3], and H_2-20/C-13 [at δ_C 27.8, J^3], H-11 [at δ_H 4.43 dd (J = 9.0, 5.0 Hz)]/C-12 [J^2], H-11/C-13 [J^3] confirmed the $\Delta^{12(20)}$ and the oxygenation of C-11 (Figure 2). Consistent with the mass spectral data and the observed up-field shift of C-11, the oxygenation of C-11 was identified as a hydroperoxide group.

The relative stereochemistry assignment was based the coupling constant of H-2 (10.1 Hz) and the vicinal coupling of H-3 (10.1 Hz) the indicated a α and *cis* orientation of H-2 [7,24,25]. NOESY correlations (Figure 3) of H-2α [δ_H 5.47 d (J = 10.1 Hz)]/ H_3-18 [δ_H 1.86 s], H-3α [δ_H 4.92 br d (J = 10.1 Hz)]/ H-5α [δ_H 2.35 dt (J = 13.0, 7.6t Hz)], and H-5α/ H-6 [δ_H 1.75 m], H_3-18/ H-6, H-5/ H-7 [δ_H 3.45 br d (J= 10.5 Hz)], H-6/ H-7, H-7/ H_3-19 [δ_H 1.26 s], H_3-19β/ H-9β [δ_H 1.51 m], H-9β/ H-11 [δ_H 4.43 dd (J = 9.0, 5.0 Hz)], H-13β [δ_H 2.25 m]/ H-identified a β orientation for H-7, H-11 and Me-19. Therefore, **5** was assigned as 7α,8α-dihydroxy-11α-hydroperoxide-16-keto-cembra-1E,3E,12(20)-triene (sarcoconvolutum E). 1D, 2D-NMR, HRMS and FTIR for all isolated secondary metabolites (1–5) were deposited in the supplementary files (see Figures S1–S50).

The initial screening of **1–5** (Figure 4) for cytotoxic activity was performed using three cancer cell lines (A549, HeLa and HSC-2) with concentrations of 100, 10 and 1 μM (Figure 4A). Compound **4** showed cytotoxic activity against cell lines A549 (Figure 4B) and HSC-2 (Figure 4C). The dose-dependent toxicity with concentrations range (0.001–100 μg/mL) was examined against A549 and HSC-2 cell lines (Figure 4). Compound **4** showed IC_{50} values of 49.70 and 53.17 μM against A549 and HSC-2 cells, respectively (Table 2, Figure 4A,B).

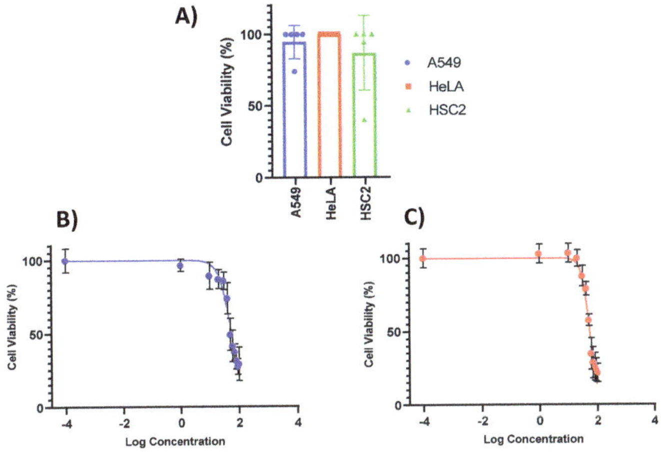

Figure 4. Cytotoxic activity: (**A**) Screening cytotoxic activity against A549, HeLa and HSC2 cell lines; (**B**) Dose-dependent toxicity with concentrations in a range from 0.001 to 100 μM for compounds **4** against A549; (**C**) Dose-dependent toxicity with concentrations in a range from 0.001 to 100 μM for compound 4 against HSC2.

Table 2. Cytotoxicity of 1-5 against cancer cell lines.

Cell Lines	(IC_{50}, μM)					
	1	2	3	4	5	Doxorubicin
A549	>100	>100	>100	49.70 ± 0.05	>100	0.42 ± 0.3
HeLa	>100	>100	>100	91.98 ± 0.15	>100	1.35 ± 0.16
HSC2	>100	>100	>100	53.17 ± 0.03	91.39 ± 0.17	0.50 ± 2.6

3. Materials and Methods

3.1. General Experimental Procedures

A JASCO P-2300 polarimeter (Tokyo, Japan) and shimazu FTIR-8400S instrument (Columbia, MD 21046, USA) was operated for optical rotation and IR spectra, respectively. Then, 1D and 2D NMR spectra were recorded on a Bruker 600 or 500 Hz NMR spectrometer (MA, USA). HR-MS spectra were obtained on a JEOL JMS-700 instrument (Tokyo, Japan). For Chromatography: column chromatography (CC) [silica gel 60 (Merck, 230–400 mesh, Merck, Darmstadt, Germany)]; TLC analysis: [precoated silica gel plates (Merck, Kieselgel 60 F_{254}, 0.25 mm, Merck, Darmstadt, Germany]. High-performance liquid chromatography (HPLC) equipped with a Jasco PU-980 pump, a Jasco UV-970 intelligent UV/VIS detector at 210 nm and a semi preparative reversed-phase column (Cosmosil C_{18} column 250 × 10 mm, 5 μm).

3.2. Coral Material

The animal soft coral *Sarcophyton convolutum* was collected from the Egyptian Red Sea (the coast of Hurghada) in March 2017 and was recognized by M Al-Hammady with a voucher specimen (08RS1071). It was deposited in the National Institute of Oceanography and Fisheries, marine biological station, Hurghada, Egypt.

3.3. Extraction and Separation

The frozen soft coral (2.5 kg, total wet weight) was chopped into small pieces and extracted with ethyl acetate at room temperature (3 L × 5 times). The collective extracts were concentrated *in vacuo* to a brown gum. The dried material (95 g) was subjected to a silica gel column (6 × 120 cm) eluting with *n*-hexane (2000 mL), followed by a gradient of *n*-hexane-EtOAc up to 100% EtOAc and EtOAc –MeOH up to 50% MeOH (3000 mL each of the solvent mixture). Fractions were collected (SC1-SC6) and monitored via TLC. Fraction (SC3; 1.4 g) was eluted step gradient with *n*-hexane-EtOAc over silica gel column afforded three main sub fractions (SC3A-C). Sub-fraction SC3A was re-purified by reversed-phase HPLC using MeOH/H_2O (6.5:3.5), 3.5 mL/min, to afford **1** (6.1 mg, t_R = 27 min), and **4** (11.6 mg, t_R = 23 min). The sub-fraction SC3B was subjected to reversed-phase HPLC using MeOH/H_2O (3:2), 3.5 mL/min, afforded **2** (10 mg, t_R = 28 min). Fraction (SC4; 1.2 g) was further fractionated over silica gel column chromatography eluted by *n*-hexane/EtOAc step gradient afforded two main sub-fractions (SC4A and B). Sub-fraction SC4A was eluted with MeOH/H_2O (1:1) over reversed-phase HPLC, 3 mL/min, to afford **3** (7.3 mg, t_R = 31 min), and **5** (9.6 mg, t_R = 32 min).

3.4. Spectral Data of Sarcoconvolutum A–E (1–5)

7,8-Dihydroxy-12-hydroxy-16-keto-cembra-1E,3E,10E-triene (Sarcoconvolutum A, **1**): yellow oil; $[\alpha]_D^{25}$ +43.0 (c 0.03, CH_3OH); FT-IR (KBr) ν_{max}: 3465, 2961, 1765, 1435, and 987 cm^{-1}; ^1H and ^{13}C NMR data ($CDCl_3$, 500 Hz), see Table 1; HRCIMS *m/z* 367.2122 (100, $[M+H]^+$); (calcd. 367.2121, for $C_{20}H_{31}O_6$).

7,8-Dihydroxy-12-hydroxy-16-keto-cembra-1E,3E,10E-triene (Sarcoconvolutum B, **2**): yellow oil; $[\alpha]_D^{25}$ +10.5 (c 0.03, CH_3OH); FT-IR (KBr) ν_{max}: 3461, 2957, 1759, 1439, and 991 cm^{-1}; ^1H and ^{13}C NMR data ($CDCl_3$, 500 Hz), see Table 1; HRCIMS *m/z* 367.2122 (100, $[M+H]^+$); (calcd. 367.2122, for $C_{20}H_{31}O_6$).

7β-Hydroxy-8α-methoxy-12α-hydroperoxide-16-keto-cembra-1E,3E,10E-triene (sarcoconvolutum C, **3**): yellow oil; $[\alpha]_D^{25}$ +37.2 (c 0.03, CH_3OH); FT-IR (KBr) ν_{max}: 3456, 2951, 1763, 1446, and 993 cm^{-1}; ^1H and ^{13}C NMR data ($CDCl_3$, 500 Hz), see Table 1; HRCIMS *m/z* 364.2258, $[M-OH+H]^+$]; (calcd. 364.2250, $[M-OH+H]^+$, for $C_{21}H_{32}O_6$).

12α-Hydroperoxide-16-keto-cembra-1E,3E,10E-triene-7α,8α-epoxide (sarcoconvolutum D, **4**): yellow oil; $[\alpha]_D^{25}$ +37.2 (c 0.03, CH_3OH); FT-IR (KBr) ν_{max}: 3456, 2958, 1763, 1442, and 996 cm^{-1}; ^1H and ^{13}C NMR data ($CDCl_3$, 500 Hz), see Table 1; HREIMS *m/z* 348.1939 $[M]^+$; (calcd. 348.1937, for $C_{20}H_{28}O_5$).

7α,8α-Dihydroxy-11α-hydroperoxide-16-keto-cembra-1E,3E,12(20)-triene (sarcoconvolutum E, **5**): yellow oil; $[\alpha]_D^{25}$ +10.5 +61.7 (c 0.03, CH_3OH); FT-IR (KBr) ν_{max}: 3464, 2955, 1759, 1433, and 997 cm^{-1}; ^1H and ^{13}C NMR data ($CDCl_3$, 500 Hz), see Table 1; HREIMS *m/z* 367.2130 (100, $[M+H]^+$); (calcd. 367.2042, for $C_{20}H_{31}O_6$).

3.5. Cell Culture and Treatment Conditions

Human cancer cell lines of non-small cell lung adenocarcinoma (A549), squamous cell carcinoma of the oral cavity (HSC-2), and human cervical cancer cell (HeLa). All cell lines were purchased from American Type Culture Collection (ATCC®) and were maintained as monolayer culture in Dulbecco's modified Eagle's medium (DMEM) supplemented with 10% FBS, 4 mM l-glutamine, 100 U/mL penicillin, and 100 μg/mL streptomycin sulfate. Monolayers were passaged at 70–90% confluence using a trypsin-EDTA solution. All cell incubations were maintained in a humidified CO_2 incubator with 5% CO_2 at 37 °C. All materials and reagents for the cell cultures were purchased from Lonza (Verviers, Belgium).

3.6. Cytotoxicity Assay

A modified MTT (3-[4,5,[4,5-dimethylthiazole-2-yl]-2,5-diphenyltetrazolium bromide) assay was used for cytotoxicity investigation were performed using based on a previously published method [26]. A549, HeLa and HSC2 cells (5000–10,000 cells/well) were seeded onto 96-well plates and incubated for 24 h with 5% CO_2 at 37 °C. The prepared tested compounds (**1–5**) were screened and the dose-dependent toxicity with concentrations range (0.001–100 μg/mL) were investigated according to our protocol [26]. Doxorubicin (2 mg/mL) was used as positive control.

3.7. Anti-Proliferation Quantitative Analysis

GraphPad Prism® v6.0 software (GraphPad Software Inc., San Diego, CA, USA) were used to calculate the concentration-response curve fit to the non-linear regression for IC_{50} values.

4. Conclusions

Five compounds, sarcoconvolutum A–E were isolated from an organic extract of *Sarcophyton convolutum* tissue. Chemical structures were elucidated based upon spectroscopic analyses. The cytotoxic activity of the isolated compounds was screened against three cancer cell lines (A549, HeLa and HSC2) and **4** was found to be the most active compound against cell lines A549 and HSC-2 with IC_{50} values of 49.70 and 53.17 μM, respectively.

Supplementary Materials: The following are available online https://www.mdpi.com/article/10.3390/md19090519/s1, Figures S1–S50: spectra for compounds **1–5**.

Author Contributions: Conceptualization, T.A.M., A.I.E., P.W.P. and M.-E.F.H.; Data curation, T.A.M., A.I.E., A.M.A.-T. and M.-E.F.H.; Formal analysis, T.A.M., A.I.E., M.M.A., P.W.P. and S.O.; Investigation, T.A.M., A.I.E. and A.M.A.-T. Methodology, M.-E.F.H.; Project administration, T.A.M. and M.-E.F.H.; Resources, T.A.M., A.I.E., A.M.A.-T. and M.-E.F.H.; Software, T.A.M. and M.-E.F.H.; Supervision, M.-E.F.H.; Visualization, T.A.M. and M.-E.F.H.; Writing—original draft, A.I.E. and M.M.A.; Writing—review and editing, T.A.M., A.I.E., A.M.A.-T., M.M.A., S.O., P.W.P. and M.-E.F.H. All authors have read and agreed to the published version of the manuscript.

Funding: This research was funded by National Research Centre, Giza, Egypt under the project title "Secondary metabolites from Egyptian Soft corals: Chemical and biological investigation against cancer cells" grant number 12060120/2019-2022.

Institutional Review Board Statement: Not applicable.

Informed Consent Statement: Not applicable.

Data Availability Statement: The data presented in this study are available in Supplementary Material.

Conflicts of Interest: The authors declare no conflict of interest.

References

1. Ahmed, A.A.; Hegazy, M.-E.F.; Hassan, N.M.; Wojcinska, M.; Karchesy, J.; Pare, P.W.; Mabry, T.J. Constituents of Chrysothamnus viscidiflorus. *Phytochemistry* **2006**, *67*, 1547–1553. [CrossRef]
2. Hegazy, M.E.F.; Mohamed, T.A.; Alhammady, M.A.; Shaheen, A.M.; Reda, E.H.; Elshamy, A.I.; Aziz, M.; Paré, P.W. Molecular architecture and biomedical leads of terpenes from red sea marine invertebrates. *Mar. Drugs* **2015**, *13*, 3154–3181. [CrossRef] [PubMed]
3. Khalifa, S.A.M.; Elias, N.; Farag, M.A.; Chen, L.; Saeed, A.; Hegazy, M.-E.F.; Moustafa, M.S.; El-Wahed, A.; Al-Mousawi, S.M.; Musharraf, S.G. Marine natural products: A source of novel anticancer drugs. *Mar. Drugs* **2019**, *17*, 491. [CrossRef] [PubMed]
4. Nweze, J.A.; Mbaoji, F.N.; Li, Y.-M.; Yang, L.-Y.; Huang, S.-S.; Chigor, V.N.; Eze, E.A.; Pan, L.-X.; Zhang, T.; Yang, D.-F. Potentials of marine natural products against malaria, leishmaniasis, and trypanosomiasis parasites: A review of recent articles. *Infect. Dis. Poverty* **2021**, *10*, 1–19. [CrossRef]
5. Hegazy, M.-E.F.; Mohamed, T.A.; Abdel-Latif, F.F.; Alsaid, M.S.; Shahat, A.A.; Pare, P.W. Trochelioid A and B, new cembranoid diterpenes from the Red Sea soft coral Sarcophyton trocheliophorum. *Phytochem. Lett.* **2013**, *6*, 383–386. [CrossRef]
6. Hegazy, M.-E.F.; Elshamy, A.I.; Mohamed, T.A.; Hamed, A.R.; Ibrahim, M.A.A.; Ohta, S.; Paré, P.W. Cembrene diterpenoids with ether linkages from Sarcophyton ehrenbergi: An anti-proliferation and molecular-docking assessment. *Mar. Drugs* **2017**, *15*, 192. [CrossRef]
7. Hegazy, M.-E.F.; Mohamed, T.A.; Elshamy, A.I.; Hamed, A.R.; Ibrahim, M.A.A.; Ohta, S.; Umeyama, A.; Paré, P.W.; Efferth, T. Sarcoehrenbergilides D–F: Cytotoxic cembrene diterpenoids from the soft coral Sarcophyton ehrenbergi. *RSC Adv.* **2019**, *9*, 27183–27189. [CrossRef]
8. Lin, W.-Y.; Su, J.-H.; Lu, Y.; Wen, Z.-H.; Dai, C.-F.; Kuo, Y.-H.; Sheu, J.-H. Cytotoxic and anti-inflammatory cembranoids from the Dongsha Atoll soft coral Sarcophyton crassocaule. *Bioorg. Med. Chem.* **2010**, *18*, 1936–1941. [CrossRef] [PubMed]
9. Liu, X.; Zhang, J.; Liu, Q.; Tang, G.; Wang, H.; Fan, C.; Yin, S. Bioactive cembranoids from the South China Sea soft coral Sarcophyton elegans. *Molecules* **2015**, *20*, 13324–13335. [CrossRef]

10. Jia, R.; Guo, Y.-W.; Chen, P.; Yang, Y.-M.; Mollo, E.; Gavagnin, M.; Cimino, G. Biscembranoids and their probable biogenetic precursor from the Hainan soft coral Sarcophyton tortuosum. *J. Nat. Prod.* **2007**, *70*, 1158–1166. [CrossRef]
11. Liang, L.F.; Guo, Y.W. Terpenes from the soft corals of the genus Sarcophyton: Chemistry and biological activities. *Chem. Biodivers.* **2013**, *10*, 2161–2196. [CrossRef] [PubMed]
12. Yasumoto, M.; Mada, K.; Ooi, T.; Kusumi, T. New terpenoid components from the volatile oils of the soft corals Clavularia viridis and Sarcophyton acutangulum. *J. Nat. Prod.* **2000**, *63*, 1534–1536. [CrossRef]
13. Anjaneyulu, A.S.R.; Rao, V.L.; Sastry, V.G.; Rao, D.V. Trocheliophorin: A novel rearranged sesquiterpenoid from the Indian Ocean soft coral Sarcophyton trocheliophorum. *J. Asian Nat. Prod. Res.* **2008**, *10*, 597–601. [CrossRef] [PubMed]
14. Cheng, S.-Y.; Wen, Z.-H.; Chiou, S.-F.; Tsai, C.-W.; Wang, S.-K.; Hsu, C.-H.; Dai, C.-F.; Chiang, M.Y.; Wang, W.-H.; Duh, C.-Y. Ceramide and cerebrosides from the octocoral Sarcophyton ehrenbergi. *J. Nat. Prod.* **2009**, *72*, 465–468. [CrossRef]
15. Anjaneyulu, A.S.R.; Krishna Murthy, M.V.R.; Gowri, P.M. Novel epoxy steroids from the Indian ocean soft coral Sarcophyton crassocaule. *J. Nat. Prod.* **2000**, *63*, 112–118. [CrossRef]
16. Wang, Z.; Tang, H.; Wang, P.; Gong, W.; Xue, M.; Zhang, H.; Liu, T.; Liu, B.; Yi, Y.; Zhang, W. Bioactive polyoxygenated steroids from the South China sea soft coral, Sarcophyton sp. *Mar. Drugs* **2013**, *11*, 775–787. [CrossRef]
17. Cheng, Z.-B.; Deng, Y.-L.; Fan, C.-Q.; Han, Q.-H.; Lin, S.-L.; Tang, G.-H.; Luo, H.-B.; Yin, S. Prostaglandin derivatives: Nonaromatic phosphodiesterase-4 inhibitors from the soft coral Sarcophyton ehrenbergi. *J. Nat. Prod.* **2014**, *77*, 1928–1936. [CrossRef]
18. Sekhar, V.C.; Rao, C.B.; Ramana, H.; Kuwar, M.M.K.; Rao, D.V. New Prostaglandins from the soft coral Sarcophyton ehrenbergi marengeller of Andaman and Nicobar Islands of Indian ocean. *Asian J. Chem.* **2010**, *22*, 5353–5358.
19. Li, Y.-X.; Wu, H.-X.; Xu, Y.; Shao, C.-L.; Wang, C.-Y.; Qian, P.-Y. Antifouling activity of secondary metabolites isolated from Chinese marine organisms. *Mar. Biotechnol.* **2013**, *15*, 552–558. [CrossRef]
20. Sun, X.-P.; Wang, C.-Y.; Shao, C.-L.; Li, L.; Li, X.-B.; Chen, M.; Qian, P.-Y. Chemical constituents of the soft coral Sarcophyton infundibuliforme from the South China Sea. *Nat. Prod. Commun.* **2010**, *5*, 1171–1174. [CrossRef]
21. Iwagawa, T.; Nakamura, S.; Masuda, T.; Okamura, H.; Nakatani, M.; Siro, M. Irregular cembranoids containing a 13-membered carbocyclic skeleton isolated from a soft coral, Sarcophyton species. *Tetrahedron* **1995**, *51*, 5291–5298. [CrossRef]
22. Badria, F.A.; Guirguis, A.N.; El-Naggar, W.A. Antibacterial and antifungal agents from Egyptian marine organisms. *Int. J. Pharmacogn.* **1997**, *35*, 284–287. [CrossRef]
23. Badria, F.A.; Guirguis, A.N.; Perovic, S.; Steffen, R.; Müller, W.E.G.; Schröder, H.C. Sarcophytolide: A new neuroprotective compound from the soft coral Sarcophyton glaucum. *Toxicology* **1998**, *131*, 133–143. [CrossRef]
24. Hegazy, M.-E.F.; Eldeen, A.M.G.; Shahat, A.A.; Abdel-Latif, F.F.; Mohamed, T.A.; Whittlesey, B.R.; Paré, P.W. Bioactive hydroperoxyl cembranoids from the Red Sea soft coral Sarcophyton glaucum. *Mar. Drugs* **2012**, *10*, 209–222. [CrossRef] [PubMed]
25. Elkhateeb, A.; El-Beih, A.A.; Gamal-Eldeen, A.M.; Alhammady, M.A.; Ohta, S.; Paré, P.W.; Hegazy, M.-E.F. New terpenes from the Egyptian soft coral Sarcophyton ehrenbergi. *Mar. Drugs* **2014**, *12*, 1977–1986. [CrossRef] [PubMed]
26. Swapana, N.; Tominaga, T.; Elshamy, A.I.; Ibrahim, M.A.A.; Hegazy, M.-E.F.; Singh, C.B.; Suenaga, M.; Imagawa, H.; Noji, M.; Umeyama, A. Kaemgalangol A: Unusual seco-isopimarane diterpenoid from aromatic ginger Kaempferia galanga. *Fitoterapia* **2018**, *129*, 47–53. [CrossRef] [PubMed]

marine drugs

MDPI

Article

Synthesis and Cytotoxicity Evaluation of Spirocyclic Bromotyrosine Clavatadine C Analogs

Piyush A. Patel [1], Tanja Bruun [1], Polina Ilina [2], Heidi Mäkkylä [2], Antti Lempinen [1], Jari Yli-Kauhaluoma [1], Päivi Tammela [2] and Paula S. Kiuru [1,*]

1 Drug Research Program, Division of Pharmaceutical Chemistry and Technology, Faculty of Pharmacy, University of Helsinki, FI-00014 Helsinki, Finland; piyushkumar.patel@helsinki.fi (P.A.P.); tanja.bruun@helsinki.fi (T.B.); antti.lempinen@helsinki.fi (A.L.); jari.yli-kauhaluoma@helsinki.fi (J.Y.-K.)

2 Drug Research Program, Division of Pharmaceutical Biosciences, Faculty of Pharmacy, University of Helsinki, FI-00014 Helsinki, Finland; polina.ilina@helsinki.fi (P.I.); heidi.makkyla@helsinki.fi (H.M.); paivi.tammela@helsinki.fi (P.T.)

* Correspondence: paula.kiuru@helsinki.fi

Abstract: Marine-originated spirocyclic bromotyrosines are considered as promising scaffolds for new anticancer drugs. In a continuation of our research to develop potent and more selective anticancer compounds, we synthesized a library of 32 spirocyclic clavatadine analogs by replacing the agmatine, i.e., 4-(aminobutyl)guanidine, side chain with different substituents. These compounds were tested for cytotoxicity against skin cancer using the human melanoma cell line (A-375) and normal human skin fibroblast cell line (Hs27). The highest cytotoxicity against the A-375 cell line was observed for dichloro compound **18** (CC_{50} 0.4 ± 0.3 μM, selectivity index (SI) 2). The variation of selectivity ranged from SI 0.4 to reach 2.4 for the pyridin-2-yl derivative **29** and hydrazide analog of 2-picoline **37**. The structure–activity relationships of the compounds in respect to cytotoxicity and selectivity toward cancer cell lines are discussed.

Keywords: Clavatadine C; spirocyclic bromotyrosines; cytotoxicity; cancer selectivity; marine compounds; melanoma A-375 cell line

Citation: Patel, P.A.; Bruun, T.; Ilina, P.; Mäkkylä, H.; Lempinen, A.; Yli-Kauhaluoma, J.; Tammela, P.; Kiuru, P.S. Synthesis and Cytotoxicity Evaluation of Spirocyclic Bromotyrosine Clavatadine C Analogs. *Mar. Drugs* **2021**, *19*, 400. https://doi.org/10.3390/md19070400

Academic Editor: Orazio Taglialatela-Scafati

Received: 8 February 2021
Accepted: 14 June 2021
Published: 20 July 2021

Publisher's Note: MDPI stays neutral with regard to jurisdictional claims in published maps and institutional affiliations.

Copyright: © 2021 by the authors. Licensee MDPI, Basel, Switzerland. This article is an open access article distributed under the terms and conditions of the Creative Commons Attribution (CC BY) license (https://creativecommons.org/licenses/by/4.0/).

1. Introduction

Natural products have a long history of use in the treatment of various diseases, including cancer [1]. Marine organisms are a rich source of novel compounds with medicinally relevant properties. Many marine-derived bioactive terpenes, alkaloids, macrolides, and other compounds isolated from aquatic fungi, cyanobacteria, algae, sponges, and tunicates have been found to exhibit anticancer activities [2,3]. To date, 15 drugs with marine origins have been approved by the U.S. Food and Drug Administration and/or European Medicines Agency. Nine of these drugs are registered for the treatment of different cancer types [4,5]. At present, 33 marine-based compounds are in clinical trials, out of which 29 are being evaluated for cancer therapy. Bromotyrosine alkaloids have acquired special importance in medicinal chemistry since the vast majority of these secondary metabolites possess potential anticancer [6], antimicrobial, antiviral, and antifungal activities [7,8]. Quinn and co-workers identified two new spirocyclic bromotyrosine compounds, clavatadine C **1** and clavatadine D **2** (Figure 1). Both were isolated as trifluoroacetic acid (TFA) salts from the marine sponge *Suberea clavata* and their anticoagulative properties were described. [9]. Furthermore, moderate activity against MCF7, MDA-MB-231 (breast), and A549 (lung) cancer cell lines have been observed for clavatadine C **1-TFA** [10]. Marine bromotyrosines with an isoxazoline moiety attached to the spiro center have exhibited anticancer properties [11,12]. The spirocyclic bromotyrosine is structurally more rigid and better occupies the chemical space than the open-chain bromotyrosine, making it an interesting scaffold for medicinal chemistry [13]. We have previously reported a set of simplified open-chain bromotyrosine analogs of purpurealidin I **3** (Figure 1) with potential antiproliferative activity [14]. As purpurealidin analogs are *E*-isomers having free rotation around the C-C σ bond, introduction of conformational restriction in the form of a spiro ring fusion offers a good strategy to improve selectivity toward the target cell of interest [15].

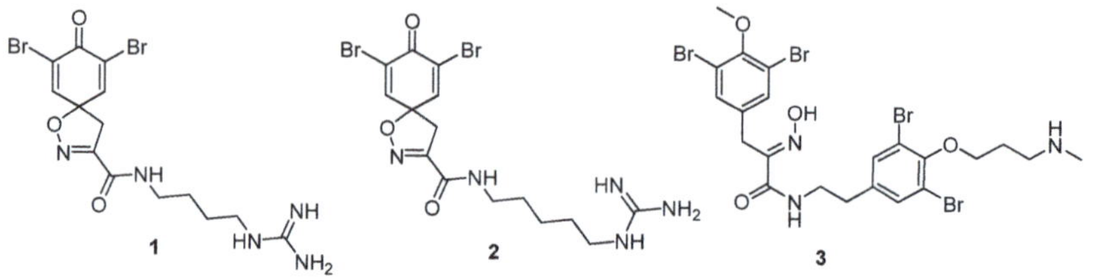

Figure 1. Clavatadine C **1**, D **2**, and purpurealidin I **3**.

Cytotoxicity toward normal cells is a major challenge with anticancer compounds. Therefore, different approaches are required to develop a target-specific anticancer treatment. The structural simplification of natural products is one of the well-known strategies to improve pharmacokinetic profiles and to reduce side effects [16]. Initially, anticancer activity of the first simplified spiroisoxazolines **4** and **5** (Figure 2) was reported in Ehrlich ascites tumor cells in mice [17,18].

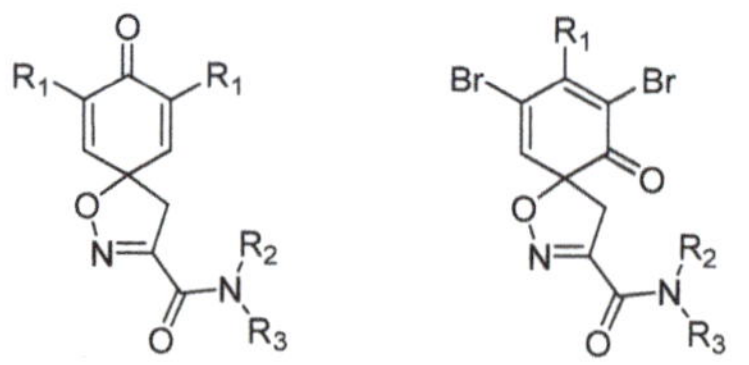

4

R_1 = H, OMe
R_2 = H, Me
R_3 = Me, Ph, aralkyl

5

R_1 = H, OMe
R_2 = H, Me
R_3 = H, Me, Ph

Figure 2. Simplified spiroisoxazoline analogs **4** [17] and **5** [18].

In order to understand the structure–activity relationships (SARs) of spirocyclic bromotyrosines as cytotoxic agents toward cancer cells, we synthesized a library of simplified spirocyclic clavatadine analogs **11–42** (Table 1). The agmatine, i.e., 4-(aminobutyl)guanidine, side chain was replaced with different amino and hydrazide substituents. These analogs were tested against a melanoma cell line (A-375) and normal human skin fibroblast cell line (Hs27) for cytotoxicity. The clavatadine scaffold was selected for the library synthesis to limit the free C-C rotation of purpurealidin analogs, to have a stereochemically simpler spiro core than the one in other spirocyclic bromotyrosines, and to build on the proven anticancer activity of simplified clavatadine analogs, such as compound **4**.

The compounds were synthesized according to the route presented in Scheme 1. Synthetic procedures and analytical data of the compounds are given in the Supporting Information.

Table 1. Structures of the target spirocyclic bromotyrosine analogs **1-TFA** and **11–42**.

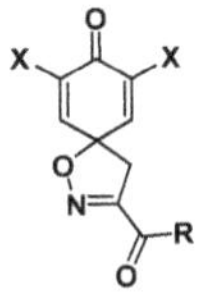

No	X	-R	No	X	-R	No	X	-R	No	X	-R
1-TFA	Br	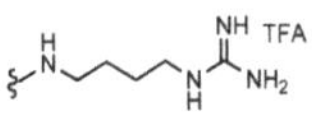	**19**	Br	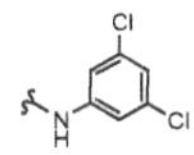	**28**	H	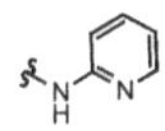	**37**	H	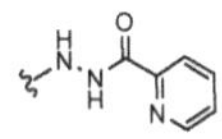
11	H	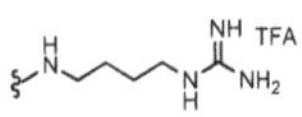	**20**	H	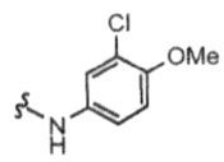	**29**	Br	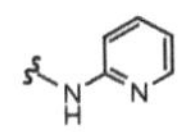	**38**	Br	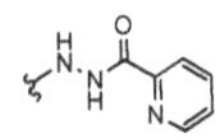
12	H	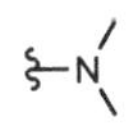	**21**	Br	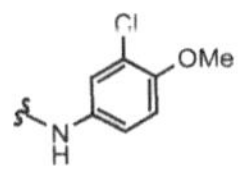	**30**	Br	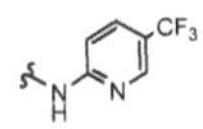	**39**	Br	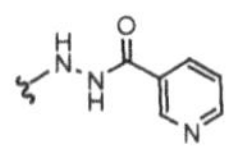
13	Br	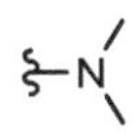	**22**	H	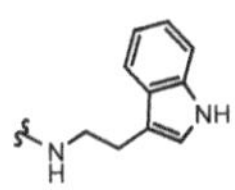	**31**	Br	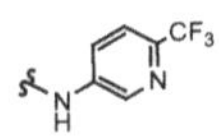	**40**	H	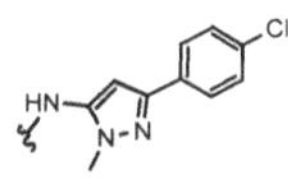
14	Br	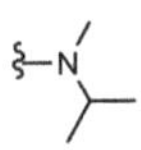	**23**	H	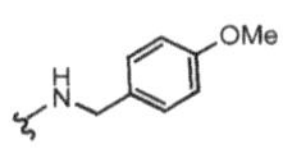	**32**	H	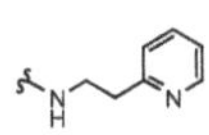	**41**	Br	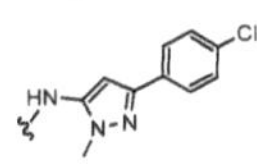
15	H	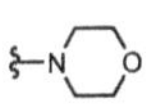	**24**	Br	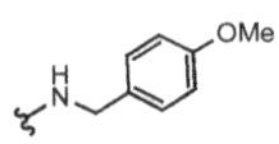	**33**	Br	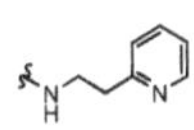	**42**	Br	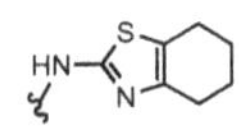
16	H	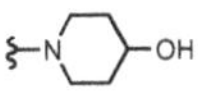	**25**	H	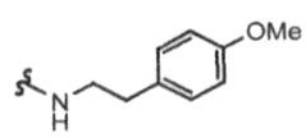	**34**	Br	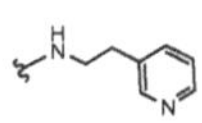			
17	H	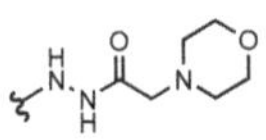	**26**	H	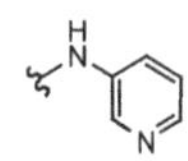	**35**	H	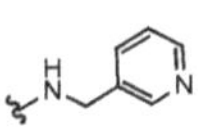			
18	H	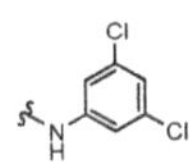	**27**	Br	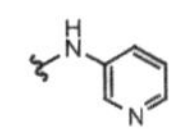	**36**	Br	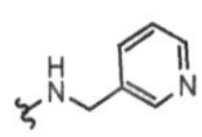			

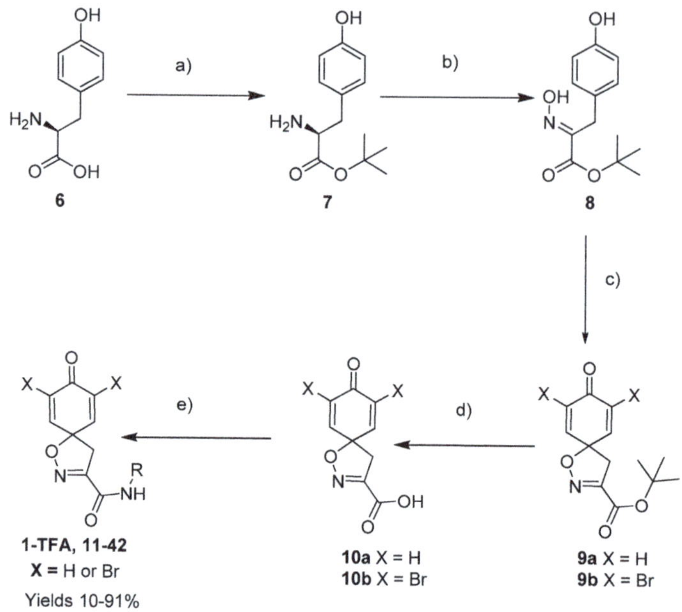

Scheme 1. General scheme for synthesis of spirocyclic bromotyrosines **1-TFA** and **11–42**. Reagents and conditions: a) $HClO_4$, *tert*-butyl acetate, 20–25 °C, 18 h; b) $Na_2WO_4{\cdot}2H_2O$, H_2O_2, EtOH, 20–25 °C, 7 h; c) PIFA, pyridine, TFE, 0 °C, 1 h, or NBS, DMF, 0 °C, 20 min; d) TFA, DCM, 20–25 °C, 6 h; e) amine, EDC·HCl, HOBt, DCM, 20–25 °C, 5–15 h. The R substituents are given in Table 1.

2. Results

2.1. Chemistry

The synthesis of the spirocyclic bromotyrosine scaffold started with esterification of L-tyrosine **6** using *tert*-butyl acetate in the presence of perchloric acid to give L-tyrosine *tert*-butyl ester **7**. The ester **7** was oxidized with sodium tungstate and H_2O_2 to give the oxime **8** [10]. This resulting oxime was subjected to oxidative spirocyclization via treatment with [bis(trifluoro-acetoxy)iodo]benzene (PIFA) in 2,2,2-trifluoroethanol (TFE) in the case of non-halogenated compounds or *N*-bromosuccinimide (NBS) in *N*,*N*-dimethylformamide (DMF) in the case of brominated compounds to provide spirocyclic esters **9a/9b**. The *tert*-butyl esters **9a/9b** were deprotected with trifluoroacetic acid in dichloromethane (DCM) to give the spirocyclic carboxyl core **10a/10b**. This spirocyclic core was coupled with various amines or hydrazides in the presence of 1-ethyl-3-(3-dimethylaminopropyl)carbodiimide hydrochloride (EDC·HCl) and 1-hydroxybenzotriazole hydrate (HOBt·H_2O) to give the target spirocyclic bromotyrosine analogs **1-TFA** and **11–42** (Table 1) with yields ranging 10–91%. We observed that the yields were typically higher in the case of dihydro carboxyl core **10a** compared to the dibromo core **10b**, and heterocyclic and aromatic amines compared to aliphatic amines and hydrazines.

2.2. Biological Activity

The cytotoxicities of the synthetic clavatadine C **1-TFA**, dihydroclavatadine C **11**, and compounds **12–42** against cancer cells were primarily evaluated in the human malignant melanoma A-375 cell line at the single concentration of 50 μM (Table 2). The compounds demonstrating over 80% cytotoxicity were selected for confirmatory dose-response experiments in the same cell line and CC_{50} (cytotoxic concentration that caused death of 50% of cells) was calculated (Table 2). The observed cytotoxicity (CC_{50}) against the A-375 melanoma cell line for the compounds **1-TFA** and **11–42** was in the range of 0.4–12.3 μM (Table 2). Furthermore, we aimed to evaluate the potential of the compounds to selectively perturb the growth of skin cancer cells. Therefore, the compounds were tested for cytotoxicity in normal human fibroblast cell line Hs27 (Table 2).

Table 2. Cytotoxicity of compounds **1-TFA** and **11–42** against human malignant melanoma cell line A-375 and normal human fibroblast Hs27 cells. Camptothecin, a compound with high selectivity to cancer cells, was used as a positive control. Purpurealidin I **3** was used as a reference compound [14]. CC_{50} = cytotoxic concentration that caused death of 50% of cells. ND = not determined. The primary screening was performed as a single experiment with three technical replicates per sample. The CC_{50} values are arithmetic means from 2–3 independent experiments performed in triplicate. The values in parentheses are standard deviations.

Compound	Primary Test Results (Cytotoxicity % at 50 μM in A-375 Cells)	CC_{50} (μM) in A-375 Cells	CC_{50} (μM) in Hs27 Cells	Selectivity Index (SI)
1-TFA	0.5	ND	ND	ND
11	−8.2	ND	ND	ND
12	95.1	2.1 (1.2)	3.8 (0.7)	1.8 (0.6)
13	99.8	3.7 (1.9)	7.2 (6.2)	1.9 (1.0)
14	99.9	7.2 (3.2)	7.8 (1.8)	1.1 (0.5)
15	96.1	3.8 (0.7)	2.5 (0.3)	0.7 (0.2)
16	97.1	4.9 (1.0)	7.4 (0.5)	1.5 (0.2)
17	20.8	ND	ND	ND
18	100.0	0.4 (0.3)	0.8 (0.2)	2.0 (0.8)
19	94.9	9.2 (2.9)	6.8 (2.8)	0.7 (0.5)
20	100.0	1.2 (0.1)	1.5 (0.7)	1.3 (0.5)
21	101.1	2.3 (0.4)	5.0 (1.1)	2.2 (0.3)
22	99.8	0.7 (0.1)	0.7 (0.2)	1.0 (0.3)
23	100.0	1.2 (0.2)	1.4 (0.8)	1.2 (0.6)
24	97.8	3.5 (1.1)	3.3 (1.1)	0.9 (0.3)
25	100.0	1.2 (0.1)	2.0 (0.6)	1.7 (0.3)
26	99.2	2.0 (1.2)	1.9 (0.9)	1.0 (0.8)
27	100.7	3.0 (0.3)	6.6 (3.1)	2.2 (0.5)
28	99.6	1.9 (0.2)	1.5 (0.6)	0.8 (0.4)
29	100.6	2.4 (0.3)	5.8 (2.5)	2.4 (0.4)
30	98.1	3.6 (0.1)	2.3 (0.4)	0.6 (0.2)
31	98.6	5.3 (0.7)	2.1 (0.1)	0.4 (0.1)
32	97.5	1.5 (1.0)	2.2 (1.3)	1.5 (0.9)
33	98.9	3.6 (1.9)	6.6 (1.3)	1.9 (0.6)
34	97.0	5.1 (2.8)	8.8 (1.8)	1.7 (0.6)
35	97.5	1.1 (0.1)	2.5 (0.2)	2.3 (0.1)
36	100.7	3.4 (0.2)	6.1 (0.9)	1.8 (0.2)
37	89.3	2.5 (0.6)	6.0 (1.3)	2.4 (0.3)
38	93.5	12.3 (1.3)	6.4 (3.0)	0.5 (0.5)
39	75.2	ND	ND	ND
40	99.9	0.5 (0.1)	0.5 (0.4)	1.0 (0.8)
41	97.6	1.3 (0.4)	1.4 (1.0)	1.1 (0.8)
42	97.5	3.5 (1.2)	4.4 (1.4)	1.3 (0.5)
Purpurealidin I **3**	98.9	3.7 (0.5)	4.7 (0.2)	1.3 (0.1)
Camptothecin	94.7	0.05 (0.02)	3.6 (1.0)	70.9 (0.5)

The degree of selectivity toward cancer cells can be expressed by the selectivity index (SI). The SI was calculated as a ratio of CC_{50} values between Hs27 fibroblasts and A-375 melanoma cells. High SI values show selectivity toward cancer cells, while values <2 show low selectivity [19] (Table 2). The highest but still moderate selectivity to cancer cells (SI 2.4, Table 2) was observed for the pyridin-2-yl compound **29** and hydrazide analog of 2-picoline **37**. To further elucidate mechanisms of cytotoxicity mediated by these compounds, we tested their ability to induce apoptosis. Apoptosis, or programmed cell death, is a mechanism utilized in the body for elimination of unwanted or damaged cells during development and aging. In cancer cells, apoptosis is typically inhibited and most selective anticancer agents act via induction of this pathway [20]. To elucidate potential effects of spirocyclic bromotyrosines on apoptosis, we tested their ability to induce the activity of caspases 3/7, a key protease involved in the apoptotic pathway. The results show that spirocyclic bromotyrosines induced the caspase pathway about twofold after 24 h, whereas no induction was observed after 48 h (Figure 3A). Treatment with a positive control camptothecin resulted in about a 20-fold caspase induction after 24 h of treatment and a nearly fivefold induction after 48 h of treatment. The data obtained correlated with microscopic observations. Cell rounding up and shrinkage, typical for apoptosis, was observed for both camptothecin-treated cells and the cells treated with spirocyclic bromotyrosines. However, for camptothecin the effect was more profound (Figure 3B–E).

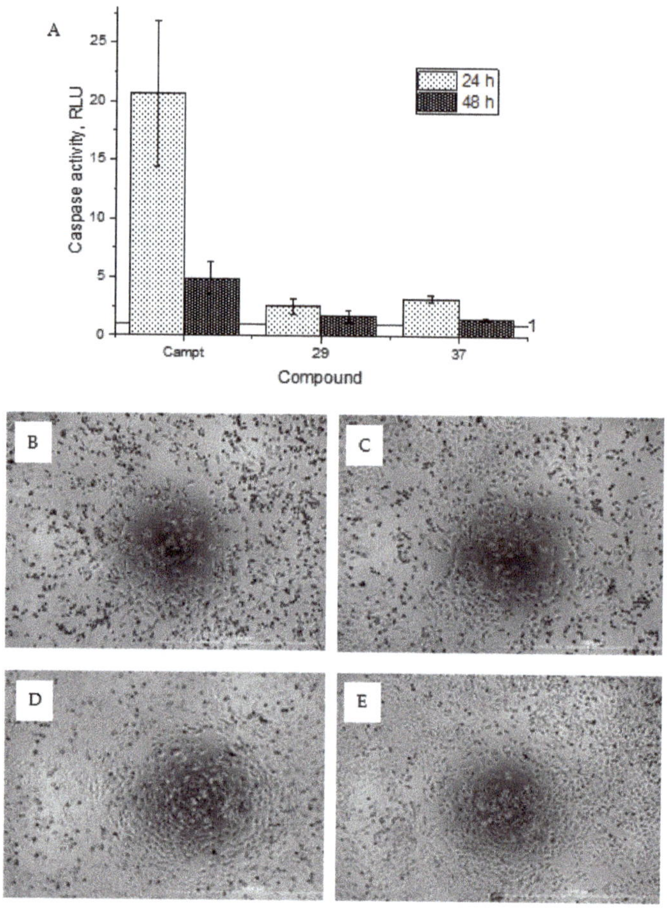

Figure 3. Induction of apoptosis in A-375 melanoma cells by compounds **29** and **37**, which demonstrated the highest selectivity, and positive control camptothecin. Cells were treated with compounds at 1 × CC_{50} concentration for 24 and 48 h. (**A**) Activity of caspase 3/7 apoptotic pathway shown as a fold change relative to DMSO-treated control, indicated with a horizontal line. Bars show mean values of two independent experiments (each performed in triplicate wells) ± SD. Representative microscopic images taken after a 24-h incubation with camptothecin (**B**), compound **29** (**C**), and **37** (**D**) show morphological changes characteristic for apoptosis; (**E**) shows cell morphology in DMSO-treated control wells. RLU = relative light units.

3. Discussion

To understand the preliminary cytotoxicity of clavatadine C **1** analogs comprised of dibromo and dihydro spirocyclic cores, we synthesized clavatadine C **1-TFA** (overall yield 38%) along with various amides **11–42** having aliphatic, aromatic, and heterocyclic substitution with or without a carbon spacer. We then evaluated their effect on cytotoxicity of the melanoma cell line A-375 and the normal skin fibroblast cell line Hs27. Though the clavatadine C **1-TFA** and its dihydro analog **11** did not show any primary cytotoxicity, its analogs showed cytotoxicity, as shown in Table 2. Clavatadine C **1-TFA,** dihydroclavatadine C **11** and aliphatic morpholinoacetyl carbohydrazide **17** showed less than 25% primary cytotoxicity (at 50 μM in A-375 cells) while the rest of the compounds had over 75% primary cytotoxicity. This result was somewhat unexpected when compared to the known activity of clavatadine C **1-TFA** against breast and colon cancer cell lines [10]. Binnewerg et al. recently found spiro-structured isofistularin-3 to display cell line dependent effects, and the three melanoma cell lines tested (SKMel-147, Mel-Juso, and Malme-3M) showed no significant decrease (and even increased in the case of SKMel-147) in cell viability, but on the contrary isofistularin-3 reduced cell viability of breast cancer cell line MCF-7 [21]. The highest cytotoxicity against the A-375 cell line was observed in dihydro 2,4-dichloro compound **18** (CC_{50} 0.4 $\pm$ 0.3 μM, with moderate SI 2). The selectivity indices of the most simplified dimethyl amides **13** and **14** were 1.8 and 1.9, respectively, and amides **14–16** containing aliphatic substituents showed low SI. While the introduction of aromatic substituent in **18–30** with or without a spacer exhibited relatively similar cytotoxicity, the 3-chloro-4-methoxyphenyl analog **21** showed a slight improvement in the selectivity index. As seen in our open chain library [14], the introduction of pyridinyl substituent **26–29** at the amide showed improvement in SI value to 2.4 in the case of pyridin-2-yl analog **29**, whereas the introduction of the pharmacologically important trifluoromethyl group [22] to pyridine in **30** and **31** lowered the selectivity. We also introduced ethylene and methylene groups as spacers in **32–36** along with hydrazide spacers in **37–39** to pyridine to evaluate their effect on selectivity and cytotoxicity. Cytotoxicity and selectivity were increased in analogs **32–36** having a spacer compared to the analogs **14–17** having aliphatic substituents. In the case of the dihydro pyridin-2-yl analogs **32** and **37**, the change of spacers to hydrazide **37** led to a modest improvement in selectivity, but in case of the corresponding bromo analogs **33** and **38** the SI was lower in hydrazide **38**. The introduction of other heterocycles **40–42** gave similar lower SIs as observed for the aliphatic analogs **14–16**. In comparison with our earlier reported open-chain bromotyrosine analogs [14], we found that most spirocyclic bromotyrosine analogs have lower CC_{50} to both cell lines tested.

Overall, the SIs for this set of compounds stayed below 2.5, indicating relatively low selectivity toward A-375 cell line. The cytotoxic effect of the two most selective compounds was partially mediated by caspase-dependent apoptosis, although the low (twofold) level of apoptosis induction at CC_{50} concentration suggests predominantly an unspecific cytotoxicity mechanism. Taking into account considerable dissimilarities in the biology of different cancer types [23], future work may include testing of the compounds in a panel of cancer cell lines representing various malignancies. In summary, biological data of synthesized spiro-structured clavatadine C **1** analogs demonstrate low selectivity toward skin cancer. However, structure–activity relationships indicate further structural optimization by modification of the side chain for potential development of these analogs into anticancer agents should be explored.

4. Materials and Methods

4.1. Materials and Methods for Biological Testing

Analysis of selectivity to cancer cells. The cells were seeded to white frame and clear bottom 96-well plates (Perkin Elmer) at a density of 10,000 cells/well for the human malignant melanoma A-375 cell line (ATCC CRL-1619) and 7500 cells/well for the human skin fibroblast Hs27 cell line (ATCC CRL-1634). The cells were grown at 37 °C, 5% CO_2 until they reached 70–80% confluence (approximately 24 h). Stock solutions of test compounds and a positive control (camptothecin, Sigma-Aldrich, St. Louis, MO, USA) were prepared in DMSO and diluted into the assay medium (growth medium with 5% FBS) to the final concentration. Final DMSO concentration was 0.5% in all samples. The culture medium was removed from the plate and compounds added, 200 μL/well. After a 48-h incubation, the amount of ATP, which is directly proportional to the number of viable cells present in culture, was quantified using CellTiter-Glo® Luminescent Cell Viability kit (Promega, Madison, WI, USA), according to manufacturer's instructions. Origin Graphing and Analysis, version 9.55 (OriginLab, Northampton, MA, USA), was used for determination of CC_{50} values. The cancer cell selectivity index was calculated as a ratio of CC_{50} values between Hs27 fibroblasts and A-375 melanoma cells. Standard deviation of selectivity indices was calculated using Equation (1)

$$\sigma\left(\frac{\bar{x}}{\bar{y}}\right) = \sqrt{\left(\frac{\sigma(x)}{\bar{x}}\right)^2 + \left(\frac{\sigma(y)}{\bar{y}}\right)^2} \quad (1)$$

In the Equation (1), $\bar{x}$ and $\bar{y}$ are average CC_{50} values in Hs27 and A-375 cells, respectively, and $\sigma(x)$ and $\sigma(y)$ are their standard deviations.

Apoptosis induction assay and imaging. A-375 cells were seeded to white 96-well plates and treated with compounds at $1 \times CC_{50}$ concentration, 100 μL/well, following the procedure described above. After 24 and 48 h, caspase-3/7 activity was measured using the ApoTox-Glo kit (Promega) following the manufacturer's instructions. The light microscopy images were taken using 4× phase contrast objective and Cytation5 automated imaging reader (Biotek).

4.2. *Synthesis Experimental*

4.2.1. General

All reactions were carried out using commercially available starting materials unless otherwise stated. The melting points were measured with a Stuart SMP40 automated melting point apparatus and were uncorrected. ^1H NMR and ^{13}C NMR spectra in $CDCl_3$, d_6-DMSO, d_6-acetone, or CD_3OD at ambient temperature were recorded on a Bruker Ascend 400 spectrometer. Chemical shifts (δ) are given in parts per million (ppm) relative to the NMR reference solvent signals ($CDCl_3$: 7.26 ppm, 77.16 ppm; CD_3OD: 3.31 ppm, 49.00 ppm; d_6-DMSO: 2.50 ppm, 39.52 ppm; d_6-acetone: 2.05 ppm, 29.84 ppm). Multiplicities are indicated by s (singlet), br s (broad singlet), d (doublet), dd (doublet of doublets), ddd (doublet of doublet of doublets), t (triplet), dt (doublet of triplets), q (quartet), p (pentet), and m (multiplet). The coupling constants *J* were quoted in hertz (Hz). LC-MS and HRMS-spectra were recorded using a Waters Acquity UPLC®-system (with Acquity UPLC® BEH C18 column, 1.7 μm, 50 mm × 2.1 mm, Waters, Milford, MA, USA) with Waters Synapt G2 HDMS with the ESI (+), high resolution mode, and PDA. The mobile phase consisted of H_2O (A) and acetonitrile (B), both containing 0.1% HCOOH. Microwave syntheses were performed in sealed tubes using a Biotage Initiator+ instrument equipped with an external IR sensor. The flash chromatography was performed with a Biotage Isolera One flash chromatography purification system with a 200–800 nm UV-VIS detector using SNAP KP-Sil 10 g, 25 g, or 50 g cartridges. The TLC plates were provided by Merck (Silica gel 60-F254) and visualization of the amine compounds was conducted using ninhydrin (a 0.2% *w*/*v* solution in a 3% solution of acetic acid in 1-butanol) staining.

4.2.2. Experimental Procedures and Characterization Data

***tert*-Butyl L-tyrosinate (7)**

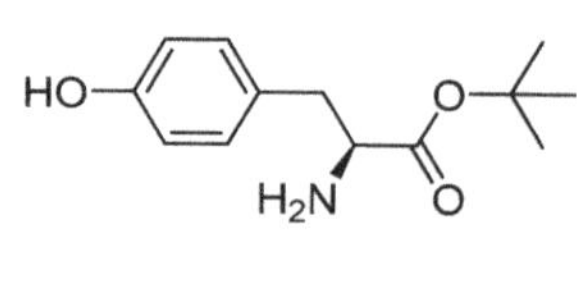

To a stirred suspension of L-tyrosine **6** (25.0 g, 0.138 mol) in *tert*-butyl acetate (100 mL) in an ice bath (0 °C), perchloric acid (15.7 mL, 0.276 mol, 2.0 equiv) was added dropwise. The reaction mixture was allowed to warm to room temperature and was stirred for 17 h. The mixture was washed with H_2O (300 mL) and a 1 M solution of HCl in H_2O (250 mL). The aqueous phase was diluted with H_2O (300 mL), followed by the addition of solid K_2CO_3 until the pH was 7. The resulting mixture was filtered, the filtrate was made alkaline (pH 9) by adding solid K_2CO_3, and then it was extracted with EtOAc (3 × 300 mL). The combined organic phases were washed with brine (300 mL), dried over anhydrous Na_2SO_4, filtered, and concentrated in vacuo to give an off-white solid; crude yield: 29 g (86%). The crude product was purified with automated flash chromatography (DCM/MeOH, gradient: 0→10%) to give the product **7** as a white solid (25 g, 76%). ^{1}H NMR (400 MHz, $CDCl_3$) δ 7.01 (d, J = 8.5 Hz, 2H), 6.65 (d, J = 8.5 Hz, 2H), 3.60 (dd, J = 7.7, 5.3 Hz, 1H), 3.00 (dd, J = 13.8, 5.3 Hz, 1H), 2.77 (dd, J = 13.8, 7.7 Hz, 1H), 1.45 (s, 9H). ^{13}C NMR (101 MHz, $CDCl_3$) δ 174.2, 155.5, 130.5, 128.2, 115.8, 81.8, 56.2, 40.0, 28.2. ^{1}H NMR is in accordance with the literature [24].

tert-Butyl (_E_)-2-(hydroxyimino)-3-(4-hydroxyphenyl)propanoate (8)

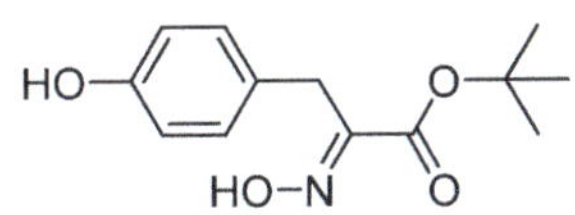

To a stirred solution of *tert*-butyl L-tyrosinate **7** (1.20 g, 5.06 mmol) in EtOH (20 mL) in an ice bath (0 °C), $Na_2WO_4{\cdot}2H_2O$ (1.83 g, 10.4 mmol, 1.1 equiv), a 30% solution of H_2O_2 in H_2O (9 mL), and H_2O (14 mL) wereadded. The resulting mixture was stirred for 8 h and slowly allowed to reach room temperature. The mixture was diluted with EtOAc (25 mL) and washed with a 10% solution of Na_2SO_3 in H_2O (2 × 15 mL), H_2O (2 × 15 mL), and brine (15 mL). The aqueous phase was extracted with EtOAc (3 × 20 mL), and the combined organic phases were washed with brine (10 mL), dried over anhydrous Na_2SO_4, filtered, and concentrated in vacuo. The crude product was purified with automated flash chromatography (*n*-heptane/EtOAc gradient: 5→50%) to give the compound **8** as a white solid (1.00 g, 79%). ^{1}H NMR (400 MHz, CD_3OD) δ 7.05 (d, J = 8.7 Hz, 2H), 6.67 (d, J = 8.6 Hz, 2H), 3.79 (s, 2H), 1.43 (s, 9H). ^{13}C NMR (101 MHz, CD_3OD) δ 164.6, 156.9, 153.6, 131.0, 128.6, 116.1, 83.3, 30.3, 28.1. ^{1}H NMR is in accordance with the literature [10].

tert-Butyl 8-oxo-1-oxa-2-azaspiro[4.5]deca-2,6,9-triene-3-carboxylate (9a)

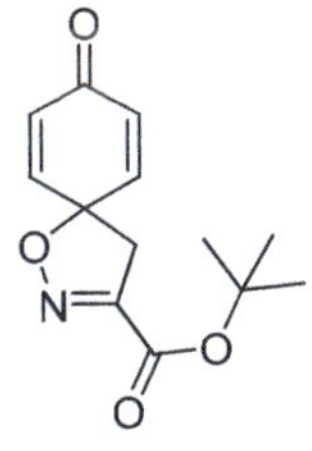

tert-Butyl (*E*)-2-(hydroxyimino)-3-(4-hydroxyphenyl)propanoate **8** (0.40 g, 1.6 mmol) was dissolved in 2,2,2-trifluoroethanol (7.7 mL), followed by the addition of anhydrous pyridine (0.39 mL, 4.8 mmol, 2 equiv). The mixture was cooled in an ice bath (0 °C) for 5 min. Phenyliodine bis(trifluoroacetate) (0.76 g, 1.8 mmol, 1.1 equiv) was added to the cooled mixture, and stirring was continued for 1.5 h. The reaction was quenched with a 10% solution of $Na_2S_2O_3$ in H_2O (13 mL), and the resulting mixture extracted with EtOAc (3 × 15 mL). The combined organic phases were washed with brine, dried over anhydrous Na_2SO_4, filtered, and concentrated in vacuo. The crude product was purified with automated flash chromatography (*n*-heptane/EtOAc gradient: 12→100%)

to give the compound **9a** as a yellow oil (0.33 g, 84%). ^{1}H NMR (400 MHz, d_6-acetone) δ 7.12–7.05 (m, 2H), 6.24–6.18 (m, 2H), 3.48 (s, 2H), 1.52 (s, 9H). ^{13}C NMR (101 MHz, d_6-acetone) δ 184.9, 159.5, 153.7, 145.7, 129.2, 83.6, 83.6, 44.3, 28.1. ^{1}H NMR is in accordance with the literature [10].

8-Oxo-1-oxa-2-azaspiro[4.5]deca-2,6,9-triene-3-carboxylic acid (10a)

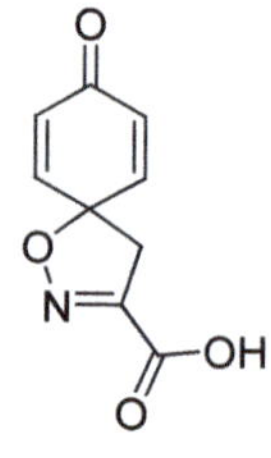

To a solution of *tert*-butyl 8-oxo-1-oxa-2-azaspiro[4.5]deca-2,6,9-triene-3-carboxylate **9a** (0.33 g, 1.3 mmol) in anhydrous DCM (10 mL), trifluoroacetic acid (5.0 mL) was added dropwise. The resulting mixture was stirred at room temperature for 3 h. The solvent was removed in vacuo to give the compound **10a** as a light brown solid (0.24 g, 93%). ^{1}H NMR (400 MHz, d_6-acetone) δ 7.15–7.08 (m, 1H), 6.26–6.19 (m, 1H), 3.51 (s, 1H). ^{13}C NMR (101 MHz, d_6-acetone) δ 184.9, 161.0, 153.0, 145.7, 129.3, 116.5, 83.8.

***tert*-Butyl 7,9-dibromo-8-oxo-1-oxa-2-azaspiro[4.5]deca-2,6,9-triene-3-carboxylate (9b)**

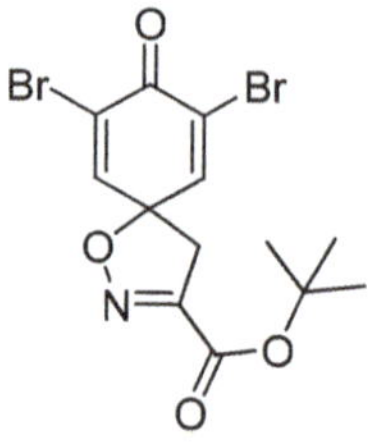

To a solution of *tert*-butyl (*E*)-2-(hydroxyimino)-3-(4-hydroxyphenyl)propanoate **8** (0.59 g, 2.348 mmol) in anhydrous DMF (10 mL) in an ice bath (0 °C), *N*-bromosuccinimide (1.35 g, 7.58 mmol, 3.25 equiv) in anhydrous DMF (5 mL) was added dropwise (15 min). The mixture was diluted with Et_2O (25 mL), and washed with H_2O (2 × 15 mL) and a 10% solution of $Na_2S_2O_3$ in H_2O (2 × 15 mL). The aqueous phase was back-extracted with Et_2O (2 × 30 mL). The combined organic phases were washed with brine (20 mL), dried over anhydrous Na_2SO_4, filtered, and concentrated in vacuo. The crude product was purified with automated flash chromatography (isocratic DCM) to give the compound **9b** as a white solid (0.58 g, 62%). ^{1}H NMR (400 MHz, $CDCl_3$) δ 7.32 (s, 2H), 3.42 (s, 2H), 1.57 (s, 9H). ^{13}C NMR (101 MHz, $CDCl_3$) δ 171.5, 158.2, 152.3, 144.1, 123.4, 85.8, 84.9, 43.2, 27.8. ^{1}H NMR is in accordance with the literature [10].

7,9-Dibromo-8-oxo-1-oxa-2-azaspiro[4.5]deca-2,6,9-triene-3-carboxylic acid (10b)

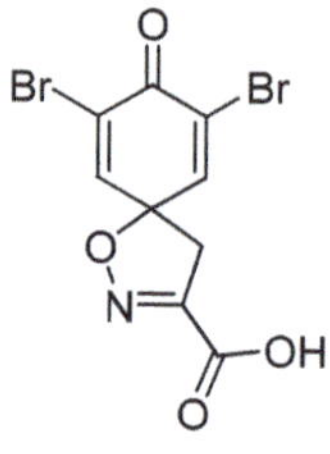

To a solution of *tert*-butyl 7,9-dibromo-8-oxo-1-oxa-2-azaspiro[4.5]deca-2,6,9-triene-3-carboxylate **9b** (0.58 g, 1.4 mmol) in anhydrous DCM (10 mL), trifluoroacetic acid (5.0 mL) was added dropwise. The resulting mixture was stirred at room temperature for 1 h, after which the solvent was removed in vacuo. The product was purified via trituration with Et_2O to give the compound **10b** as a white solid (0.50 g, 98%). ^{1}H NMR (400 MHz, d_6-DMSO) δ 7.81 (s, 2H), 3.52 (s, 2H). ^{1}H NMR is in accordance with the literature [22]. ^{13}C NMR (101 MHz, d_6-acetone) δ 172.3, 160.7, 153.6, 146.8, 123.2, 87.3, 43.7. HRMS (ESI-): calculated 303.8609 ($C_8H_4Br_2NO_2$), found 303.8609. LC-MS: $[M\text{-}CO_2]^-$ m/z 304 (t_R = 2.12 min), >99%. Mp: 174–175 °C, (Lit. Mp: 167–168 °C) [10].

The spiro carboxylate core was mainly constructed using the synthetic method given below, followed by *N*-(3-dimethylaminopropyl)-*N*′-ethylcarbodiimide (EDC)-mediated coupling (General procedures for coupling A and B) to give the corresponding product. Some compounds were deprotected with trifluoroacetic acid to give the corresponding trifluoroacetate salts (General procedure C).

General procedure for EDC-mediated coupling (A). To a stirred solution of carboxylic acid **10a** or **10b** (0.36 mmol) in DCM (5 mL), 1-hydroxybenzotriazole (HOBt) hydrate (0.036 mmol, 0.1 equiv) and *N*-(3-dimethylaminopropyl)-*N*′-ethylcarbodiimide (EDC) hydrochloride (0.39 mmol, 1.1 equiv) at 0–5 °C were added and stirred for 15 min. After this, the amine/hydrazide (0.36 mmol, 1.0 equiv) was added. The reaction mixture was allowed to reach room temperature and was stirred for a further 8–16 h. The mixture was diluted with DCM (10 mL) and washed with 1 M hydrochloric acid (5 mL), a saturated solution of $NaHCO_3$ in H_2O (5 mL), and brine (5 mL). The organic layer was dried over anhydrous Na_2SO_4, filtered, and concentrated in vacuo. The crude product was purified by automated flash chromatography (*n*-heptane/EtOAc gradient: 0→100%) to give the pure product.

General procedure for EDC-mediated coupling (B). Carboxylic acid **10a** or **10b** (0.3 mmol), amine (0.45 mmol, 1.5 equiv), HOBt hydrate (0.45 mmol, 1.5 equiv), and EDC·HCl (0.45 mmol, 1.5 equiv) were dissolved in anhydrous DCM (3 mL). The mixture was irradiated under microwave conditions at 60 °C for 2 h, after which it was diluted with DCM (10 mL). The solution was washed with a saturated solution of NH_4Cl in H_2O, water, and brine. The organic phase was dried over anhydrous Na_2SO_4, filtered, and concentrated in vacuo. The crude product was purified with automated flash column chromatography (*n*-heptane/EtOAc-EtOH 3:1 (12→100%) to give the pure product.

General procedure for deprotection of the Boc groups (C). To a solution of clavatadine bis-Boc-derivative (0.28 mmol) in DCM (2 mL), TFA (1 mL) at 0–5 °C was added dropwise. The reaction mixture was allowed to reach room temperature. The resulting mixture was stirred for 3 h at room temperature. The solvent was removed in vacuo to give the crude product, which was triturated in Et_2O to give a solid trifluoroacetate salt.

7,9-Dibromo-N-(4-guanidinobutyl)-8-oxo-1-oxa-2-azaspiro[4.5]deca-2,6,9-triene-3-carboxamide TFA salt (1-TFA)

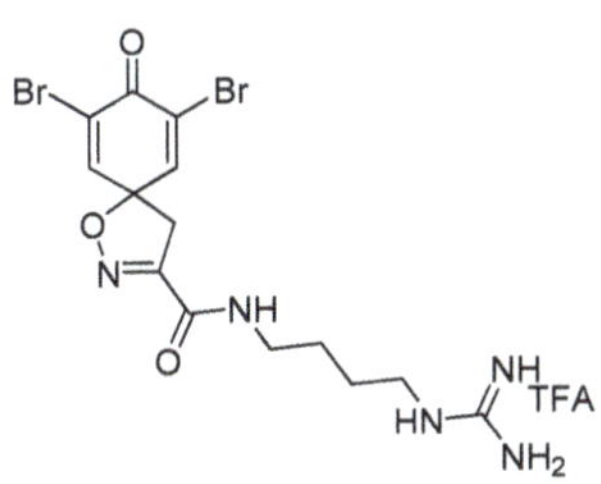

General procedures **A** and **C** were followed to give the clavatadine C TFA salt **12** as an off-white solid (0.10 g, 77%). ^{1}H NMR (400 MHz, d_6-DMSO) δ 8.65 (t, J = 5.9 Hz, 1H), 7.80 (s, 2H), 7.59 (t, J = 5.7 Hz, 1H), 3.55 (s, 2H), 3.23–3.06 (m, 4H), 1.48 (m, 4H). ^{13}C NMR (101 MHz, d_6-DMSO) δ 171.6, 158.2, 156.7, 155.0, 146.7, 121.6, 85.2, 43.2, 40.4, 38.4, 26.0,

25.9. Spectra are in accordance with the literature [10]. HRMS (ESI$^+$): Calculated 463.9757 ($C_{14}H_{18}Br_2N_5O_3$), found 463.9755. LC-MS: [M + H]$^+$ m/z 464 (t_R = 2.25 min), >91%. Mp:115–118 °C, decomp. (Lit. Mp: 130–140 °C, decomp.) [10].

N-(4-Guanidinobutyl)-8-oxo-1-oxa-2-azaspiro[4.5]deca-2,6,9-triene-3-carboxamide TFA salt (11)

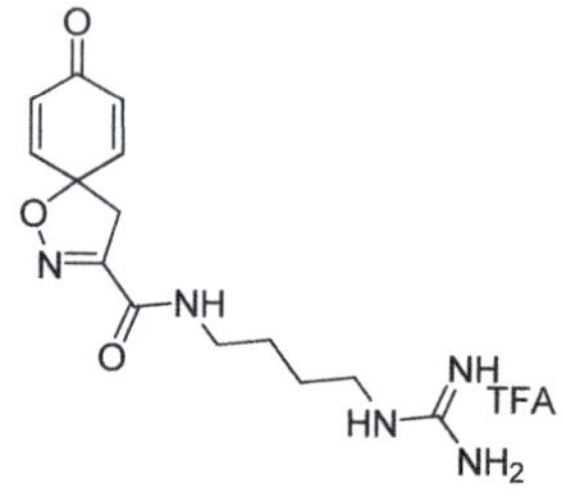

General procedures **A** and **C** were followed to give the compound **11** as an off-white solid (0.11 g, 34%). ^{1}H NMR (400 MHz, CD_3OD) δ 7.04–7.00 (m, 2H), 6.26–6.22 (m, 2H), 3.44 (s, 2H), 3.36–3.34 (m, 2H), 3.23–3.20 (m, 2H), 1.64 (m, 4H). ^{13}C NMR (101 MHz, CD_3OD) δ 186.4, 161.3, 158.6, 153.3, 146.7, 129.4, 83.6, 44.4, 42.0, 39.8, 27.5, 27.1. HRMS (ESI$^+$): calculated 306.1566 ($C_{14}H_{20}N_5O_3$), found 306.1567. LC-MS: [M + H]$^+$ m/z 306 (t_R = 0.92 min), >98%. Mp: 170–173 °C.

N,N-Dimethyl-8-oxo-1-oxa-2-azaspiro[4.5]deca-2,6,9-triene-3-carboxamide (12)

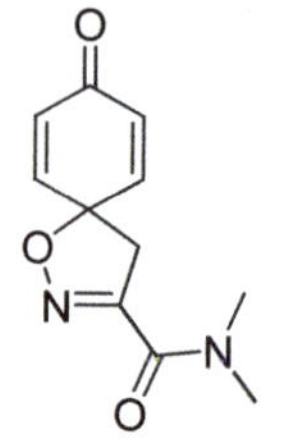

General procedure **A** was followed to give the compound **12** as an off-white amorphous solid (0.011 g, 28%). ^{1}H NMR (400 MHz, CD_3OD) δ 7.05 (d, J = 10.1 Hz, 2H), 6.25 (d, J = 10.1 Hz, 2H), 3.50 (s, 2H), 3.28 (s, 3H), 3.06 (s, 3H). ^{13}C NMR (101 MHz, CD_3OD) δ 185.1, 160.7, 153.4, 145.5, 128.7, 80.6, 45.2, 37.6, 34.7. HRMS (ESI$^+$): calculated 221.0926 ($C_{11}H_{13}N_2O_3$), found 221.0927. LC-MS: [M + H]$^+$ m/z 221 (t_R = 1.85 min), >99%.

7,9-Dibromo-N,N-dimethyl-8-oxo-1-oxa-2-azaspiro[4.5]deca-2,6,9-triene-3-carboxamide (13)

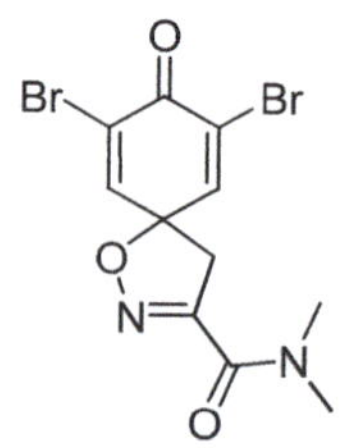

General procedure **A** was followed to give the compound **13** as a white amorphous solid (0.12 g, 37%). ^{1}H NMR (400 MHz, CDCl3) δ 7.32 (s, 2H), 3.55 (s, 2H), 3.32 (s, 3H), 3.09 (s, 3H). ^{13}C NMR (101 MHz, $CDCl_3$) δ 171.6, 159.3, 153.7, 144.9, 123.8, 84.1, 45.8, 38.8, 36.5. HRMS (ESI$^+$): calculated 378.9117 ($C_{11}H_{11}Br_2N_2O_3$), found 378.9119.

7,9-Dibromo-*N*-isopropyl-*N*-methyl-8-oxo-1-oxa-2-azaspiro[4.5]deca-2,6,9-triene-3-carboxamide (14)

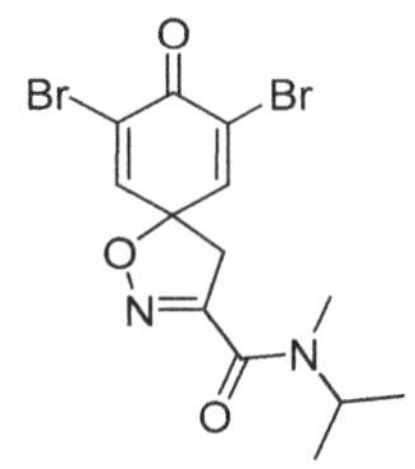

General procedure **A** was followed to give the compound **14** as an off-white amorphous solid (0.061 g, 35%). ^{1}H NMR (400 MHz, $CDCl_3$) (1:1 mixture of rotamers) δ 7.33 (7.32) (s, 2H), 4.84 (4.66) (p, *J* = 6.8 Hz, 1H), 3.56 (3.55) (s, 2H), 3.10 (2.92) (s, 3H), 1.26 (1.19) (d, *J* = 6.8 Hz, 6H) ^{13}C NMR (101 MHz, $CDCl_3$) δ 171.6, 159.0 (158.9), 154.2 (153.5), 144.98 (144.96), 123.71 (123.69), 84.0 (83.9), 49.6 (45.9), 46.03 (45.97), 30.1 (27.0), 20.9 (19.3). HRMS (ESI$^+$): calculated 406.9430 ($C_{13}H_{15}Br_2N_2O_3$), found 406.9426. LC-MS: $[M + H]^+$ m/z 407 (t_R = 4.31 min), >99%. Mp: 148–153 °C.

3-(Morpholine-4-carbonyl)-1-oxa-2-azaspiro[4.5]deca-2,6,9-trien-8-one (15)

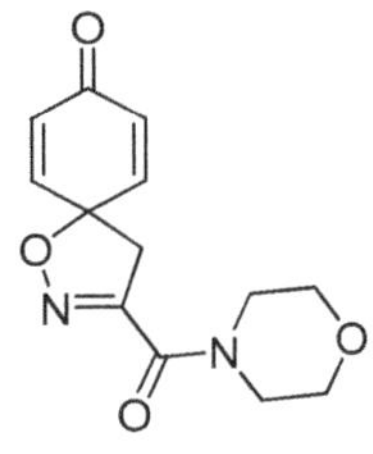

General procedure **A** was followed to give the compound **15** as an off-white amorphous solid (0.012 g, 12%). ^{1}H NMR (400 MHz, $CDCl_3$) δ 6.90–6.81 (m, 2H), 6.33–6.25 (m, 2H), 4.02–3.95 (m, 2H), 3.80–3.70 (m, 6H), 3.48 (s, 2H). ^{13}C NMR (101 MHz, $CDCl_3$) δ 184.5, 158.9, 153.2, 144.1, 129.5, 80.9, 67.1, 66.8, 47.4, 46.2, 43.3. HRMS (ESI$^+$): calculated 263.1032 ($C_{13}H_{1}5N_2O_4$), found 263.1036. LC-MS: $[M + H]^+$ m/z 442 (t_R = 5.39 min), >99%.

3-(4-Hydroxypiperidine-1-carbonyl)-1-oxa-2-azaspiro[4.5]deca-2,6,9-trien-8-one (16)

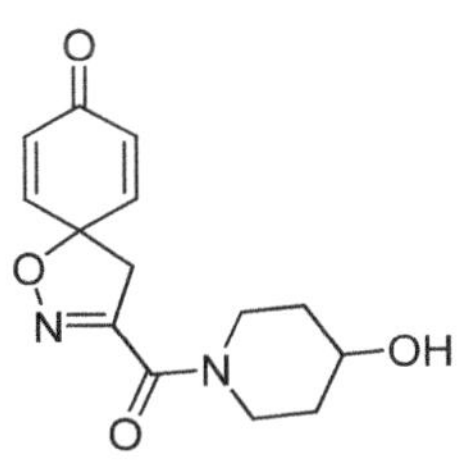

General procedure **A** was followed to give the compound **16** as an off-white amorphous solid (0.024 g, 24%). ^{1}H NMR (400 MHz, $CDCl_3$): δ 6.92–6.83 (m, 2H), 6.33–6.24 (m, 2H), 4.23–4.14 (m, 1H), 4.08–4.00 (m, 2H), 3.72–3.60 (m, 1H), 3.53–3.42 (m, 3H), 2.02–1.90 (m, 2H), 1.69–1.59 (m, 2H), 1.57 (br s, 1H). ^{13}C NMR (101 MHz, $CDCl_3$) δ 184.5, 158.4, 153.2, 144.3, 129.4, 80.8, 66.7, 46.3, 39.9, 34.7, 33.8. HRMS (ESI$^+$): calculated 277.1188 ($C_{14}H_{17}N_2O_4$), found 277.1187. LC-MS: $[M + H]^+$ m/z 277 (t_R = 1.61 min), >99%.

N′-(2-Morpholinoacetyl)-8-oxo-1-oxa-2-azaspiro[4.5]deca-2,6,9-triene-3-carbohydrazide (17)

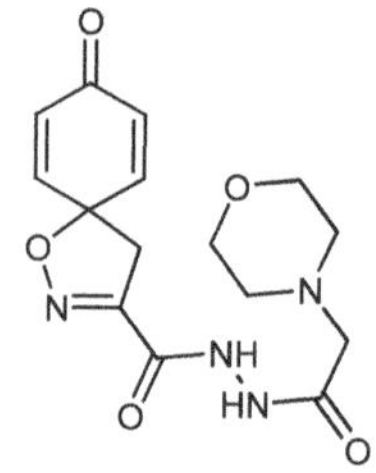

General procedure **A** was followed to give the compound **17** as an amorphous off-white solid (0.030 g, 17%). ^{1}H NMR (400 MHz, CD_3OD) δ 7.09–7.00 (m, 2H), 6.29–6.20 (m, 2H), 3.77–3.61 (m, 4H), 3.47 (s, 2H), 3.17 (s, 2H), 2.68–2.55 (m, 4H). ^{13}C NMR (101 MHz, CD_3OD) δ 186.4, 171.6, 160.2, 154.3, 146.6, 129.5, 83.5, 67.7, 61.5, 54.7, 44.4. HRMS (ESI^{+}): calculated 335.1356 ($C_{15}H_{19}N_4O_5$), found 335.1354. LC-MS: $[M + H]^+$ m/z 335 (t_R = 0.53 min), >96%.

N-(3,5-Dichlorophenyl)-8-oxo-1-oxa-2-azaspiro[4.5]deca-2,6,9-triene-3-carboxamide (18)

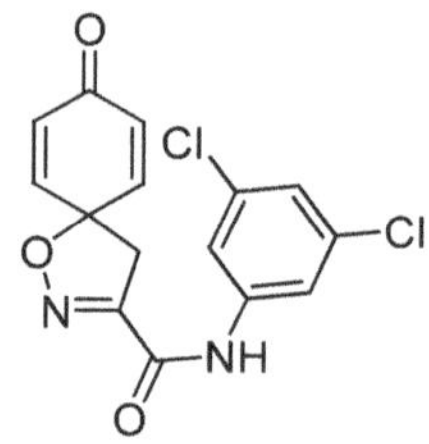

General procedure **A** was followed to give the compound **18** as an off-white amorphous solid (0.098 g, 51%). ^{1}H NMR (400 MHz, $CDCl_3$) δ 8.36 (br s, 1H), 7.56 (d, J = 1.8 Hz, 2H), 7.17 (t, J = 1.8 Hz, 1H), 6.89–6.84 (m, 2H), 6.35–6.29 (m, 2H), 3.45 (s, 2H). ^{13}C NMR (101 MHz, $CDCl_3$) δ 183.9, 156.3, 153.4, 143.1, 138.2, 135.4, 129.4, 125.0, 117.9, 83.6, 42.7. HRMS (ESI^{+}): calculated 337.0147 ($C_{15}H_{11}Cl_2N_2O_3$), found 337.0148. LC-MS: $[M + H]^+$ m/z 337. (t_R = 4.81 min), >91%.

7,9-Dibromo-N-(3,5-dichlorophenyl)-8-oxo-1-oxa-2-azaspiro[4.5]deca-2,6,9-triene-3-carboxamide (19)

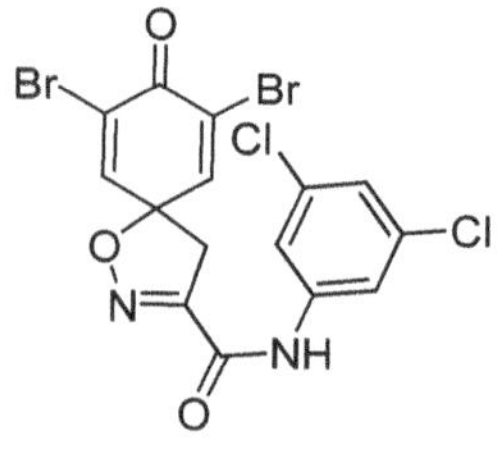

General procedure **B** was followed to give the compound **19** as a white amorphous solid (0.0045 g, 13%). ^{1}H NMR (400 MHz, d_6-acetone) δ 9.78 (br s, 1H), 7.93 (d, J = 1.9 Hz, 2H), 7.77 (s, 2H), 7.26 (t, J = 1.8 Hz, 1H), 3.76 (s, 2H). ^{13}C NMR (101 MHz, d_6-acetone) δ 172.2, 158.3, 155.8, 146.7, 141.3, 135.7, 124.7, 123.3, 119.1, 119.0, 87.4, 43.4. HRMS (ESI^{-}): calculated 490.8200 ($C_{15}H_9Br_2Cl_2N_2O_3$), found 490.8198. LC-MS: $[M-H]^-$ m/z 491 (t_R = 5.84 min), >99%.

N-(3-Chloro-4-methoxyphenyl)-8-oxo-1-oxa-2-azaspiro[4.5]deca-2,6,9-triene-3-carboxamide (20)

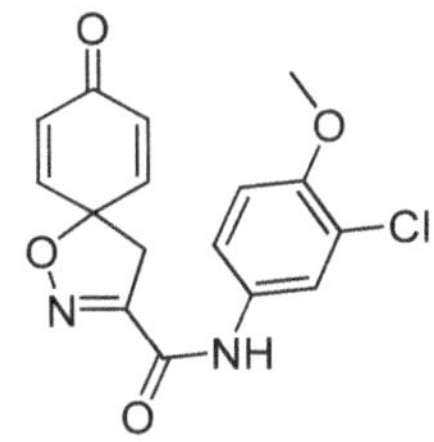

General procedure **A** was followed to give the compound **20** as an off-white amorphous solid (0.025 g, 13%). ^{1}H NMR (400 MHz, $CDCl_3$) δ 8.23 (br s, 1H), 7.68 (d, J = 2.6 Hz, 1H), 7.43 (dd, J = 8.9, 2.6 Hz, 1H), 6.92 (d, J = 8.9 Hz, 1H), 6.90–6.85 (m, 2H), 6.34–6.28 (m, 2H), 3.91 (s, 3H), 3.46 (s, 2H). ^{13}C NMR (101 MHz, $CDCl_3$) δ 184.3, 156.4, 154.0, 152.7, 143.7, 130.2, 129.6, 123.0, 122.5, 119.6, 112.4, 83.5, 56.5, 43.3. HRMS (ESI$^+$): calculated 333.0642 ($C_{16}H_{14}ClN_2O_4$), found 333.0639. LC-MS: $[M + H]^+$ m/z 333 (t_R = 3.68 min), >99%.

7,9-Dibromo-N-(3-chloro-4-methoxyphenyl)-8-oxo-1-oxa-2-azaspiro[4.5]deca-2,6,9-triene-3-carboxamide (21)

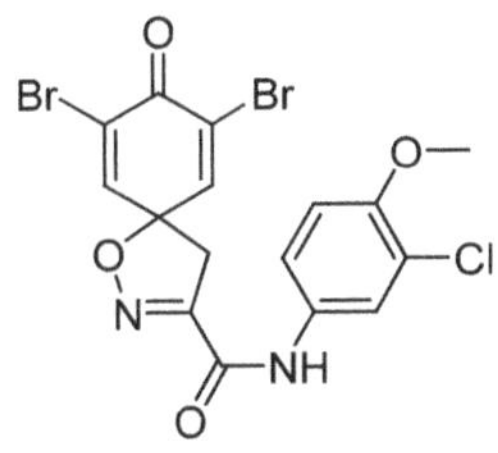

General procedure **B** was followed to give the compound **21** as a white amorphous solid (0.037 g, 18%). ^{1}H NMR (400 MHz, d_6-DMSO) δ 10.59 (br s, 1H), 7.88 (d, J = 2.6 Hz, 1H), 7.85 (s, 2H), 7.68 (dd, J = 9.0, 2.6 Hz, 1H), 7.15 (d, J = 9.1 Hz, 1H), 3.83 (s, 3H), 3.65 (s, 2H). ^{13}C NMR (101 MHz, d_6-DMSO) δ 171.6, 156.8, 155.4, 151.2, 146.5, 131.6, 121.8, 121.8, 120.5, 120.2, 112.8, 85.6, 56.2, 43.0. HRMS (ESI$^+$): calculated 486.8696 ($C_{16}H_{11}Br_2ClN_2O_4$), found 486.8696. LC-MS: $[M-H]^-$ m/z 487 (t_R = 4.95 min), >94%.

N-[2-(1H-Indol-3-yl)ethyl]-8-oxo-1-oxa-2-azaspiro[4.5]deca-2,6,9-triene-3-carboxamide (22)

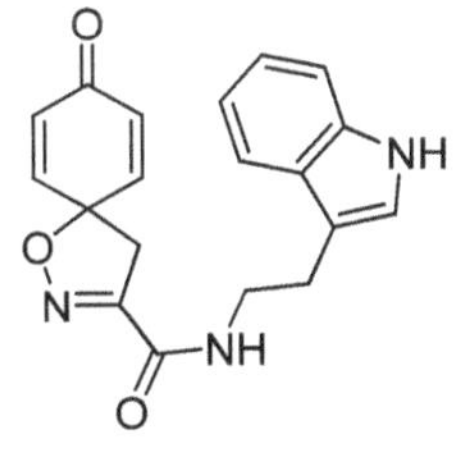

General procedure **A** was followed to give the compound **22** as a white amorphous solid (0.058 g, 56%). ^{1}H NMR (400 MHz, $CDCl_3$) δ 8.12 (br s, 1H), 7.65–7.59 (m, 1H), 7.39 (m, 1H), 7.23 (ddd, J = 8.2, 7.2, 1.1 Hz, 1H), 7.15 (ddd, J = 8.0, 7.1, 1.0 Hz, 1H), 7.08 (d, J = 2.3 Hz, 1H), 6.84–6.78 (m, 2H), 6.67 (br s, 1H), 6.30–6.23 (m, 2H), 3.71 (q, J = 6.8 Hz, 2H), 3.36 (s, 2H), 3.06 (t, J = 6.8 Hz, 2H). ^{13}C NMR (101 MHz, $CDCl_3$) δ 184.4, 158.7, 153.8, 144.0, 136.5, 129.3, 127.2, 122.5, 122.2, 119.7, 118.8, 112.5, 111.4, 82.7, 43.7, 39.8. HRMS (ESI$^+$): calculated 336.1348 ($C_{19}H_{18}N_3O_3$), found 336.1349. LC-MS: $[M-H]^-$ m/z 336 (t_R = 4.95 min), >99%.

N-(4-Methoxybenzyl)-8-oxo-1-oxa-2-azaspiro[4.5]deca-2,6,9-triene-3-carboxamide (23)

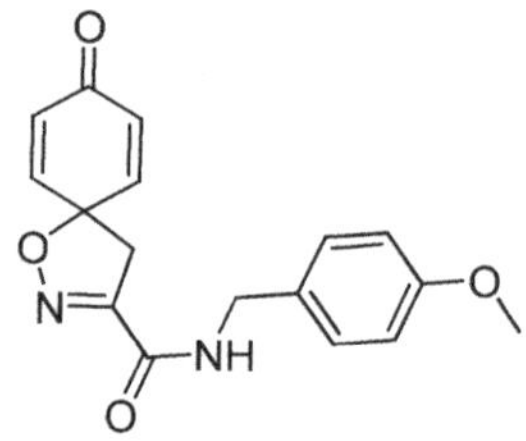

General procedure **A** was followed to give the compound **23** as an off-white amorphous solid (0.13 g, 67%). ^{1}H NMR (400 MHz, $CDCl_3$) δ 7.27–7.22 (m, 2H), 6.91–6.87 (m, 3H), 6.86–6.81 (m, 2H), 6.30–6.24 (m, 2H), 4.48 (d, J = 5.9 Hz, 2H), 3.81 (s, 3H), 3.41 (s, 2H). ^{13}C NMR (101 MHz, $CDCl_3$) δ 184.4, 159.5, 158.5, 153.7, 143.9, 129.5, 129.4, 114.5, 114.4, 82.9, 55.4, 43.6, 43.3. HRMS (ESI$^+$): calculated 313.1188 ($C_{17}H_{17}N_2O_4$), found 313.1191. LC-MS: $[M + H]^+$ m/z 313 (t_R = 3.06 min), >99%.

7,9-Dibromo-N-(4-methoxybenzyl)-8-oxo-1-oxa-2-azaspiro[4.5]deca-2,6,9-triene-3-carboxamide (24)

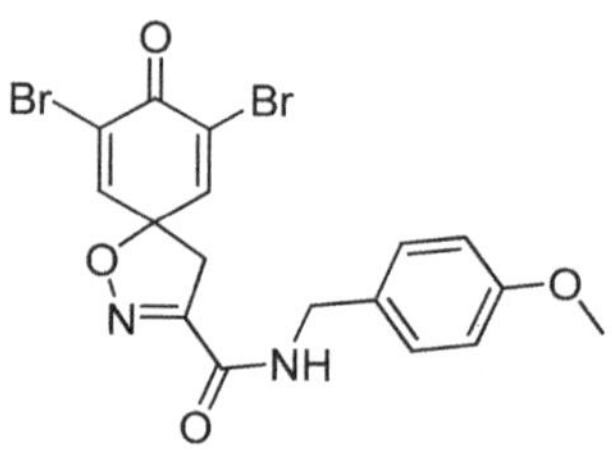

General procedure **A** was followed to give the compound **24** as an off-white amorphous solid (0.022 g, 20%). ^{1}H NMR (400 MHz, d_6-DMSO) δ 9.07 (t, J = 6.2 Hz, 1H), 7.82 (s, 2H), 7.28–7.19 (m, 2H), 6.93–6.84 (m, 2H), 4.29 (d, J = 6.2 Hz, 2H), 3.73 (s, 3H), 3.56 (s, 2H). ^{13}C NMR (101 MHz, d_6-DMSO) δ 171.6, 158.3, 158.1, 155.0, 146.7, 130.8, 128.8, 121.5, 113.6, 85.2, 55.0, 43.1, 41.7. HRMS (ESI$^+$Na$^+$): calculated 492.9199 ($C_{17}H_{15}Br_2N_2O_4Na$), found 492.9197.

N-(4-Methoxyphenethyl)-8-oxo-1-oxa-2-azaspiro[4.5]deca-2,6,9-triene-3-carboxamide (25)

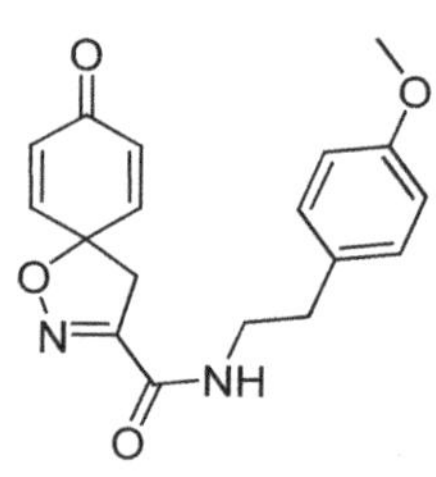

General procedure **A** was followed to give the compound **25** as an off-white amorphous solid (0.042 g, 41%). ^{1}H NMR (400 MHz, $CDCl_3$) δ 7.15–7.11 (m, 2H), 6.89–6.85 (m, 2H), 6.85–6.81 (m, 2H), 6.63 (app. t, 1H), 6.31–6.24 (m, 2H), 3.80 (s, 3H), 3.60 (q, J = 7.0 Hz, 2H), 3.38 (s, 2H), 2.83 (t, J = 7.0 Hz, 2H). ^{13}C NMR (101 MHz, $CDCl_3$) δ 184.4, 158.6, 158.6, 153.8, 143.9, 130.2, 129.7, 129.4, 114.3, 82.8, 55.4, 43.6, 41.0, 34.8. HRMS (ESI$^+$): calculated 327.1345 ($C_{18}H_{19}N_2O_4$), found 327.1348. LC-MS: $[M + H]^+$ m/z 327 (t_R = 3.35 min), >99%.

8-Oxo-*N*-(pyridin-3-yl)-1-oxa-2-azaspiro[4.5]deca-2,6,9-triene-3-carboxamide (26)

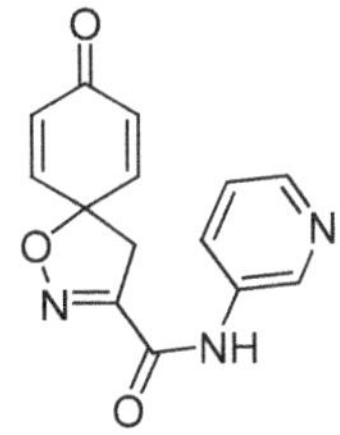

General procedure **A** was followed to give the compound **26** as an off-white amorphous solid (0.047 g, 68%). ^{1}H NMR (400 MHz, $CDCl_3$) δ 8.72 (d, J = 2.5 Hz, 1H), 8.44 (dd, J = 4.7, 1.4 Hz, 1H), 8.40 (br s, 1H), 8.14 (m, 1H), 7.33 (dd, J = 8.3, 4.7 Hz, 1H), 6.91–6.86 (m, 2H), 6.35–6.30 (m, 2H), 3.47 (s, 2H). ^{13}C NMR (101 MHz, $CDCl_3$) δ 184.2, 157.0, 153.8, 146.4, 143.5, 141.5, 133.7, 129.7, 127.2, 124.0, 83.8, 43.1. HRMS (ESI$^+$): calculated 270.0879 ($C_{14}H_{12}N_3O_3$), found 270.0876. LC-MS: $[M + H]^+$ m/z 270 (t_R = 1.03 min), >92%.

7,9-Dibromo-8-oxo-*N*-(pyridin-3-yl)-1-oxa-2-azaspiro[4.5]deca-2,6,9-triene-3-carboxamide (27)

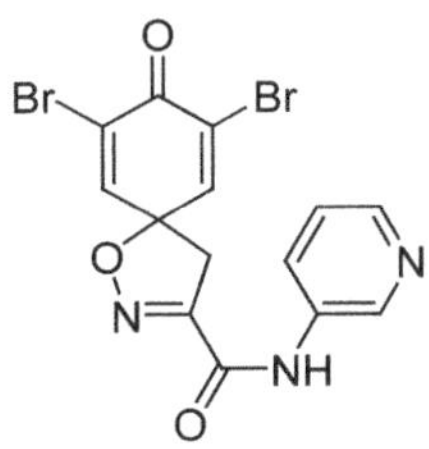

General procedure **B** was followed to give the compound **27** as a white amorphous solid (0.042 g, 34%). ^{1}H NMR (400 MHz, d_6-DMSO) δ 10.81 (br s, 1H), 8.93 (dd, J = 2.6, 0.8 Hz, 1H), 8.33 (dd, J = 4.7, 1.5 Hz, 1H), 8.14 (ddd, J = 8.4, 2.6, 1.5 Hz, 1H), 7.86 (s, 2H), 7.40 (ddd, J = 8.3, 4.7, 0.8 Hz, 1H), 3.66 (s, 2H). ^{13}C NMR (101 MHz, d_6-DMSO) δ 171.6, 157.4, 155.2, 146.4, 145.1, 142.0, 134.9, 127.4, 123.6, 121.8, 85.8, 42.9. HRMS (ESI$^+$): calculated 425.9089 ($C_{14}H_{10}Br_2N_3O_3$), found 425.9090. LC-MS: $[M + H]^+$ m/z 426 (t_R = 2.49 min), >99%.

8-Oxo-*N*-(pyridin-2-yl)-1-oxa-2-azaspiro[4.5]deca-2,6,9-triene-3-carboxamide (28)

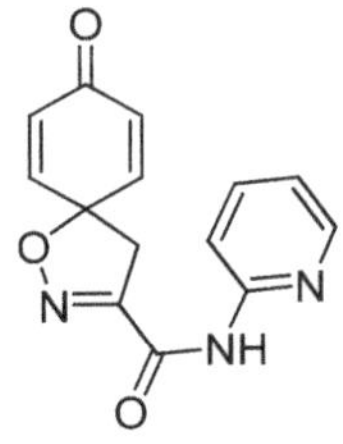

General procedure **A** was followed to give the compound **28** as an off-white amorphous solid (0.040 g, 53%). ^{1}H NMR (400 MHz, $CDCl_3$) δ 9.01 (br s, 1H), 8.35 (ddd, J = 5.0, 1.9, 1.0 Hz, 1H), 8.18–8.16 (m, 1H), 7.76 (ddd, J = 8.4, 7.4, 1.9 Hz, 1H), 7.12 (ddd, J = 7.4, 5.0, 1.0 Hz, 1H), 6.92–6.85 (m, 2H), 6.35–6.28 (m, 2H), 3.46 (s, 2H). ^{13}C NMR (101 MHz, $CDCl_3$) δ 184.3, 156.9, 153.7, 150.2, 148.4, 143.7, 138.7, 129.5, 120.7, 114.2, 83.6, 43.1. HRMS (ESI$^+$): calculated 270.0879 ($C_{14}H_{12}N_3O_3$), found 270.0881. LC-MS: $[M + H]^+$ m/z 270 (t_R = 2.11 min), >99%.

7,9-Dibromo-8-oxo-*N*-(pyridin-2-yl)-1-oxa-2-azaspiro[4.5]deca-2,6,9-triene-3-carboxamide (29)

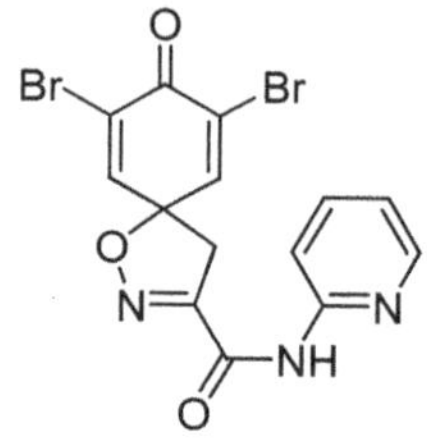

General procedure **B** was followed to give the compound **29** as a white amorphous solid (0.016 g, 13%). ^{1}H NMR (400 MHz, d_6-acetone) δ 9.22 (br s, 1H), 8.36 (ddd, J = 4.9, 1.9, 0.9 Hz, 1H), 8.15 (dt, J = 8.3, 1.0 Hz, 1H), 7.85 (ddd, J = 8.3, 7.4, 1.9 Hz, 1H), 7.80 (s, 2H), 7.19 (ddd, J = 7.4, 4.9, 1.0 Hz, 1H), 3.80 (s, 2H). ^{13}C NMR (101 MHz, d_6-acetone) δ 172.3, 157.9, 155.9, 151.6, 150.7, 149.4, 146.7, 139.3, 123.3, 121.3, 114.5, 87.5, 43.3. HRMS (ESI$^+$): calculated 427.9245 ($C_{14}H_{12}Br_2N_3O_3$), found 427.9243. LC-MS: $[M + H]^+$ m/z 426 (t_R = 3.92 min), >95%.

7,9-Dibromo-8-oxo-*N*-[5-(trifluoromethyl)pyridin-2-yl]-1-oxa-2-azaspiro[4.5]-deca-2,6,9-triene-3-carboxamide (30)

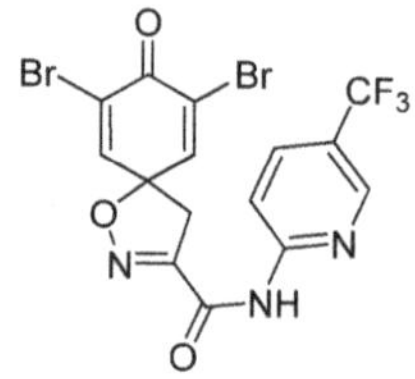

General procedure **A** was followed to give the compound **30** as an off-white amorphous solid (0.012 g, 10%). ^{1}H NMR (400 MHz, $CDCl_3$) δ 9.14 (br s, 1H), 8.62 (d, J = 2.3 Hz, 1H), 8.32 (d, J = 8.7 Hz, 1H), 7.99 (dd, J = 8.7, 2.4 Hz, 1H), 7.34 (s, 2H), 3.56 (s, 2H). ^{13}C NMR (101 MHz, $CDCl_3$) δ 171.3, 156.7, 153.6, 152.6, 146.0, 144.5 (q, $J_{C,F}$ = 40.4 Hz), 143.9, 136.2 (q, $J_{C,F}$ = 33.3 Hz), 124.3, 123.9, 113.6, 87.0, 42.4. HRMS (ESI$^+$): calculated 495.8643 ($C_{15}H_9Br_2F_3N_3O_3$), found 495.8941. LC-MS: $[M + H]^+$ m/z 496 and 498 (t_R = 5.30 and 5.15 min), >97%.

7,9-Dibromo-8-oxo-*N*-[6-(trifluoromethyl)pyridin-3-yl]-1-oxa-2-azaspiro[4.5] deca-2,6,9-triene-3-carboxamide (31)

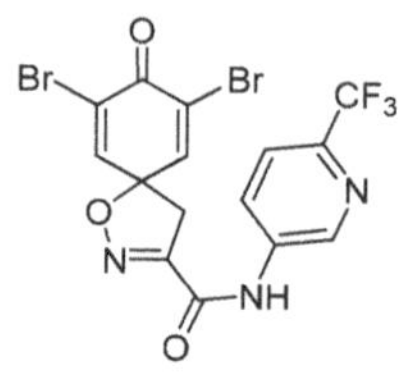

General procedure **A** was followed to give the compound **31** as an off-white amorphous solid (0.015 g, 13%). ^{1}H NMR (400 MHz, d_6-acetone) δ 10.09 (br s, 1H), 9.14 (d, J = 2.4 Hz, 1H), 8.55 (dd, J = 8.7, 2.5 Hz, 1H), 7.87 (d, J = 8.6 Hz, 1H), 7.78 (s, 2H), 3.80 (s, 2H). ^{13}C NMR (101 MHz, d_6-acetone) δ 172.3, 158.7 (m), 155.8 (m), 146.7, 143.4 (q, $J_{C,F}$ = 34.7 Hz), 142.6 (m), 138.5 (m), 128.4 (m), 123.4, 122.8 (q, $J_{C,F}$ = 272.6 Hz), 121.9 (q, $J_{C,F}$ = 2.9 Hz), 87.5, 43.4. HRMS (ESI$^+$): calculated 495.8943 ($C_{15}H_9Br_2F_3N_3O_3$), found 495.8948. LC-MS: $[M + H]^+$ m/z 496 and 498 (t_R = 4.80 and 4.72 min), >91%.

8-Oxo-*N*-[2-(pyridin-2-yl)ethyl]-1-oxa-2-azaspiro[4.5]deca-2,6,9-triene-3-carboxamide (32)

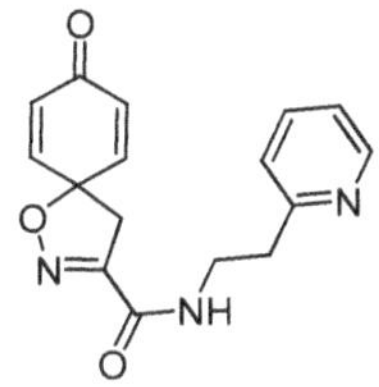

General procedure **A** was followed to give the compound **32** as an off-white amorphous solid (0.076 g, 91%). ^{1}H NMR (400 MHz, $CDCl_3$) δ 8.59–8.54 (m, 1H), 7.71 (app. t, 1H), 7.65 (td, J = 7.7, 1.8 Hz, 1H), 7.21–7.19 (m, 1H), 7.19–7.16 (m, 1H), 6.87–6.81 (m, 2H), 6.29–6.23 (m, 2H), 3.81 (dt, J = 6.8, 5.9 Hz, 2H), 3.39 (s, 2H), 3.07 (t, J = 6.3 Hz, 2H). ^{13}C NMR (101 MHz, $CDCl_3$) δ 184.5, 159.0, 158.6, 153.9, 149.4, 144.1, 137.0, 129.3, 123.6, 121.9, 82.7, 43.8, 38.6, 36.5. HRMS (ESI$^+$): calculated 298.1192 ($C_{16}H_{16}N_3O_3$), found 298.1191. LC-MS: $[M + H]^+$ m/z 298 (t_R = 0.74, salt and 1.15 min), >99%.

7,9-Dibromo-8-oxo-*N*-[2-(pyridin-2-yl)ethyl]-1-oxa-2-azaspiro[4.5]deca-2,6,9-triene-3-carboxamide (33)

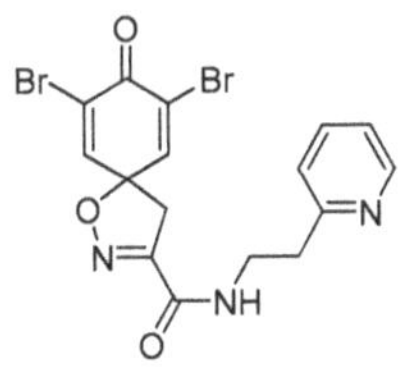

General procedure **B** was followed to give the compound **33** as a white amorphous solid (0.062 g, 24%). ^{1}H NMR (400 MHz, $CDCl_3$) δ 8.59–8.54 (m, 1H), 7.79 (app. t, 1H), 7.64 (td, J = 7.7, 1.8 Hz, 1H), 7.30 (s, 2H), 7.21–7.15 (m, 2H), 3.81 (q, J = 6.0 Hz, 2H), 3.47 (s, 2H), 3.06 (t, J = 6.2 Hz, 2H). ^{13}C NMR (101 MHz, $CDCl_3$) δ 171.5, 159.1, 158.0, 154.1, 149.5, 144.6, 136.9, 123.8, 123.5, 122.0, 85.8, 43.4, 38.7, 36.4. HRMS (ESI$^+$): calculated 453.9402 ($C_{16}H_{14}Br_2N_3O_3$), found 453.9403. LC-MS: $[M + H]^+$ m/z 454 (t_R = 2.27 min), >90%.

7,9-Dibromo-8-oxo-*N*-[2-(pyridin-3-yl)ethyl]-1-oxa-2-azaspiro[4.5]deca-2,6,9-triene-3-carboxamide (34)

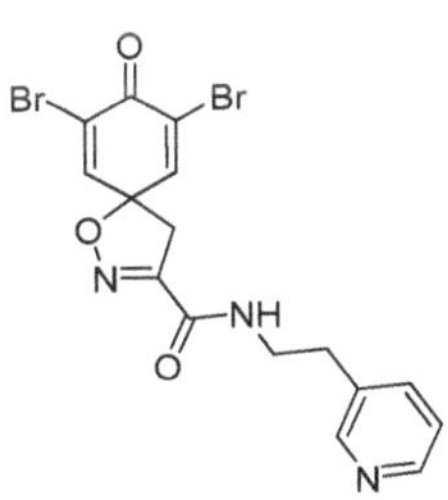

General procedure **A** was followed to give the compound **34** as an off-white solid (0.075 g, 39%). ^{1}H NMR (400 MHz, d_6-DMSO) δ 8.72 (t, J = 5.8 Hz, 1H), 8.44 (dq, J = 6.5, 2.6, 1.7 Hz, 2H), 7.80 (s, 2H), 7.66 (dt, J = 7.8, 2.0 Hz, 1H), 7.33 (ddd, J = 7.8, 4.8, 0.9 Hz, 1H), 3.54 (s, 2H), 3.48–3.38 (m, 2H), 2.83 (t, J = 7.2 Hz, 2H). ^{13}C NMR (101 MHz, d_6-DMSO) δ 171.6, 158.2, 154.9, 149.8, 147.5, 146.7, 146.7, 136.1, 134.6, 123.4, 121.6, 85.2, 43.1, 31.7. HRMS (ESI$^+$): calculated 492.9199 ($C_{16}H_{14}Br_2N_3O_3$), found 492.9197. Mp: 202–205 °C.

8-Oxo-*N*-(pyridin-3-ylmethyl)-1-oxa-2-azaspiro[4.5]deca-2,6,9-triene-3-carboxamide (35)

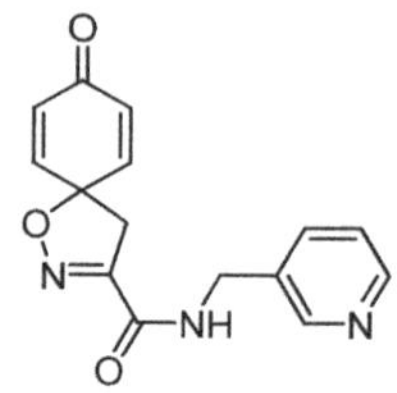

General procedure **B** was followed to give the compound **35** as a white amorphous solid (0.13 g, 61%). ^{1}H NMR (400 MHz, d_6-acetone) δ 8.59 (dd, J = 2.3, 0.9 Hz, 1H), 8.48 (dd, J = 4.8, 1.7 Hz, 1H), 8.36 (br s, 1H), 7.80–7.75 (m, 1H), 7.32 (ddd, J = 7.9, 4.8, 0.9 Hz, 1H), 7.14–7.05 (m, 2H), 6.25–6.15 (m, 2H), 4.55 (d, J = 6.3 Hz, 2H), 3.50 (s, 2H). ^{13}C NMR (101 MHz, d_6-acetone) δ 184.9, 159.9, 155.1, 150.3, 149.4, 145.9, 136.1, 135.4, 129.2, 124.2, 83.2, 44.2, 41.2. HRMS (ESI$^+$): calculated 284.1035 ($C_{15}H_{14}N_3O_3$), found 284.1032. LC-MS: $[M + H]^+$ m/z 284 (t_R = 0.68 min), >99%.

7,9-Dibromo-8-oxo-*N*-(pyridin-3-ylmethyl)-1-oxa-2-azaspiro[4.5]deca-2,6,9-triene-3-carboxamide (36)

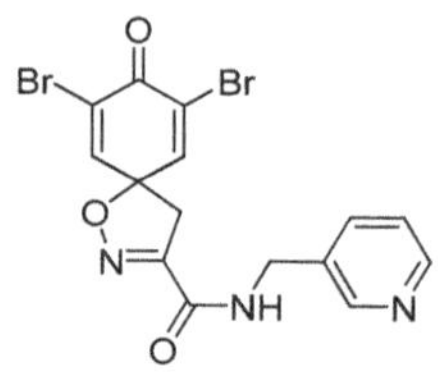

General procedure **B** was followed to give **36** as a white amorphous solid (0.068 g, 55%). ^{1}H NMR (400 MHz, d_6-DMSO) δ 8.53 (dd, J = 2.3, 0.9 Hz, 1H), 8.47 (dd, J = 4.8, 1.7 Hz, 1H), 7.83 (s, 2H), 7.74–7.68 (m, 1H), 7.36 (ddd, J = 7.8, 4.8, 0.9 Hz, 1H), 4.39 (s, 2H), 3.57 (s, 2H). ^{13}C NMR (101 MHz, d_6-DMSO) δ 171.6, 158.4, 158.4, 154.9, 154.8, 148.9, 148.2, 146.7, 135.3, 134.3, 134.3, 123.4, 121.6, 85.4, 43.0, 40.0. HRMS (ESI$^+$): calculated 439.9245 ($C_{15}H_{12}Br_2N_3O_3$), found 439.9244. LC-MS: $[M + H]^+$ m/z 440 (t_R = 2.08 min), >94%.

8-Oxo-*N'*-picolinoyl-1-oxa-2-azaspiro[4.5]deca-2,6,9-triene-3-carbohydrazide (37)

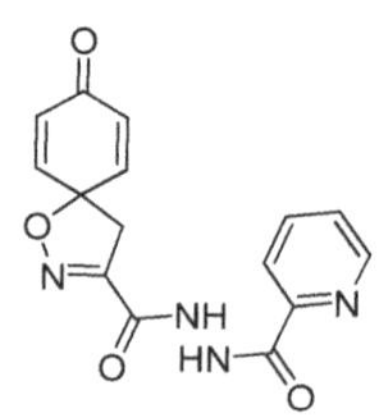

General procedure **A** was followed to give the compound **37** as an off-white solid (0.025 g, 16%). ^{1}H NMR (400 MHz, d_6-DMSO) δ 10.71 (br s, 1H), 10.65 (br s, 1H), 8.75–8.67 (m, 1H), 8.10–8.00 (m, 2H), 7.69–7.63 (m, 1H), 7.22–7.13 (m, 2H), 6.31–6.22 (m, 2H), 3.54 (s, 2H). ^{13}C NMR (101 MHz, d_6-DMSO) δ 184.5, 163.0, 157.8, 153.2, 149.1, 148.7, 145.6, 137.9, 128.2, 127.1, 122.5, 81.6, 43.3. HRMS (ESI$^+$): calculated 313.0937 ($C_{15}H_{13}N_4O_4$), found 313.0937. LC-MS: [M + H]+ m/z 313 (t_R = 1.51 min), >93%. Mp: 191–193 °C.

7,9-Dibromo-8-oxo-N′-picolinoyl-1-oxa-2-azaspiro[4.5]deca-2,6,9-triene-3-carbohydrazide (38)

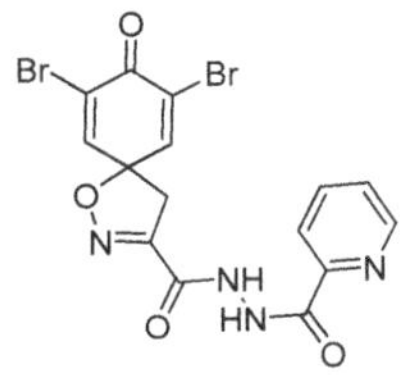

General procedure **A** was followed to give the compound **38** as an off-white solid (0.1 g, 50%). ^{1}H NMR (400 MHz, d_6-DMSO) δ 10.74 (s, 1H), 10.65 (s, 1H), 8.70 (dt, J = 4.7, 1.4 Hz, 1H), 8.08–7.99 (m, 2H), 7.88 (s, 2H), 7.71–7.63 (m, 1H), 3.63 (s, 2H). ^{13}C NMR (101 MHz, d_6-DMSO) δ 171.7, 163.0, 157.5, 153.6, 149.0, 148.6, 146.7, 137.9, 127.1, 122.5, 121.7, 85.2, 43.5. HRMS (ESI$^+$): calculated 470.9128 ($C_{15}H_{11}Br_2N_4O_4$), found 470.9129. LC-MS: [M + H]$^+$ m/z 471 and 473 (t_R = 3.14 and 3.11 min), >98%. Mp: 199–202 °C.

7,9-Dibromo-8-oxo-N′-picolinoyl-1-oxa-2-azaspiro[4.5]deca-2,6,9-triene-3-carbohydrazide (39)

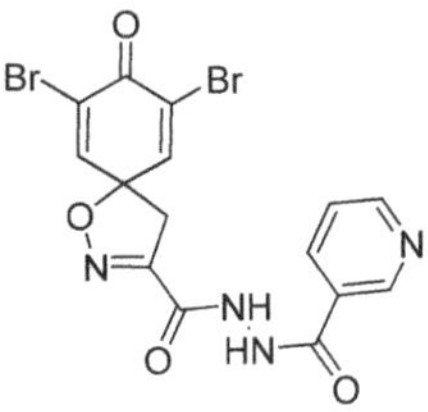

General procedure **A** was followed to give the compound **39** as an off-white solid (0.025 g, 14%). ^{1}H NMR (400 MHz, d_6-DMSO) δ 10.73 (br s, 2H), 9.06–9.01 (m, 1H), 8.78 (dd, J = 4.9, 1.7 Hz, 1H), 8.23 (ddd, J = 8.0, 2.3, 1.7 Hz, 1H), 7.88 (s, 2H), 7.62–7.53 (m, 1H), 3.64 (s, 2H). ^{13}C NMR (101 MHz, d_6-DMSO) δ 171.6, 164.1, 157.7, 153.5, 152.6, 148.4, 146.6, 135.2, 128.0, 123.7, 121.77, 85.2, 43.0. HRMS (ESI$^+$): calculated 470.9128 ($C_{15}H_{11}Br_2N_4O_4$), found 470.9127. LC-MS: [M + H]$^+$ m/z 471 and 473 (t_R = 2.48 and 2.37 min), >99%. Mp: 163–166 °C.

N-[3-(4-Chlorophenyl)-1-methyl-1H-pyrazol-5-yl]-8-oxo-1-oxa-2-azaspiro[4.5]deca-2,6,9-triene-3-carboxamide (40)

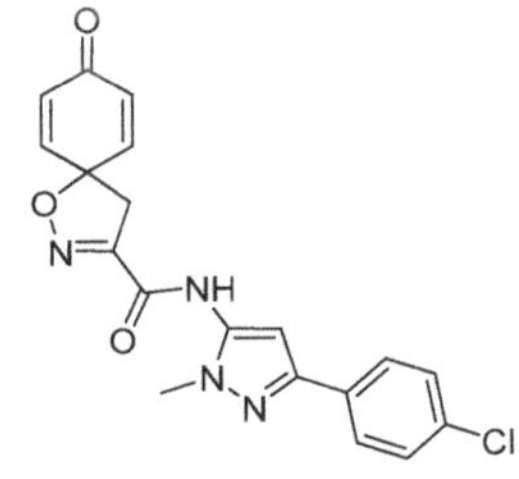

General procedure **A** was followed to give the compound **40** as an off-white solid (0.021 g, 18%). ^{1}H NMR (400 MHz, $CDCl_3$) δ 8.25 (br s, 1H), 7.74–7.68 (m, 2H), 7.40–7.33 (m, 2H), 6.91–6.87 (m, 2H), 6.67 (s, 1H), 6.36–6.31 (m, 2H), 3.86 (s, 3H), 3.48 (s, 2H). ^{13}C NMR (101 MHz, $CDCl_3$) δ 184.0, 156.2, 152.9, 149.2, 143.1, 134.9, 133.7, 131.5, 129.6, 128.8, 126.6, 96.9, 83.8, 42.8, 35.8. HRMS (ESI$^+$): calculated 383.0911 ($C_{19}H_{16}ClN_4O_3$), found 383.0911. LC-MS: [M + H]$^+$ m/z 383 and 385 (t_R = 4.21 and 4.14min), >99%.

7,9-Dibromo-*N*-[3-(4-chlorophenyl)-1-methyl-1*H*-pyrazol-5-yl]-8-oxo-1-oxa-2-azaspiro[4.5] deca-2,6,9-triene-3-carboxamide (41)

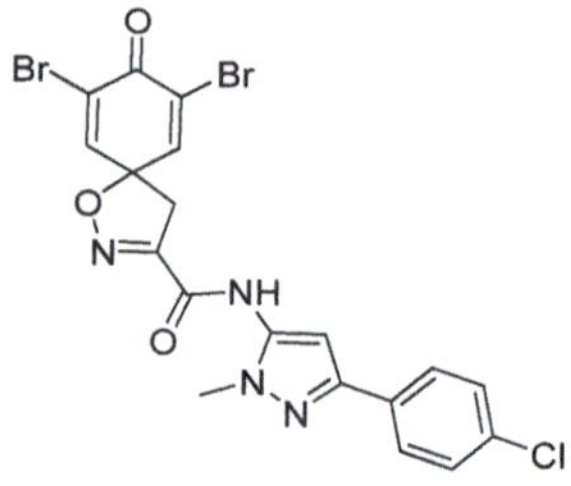

General procedure **A** was followed to give the compound **41** as an off-white solid (0.075 g, 35%). ^{1}H NMR (400 MHz, d_6-DMSO) δ 10.74 (br s, 1H), 7.88 (s, 2H), 7.85–7.76 (m, 2H), 7.50–7.42 (m, 2H), 3.74 (s, 3H), 3.65 (s, 2H). ^{13}C NMR (101 MHz, d_6-DMSO) δ 171.6, 157.6, 154.6, 147.1, 146.4, 136.4, 132.0, 132.0, 128.7, 126.5, 121.9, 98.3, 85.9, 42.8, 36.0. Mp: 251–254 °C. HRMS (ESI$^+$): calculated 538.9121 ($C_{19}H_{14}Br_2ClN_4O_3$), found 538.9120. LC-MS: $[M + H]^+$ m/z 541 (t_R = 5.29 min), >99%.

7,9-Dibromo-8-oxo-*N*-(4,5,6,7-tetrahydrobenzo[d]thiazol-2-yl)-1-oxa-2-azaspiro[4.5]deca-2,6,9-triene-3-carboxamide (42)

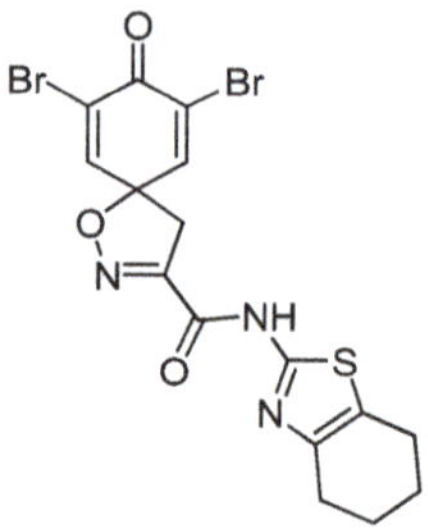

General procedure **A** was followed to give the compound **42** as a pale yellow solid (0.085 g, 40%). ^{1}H NMR (400 MHz, d_6-acetone) δ 10.92 (br s, 1H), 7.78 (s, 2H), 3.79 (s, 2H), 2.72–2.69 (m, 2H), 2.62–2.59 (m, 2H), 1.84 (p, J = 3.2 Hz, 4H). ^{13}C NMR (101 MHz, d_6-acetone) δ 172.29, 157.75, 155.14, 155.10, 146.75, 145.21, 123.69, 123.34, 87.35, 43.40, 29.84, 26.92, 24.02, 23.67, 23.33. HRMS (ESI$^+$): calculated 487.9102 ($C_{16}H_{14}Br_2N_3O_3S$), found 487.9109. LC-MS: $[M + H]^+$ m/z 488 and 490 (t_R = 4.92 and 5.03 min), >99%. Mp: 185–190 °C.

5. Conclusions

In summary, the highest cytotoxicity against the A-375 cell line was observed in 2,4-dichloro compound **18** (CC_{50} 0.4 ± 0.3 µM, SI 2) and the highest SI (2.4) was observed for the pyridin-2-yl derivative **29** and hydrazide analog of 2-picoline **37**. The results of these spirocyclic clavatadine analogs provide a path for further mechanistic studies and optimization of simplified spirocyclic bromotyrosine derivatives to understand the elements of their SARs and improve the selectivity.

Supplementary Materials: The following are available online at https://www.mdpi.com/article/10.3390/md19070400/s1. Experimental data: ^{1}H and ^{13}C spectra of all compounds.

Author Contributions: The manuscript was written with contributions from all authors. Conceptualization; P.S.K., P.A.P., P.T., T.B. and P.I.; synthesis, P.A.P., T.B. and A.L.; biological screening, P.I., H.M. and T.B.; writing—original draft preparation, P.A.P., P.S.K., P.I. and T.B.; writing—review and editing, P.S.K., P.A.P., P.I., T.B., J.Y.-K. and P.T.; supervision, P.S.K. and P.T.; funding acquisition: P.S.K., P.T. and J.Y.-K. All authors have read and agreed to the published version of the manuscript.

Funding: This research was supported by the Academy of Finland (Grant Nos. 307464 and 315937). We confirm we support the Open access funding provided by University of Helsinki.

Institutional Review Board Statement: Not applicable.

Data Availability Statement: Data is contained within the article and Supplementary Material.

Acknowledgments: We thank Andrew Neal for revising the language, Antti Lehtinen for the synthesis assistance, Nina Sipari from the Viikki Metabolomics Unit (Helsinki Institute of Life Science, University of Helsinki; Biocenter Finland) for her expertise with the LC-MS analyses, and the DDCB core facility supported by the University of Helsinki (HiLIFE) and Biocenter Finland for access to bioactivity testing facilities. We confirm we support the Open access funding provided by University of Helsinki.

Conflicts of Interest: The authors declare no competing financial interest.

References

1. Newman, D.J.; Cragg, G.M.J. Natural Products as Sources of New Drugs over the Nearly Four Decades from 01/1981 to 09/2019. *J. Nat. Prod.* **2020**, *83*, 770–803. [CrossRef] [PubMed]
2. Kiuru, P.; D'Auria, V.M.; Muller, C.D.; Tammela, P.; Vuorela, H.; Yli-Kauhaluoma, J. Exploring Marine Resources for Bioactive Compounds. *Planta Med.* **2014**, *80*, 1234–1246. [CrossRef] [PubMed]
3. Khalifa, S.M.; Elias, N.; Farag, M.A.; Chen, L.; Saeed, A.; Hegazy, M.F.; Moustafa, M.S.; Abd El-Wahed, A.; Al-Mousawi, S.M.; Musharraf, S.G.; et al. Marine Natural Products: A Source of Novel Anticancer Drugs. *Mar. Drugs* **2019**, *17*, 491. [CrossRef] [PubMed]
4. Jimenez, P.C.; Wilke, D.V.; Branco, P.C.; Bauermeister, A.; Rezende-Teixeira, P.; Gaudêncio, S.P.; Costa-Lotufo, L.V. Enriching Cancer Pharmacology with Drugs of Marine Origin. *Brit. J. Pharmacol.* **2020**, *177*, 3–27. [CrossRef] [PubMed]
5. Marine Pharmacology, Approved Marine Drugs. Available online: https://www.marinepharmacology.org/approved (accessed on 26 May 2021).
6. Calcabrini, C.; Catanzaro, E.; Bishayee, A.; Turrini, E.; Fimognari, C. Marine Sponge Natural Products with Anticancer Potential: An Updated Review. *Mar. Drugs* **2017**, *15*, 310. [CrossRef] [PubMed]
7. Peng, J.; Li, J.; Hamann, M.T. The Marine Bromotyrosine Derivatives. In *The Alkaloids: Chemistry and Biology*; Cordell, G.A., Ed.; Elsevier: Amsterdam, The Netherlands, 2007; Volume 61, pp. 59–262.
8. Niemann, H.; Marmann, A.; Lin, W.; Proksch, P. Sponge Derived Bromotyrosines: Structural Diversity through Natural Combinatorial Chemistry. *Nat. Prod. Commun.* **2015**, *10*. [CrossRef]
9. Buchanan, M.; Carroll, A.; Wessling, D.; Hooper, J.; Quinn, R.J. Clavatadines C–E, Guanidine Alkaloids from the Australian Sponge *Suberea clavata*. *J. Nat. Prod.* **2009**, *72*, 973–975. [CrossRef] [PubMed]
10. Badart, M.; Squires, C.; Baird, S.; Hawkins, B. The Synthesis of Clavatadine C. *Tetrahedron Lett.* **2016**, *57*, 5108–5111. [CrossRef]
11. Kaur, K.; Kumar, V.; Sharma, A.K.; Gupta, G.K. Isoxazoline Containing Natural Products as Anticancer Agents: A Review. *Eur. J. Med. Chem.* **2014**, *77*, 121–133. [CrossRef] [PubMed]
12. Drechsel, A.; Helm, J.; Ehrlich, H.; Pantovic, S.; Bornstein, S.R.; Bechmann, N. Anti-Tumor Activity vs. Normal Cell Toxicity: Therapeutic Potential of the Bromotyrosines Aerothionin and Homoaerothionin In Vitro. *Mar. Drugs* **2020**, *18*, 236. [CrossRef] [PubMed]
13. Zheng, Y.J.; Tice, C.M. The Utilization of Spirocyclic Scaffolds in Novel Drug Discovery. *Expert Opin. Drug Dis.* **2016**, *11*, 831–834. [CrossRef] [PubMed]
14. Bhat, C.; Ilina, P.; Tilli, I.; Voráčová, M.; Bruun, T.; Barba, V.; Hribernik, N.; Lillsunde, K.-E.; Mäki-Lohiluoma, E.; Rüffer, T.; et al. Synthesis and Antiproliferative Activity of Marine Bromotyrosine Purpurealidin I and Its Derivatives. *Mar. Drugs* **2018**, *16*, 481. [CrossRef] [PubMed]
15. Yajun, Z.; Tice, C.; Singh, S. The Use of Spirocyclic Scaffolds in Drug Discovery. *Bioorg. Med. Chem. Lett.* **2014**, *24*, 3673–3682. [CrossRef]
16. Wang, S.; Dong, G.; Sheng, C. Structural Simplification: An Efficient Strategy in Lead Optimization. *Acta Pharm. Sin. B* **2019**, *9*, 880–901. [CrossRef]
17. Banyu Pharmaceutical Co., Ltd. Spiroisoxazoline Derivatives. Japanese Patent JP 59176268 A, 28 March 1983.
18. Banyu Pharmaceutical Co., Ltd. Spiroisoxazoline Derivatives. Japanese Patent JP 59190978 A, 13 April 1983.
19. Badisa, R.B.; Darling-Reed, S.F.; Joseph, P.; Cooperwood, J.S.; Latinwo, L.M.; Goodman, C.B. Selective Cytotoxic Activities of Two Novel Synthetic Drugs on Human Breast Carcinoma MCF-7 Cells. *Anticancer Res.* **2009**, *29*, 2993–2996. [PubMed]
20. Fulda, S.; Debatin, K.M. Extrinsic versus Intrinsic Apoptosis Pathways in Anticancer Chemotherapy. *Oncogene* **2006**, *25*, 4798–4811. [CrossRef] [PubMed]
21. Binnewerg, B.; Schubert, M.; Voronkina, A.; Muzychka, L.; Wysokowski, M.; Petrenko, I.; Djurović, M.; Kovalchuk, V.; Tsurkan, M.; Martinovic, R.; et al. Biomaterials: Biomimetic and Pharmacological Potential of Cultivated *Aplysina aerophoba* Marine Demosponge. *Mater. Sci. Eng. C* **2020**, *109*, 110566. [CrossRef] [PubMed]

22. Bassetto, M.; Ferla, S.; Pertusati, F. Polyfluorinated Groups in Medicinal Chemistry. *Future Med. Chem.* **2015**, *7*, 527–546. [CrossRef] [PubMed]
23. López-Lázaro, M. A Simple and Reliable Approach for Assessing Anticancer Activity In Vitro. *Curr. Med. Chem.* **2015**, *22*, 1324–1334. [CrossRef] [PubMed]
24. Rerat, V.; Dive, G.; Cordi, A.; Tucker, G.; Bareille, R.; Amedee, J.; Bordenave, L.; Marchand-Brynaert, J. αvβ3 Integrin-targeting Arg-Gly-Asp (RGD) Peptidomimetics Containing Oligoethylene Glycol (OEG) Spacers. *J. Med. Chem.* **2009**, *52*, 7029–7043. [CrossRef] [PubMed]

marine drugs

MDPI

Article

Semi-Synthesis, Cytotoxic Evaluation, and Structure—Activity Relationships of Brefeldin A Derivatives with Antileukemia Activity

Xu-Xiu Lu [1,2,†], Yao-Yao Jiang [1,2,†], Yan-Wei Wu [1,2], Guang-Ying Chen [3], Chang-Lun Shao [1,2], Yu-Cheng Gu [4], Ming Liu [1,2,5,*] and Mei-Yan Wei [1,6,*]

1 Key Laboratory of Marine Drugs, The Ministry of Education of China, School of Medicine and Pharmacy, Ocean University of China, Qingdao 266003, China; xuxiulu@126.com (X.-X.L.); jiangyaoyao1226@163.com (Y.-Y.J.); wuyanwei1214@163.com (Y.-W.W.); shaochanglun@163.com (C.-L.S.)

2 Laboratory for Marine Drugs and Bioproducts, Qingdao National Laboratory for Marine Science and Technology, Qingdao 266200, China

3 Key Laboratory of Tropical Medicinal Resource Chemistry of Ministry of Education, College of Chemistry and Chemical Engineering, Hainan Normal University, Haikou 571158, China; chgying123@163.com

4 Syngenta Jealott's Hill International Research Centre, Bracknell RG42 6EY, UK; yucheng.gu@syngenta.com

5 State Key Laboratory for Chemistry and Molecular Engineering of Medicinal Resources, Guangxi Normal University, Guilin 541001, China

6 College of Food Science and Engineering, Ocean University of China, Qingdao 266003, China

* Correspondence: lmouc@ouc.edu.cn (M.L.); mywei95@126.com (M.-Y.W.); Tel.: +86-532-8203-1980 (M.L.); +86-532-8203-1381 (M.-Y.W.)

† These authors contributed equally to this work.

Citation: Lu, X.-X.; Jiang, Y.-Y.; Wu, Y.-W.; Chen, G.-Y.; Shao, C.-L.; Gu, Y.-C.; Liu, M.; Wei, M.-Y. Semi-Synthesis, Cytotoxic Evaluation, and Structure—Activity Relationships of Brefeldin A Derivatives with Antileukemia Activity. *Mar. Drugs* **2022**, *20*, 26. https://doi.org/10.3390/md20010026

Academic Editors: Marc Diederich and Celso Alves

Received: 14 November 2021
Accepted: 22 December 2021
Published: 24 December 2021

Publisher's Note: MDPI stays neutral with regard to jurisdictional claims in published maps and institutional affiliations.

Copyright: © 2021 by the authors. Licensee MDPI, Basel, Switzerland. This article is an open access article distributed under the terms and conditions of the Creative Commons Attribution (CC BY) license (https://creativecommons.org/licenses/by/4.0/).

Abstract: Brefeldin A (**1**), a potent cytotoxic natural macrolactone, was produced by the marine fungus *Penicillium* sp. (HS-N-29) from the medicinal mangrove *Acanthus ilicifolius*. Series of its ester derivatives **2–16** were designed and semi-synthesized, and their structures were characterized by spectroscopic methods. Their cytotoxic activities were evaluated against human chronic myelogenous leukemia K562 cell line in vitro, and the preliminary structure–activity relationships revealed that the hydroxy group played an important role. Moreover, the monoester derivatives exhibited stronger cytotoxic activity than the diester derivatives. Among them, brefeldin A 7-*O*-2-chloro-4,5-difluorobenzoate (**7**) exhibited the strongest inhibitory effect on the proliferation of K562 cells with an IC_{50} value of 0.84 μM. Further evaluations indicated that **7** induced cell cycle arrest, stimulated cell apoptosis, inhibited phosphorylation of BCR-ABL, and thereby inactivated its downstream AKT signaling pathway. The expression of downstream signaling molecules in the AKT pathway, including mTOR and p70S6K, was also attenuated after **7**-treatment in a dose-dependent manner. Furthermore, molecular modeling of **7** docked into **1** binding site of an ARF1–GDP-GEF complex represented well-tolerance. Taken together, **7** had the potential to be served as an effective antileukemia agent or lead compound for further exploration.

Keywords: brefeldin A; ester derivative; chronic myelogenous leukemia; BCR-ABL; proliferation inhibition; molecular modeling

1. Introduction

Chronic myelogenous leukemia (CML) is characterized by the translocation of chromosomes 9 and 22, which generates the BCR-ABL fusion oncogene with constitutively active tyrosine kinase [1]. This aberrant tyrosine kinase exerts its oncogenic function for malignant transformation mainly by activating multiple cellular signaling pathways, including the PI3K/AKT, MAPK/ERK, and JAK-STAT, which also contributes to the insensitivity of chemotherapy drugs [2,3]. Imatinib mesylate (Gleevec) was selected as the first tyrosine kinase inhibitor (TKI) that has been proven to be an effective agent in CML treatment.

However, the emergence of drug resistance is becoming a common problem for the failure of imatinib treatment [4]. The second-generation TKIs, such as nilotinib, dasatinib, and bosutinib, were then employed to overcome acquired resistance to imatinib [5–7]. Though they show a significant effect on imatinib-resistant patients, the effect on those patients carrying T315I mutation is limited [8]. Therefore, novel agents to improve therapeutic outcomes of CML are needed urgently.

Marine secondary metabolites with novel structures and wide-ranging biological activities have been proven to be rich sources of chemical entities for drug discovery [9,10]. Brefeldin A (BFA, **1**, Figure 1), a 13-membered macrolactone with a cyclopentane substituent, was first isolated from *Penicillium decumbens* in 1958 [11] and subsequently identified as a metabolite from the marine-derived fungus *Penicillium* sp. PSU-F44 [12], *Penicillium janthinellum* DT-F29 [13,14], as well as *Penicillium* sp. (CGMCC No.17193) recently published by our group [15], which is the same as marine fungus *Penicillium* sp. (HS-N-29) described here. BFA (**1**) impairs the small G-protein ARF1 (ADP ribosylation factor 1) activation by hindering its association with its large guanine nucleotide exchange factor (GEF) enzyme [16,17], which induces the breakdown of vesicle-mediated protein transport, thus, causes the Golgi complex redistributing into the endoplasmic reticulum (ER) [18–20]. Structural insights into the uncompetitive inhibitory mechanism of **1** conduct to an abortive pentameric ARF1–Mg^{2+}–GDP–BFA–Sec7 complex, and **1** was described as an interfacial inhibitor [21]. Previous studies reported that **1** showed obvious anticancer activity in a variety of cancers, including colorectal, prostate, lung, and breast cancers [22,23], which has been touted as a promising lead molecule for anticancer drug development. However, **1** showed some undesirable limitations due to its low bioavailability, high toxicity, and poor pharmacokinetics [24,25]. Therefore, it is of great necessity to synthesize the derivatives of **1** with kept or enhanced potency and decreased toxicity simultaneously. In fact, a number of derivatives of **1** have been reported in conjunction with anticancer investigations [25–31]. The existing information on structure–activity relationships (SARs) of **1** indicated the significant influences of α, β-unsaturated lactone, alkenes, and conformational rigidity of the molecule on its cytotoxicity [26,30]. Most of the derivatives generated in the way that alters the above moiety of the structure showed no or reduced biological activity compared with **1** [27,28]. However, sulfide and sulfoxide prodrugs of **1** showed promising antitumor effects both in vitro and in vivo due to its yield of an intact pharmacophore of **1** after drug metabolism [29]. Moreover, C15-substituted analogs were also reported to exhibit significant activities tested at the NCI [31]. Previous studies outlined the ester derivatives at 4-OH or 7-OH group of **1** generally displayed excellent cytotoxicity against different cancer cell lines [23,25]. However, the lack of a clear understanding of **1** and its derivatives in CML cells inhibition limits its usefulness as a lead compound for antileukemia agents. The detailed mechanism supporting the antileukemia effect of **1** and its derivatives needs to be further elucidated. That provides a rational and effective strategy for structure modification and mechanism study.

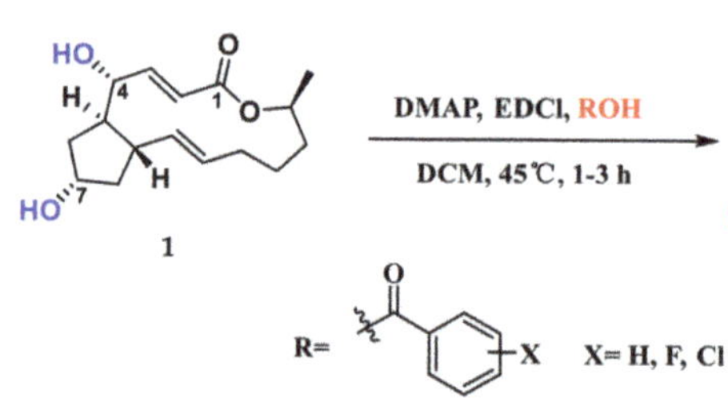

Figure 1. Synthesis of the derivatives **2–16** of brefeldin A (**1**).

In the present study, the crude extracts of 55 marine fungal strains from the medicinal mangrove *Acanthus ilicifolius* were evaluated, and the potent natural compound **1** was discovered in the extract of the *Penicillium* sp. (HS-N-29) strain under the guidance of cytotoxic activity. Our focus was to design and synthesize a series of new derivatives (**2–16**) of **1**, and evaluate their cytotoxicities against K562 cells. Of them, compound 7, the most active one, arrested cell cycle at G0/G1 phase, stimulated caspase-dependent cell apoptosis, inhibited phosphorylation of BCR-ABL, and thereby inactivated its downstream AKT signaling pathway. The present results provided evidence that **7** exhibited the great potential to be developed as an antileukemia agent.

2. Results and Discussion

2.1. Chemistry

The excellent cytotoxic activity, along with poor pharmacokinetic properties of **1**, prompted us to semi-synthesize a series of derivatives to explore the potency of this class of molecules. Natural **1** was obtained by fermentation of the *Penicillium* sp. (HS-N-29) strain. Detailly, the fungal strain HS-N-29 was cultivated in a PDB medium (200.0 g of potato, 20.0 g of glucose in 1 L of seawater) at 28 °C with shaking for 2 weeks, and subsequently extracted with EtOAc. The EtOAc extract was subjected to silica gel and then recrystallized to produce compound 1. The structure of 1 was confirmed by NMR data analysis compared with the literature [30] and single-crystal X-ray diffraction analysis.

Given that both the aryl esters and C15-aryl-substituted analogs of **1** displayed efficient cytotoxicities [25,31], as well as halogen substitution played an important role in the regulation of diverse bioactivities of compounds [32,33], the semi-synthesis of various halogenated benzoic acids of **1** was carried out and outlined in Figure 1. Simply, compound **1** reacted with different halogen-substituted benzoic acids in the presence of 4-dimethylaminopyridine (DMAP, catalyst) and 1-ethyl-3-(3-dimethylaminopropyl) carbodiimide hydrochloride (EDCl, dehydrating agent) afforded thirteen new ester derivatives **4–16** and two known derivatives **2–3**. All of them were separated by using repeated reversed-phase silica column chromatography combined with semi-preparative HPLC. The structures of new compounds were characterized by ^{1}H NMR, ^{13}C NMR, and HRESIMS. It is worth noting that the position of esterification at 4-OH or 7-OH was the key point to structural identification, which was distinguished by the changes of their corresponding chemical shift (δ) values of H-4 or H-7. It followed such a regular pattern that the δ value of H-4 or H-7 shifted by nearly 1–1.5 ppm downfield after esterification. Three corresponding derivatives **7**, **8**, and **9** of 2-chloro-4,5-difluorobenzoic acid were used to illustrate the detailed structural determination (Figure 2). In detail, comparisons of their partial ^{1}H NMR spectra with that of **1** in the interval of δ_H 4.0–8.0 ppm, where the key proton signals appeared, the chemical shift of H-7 in 7-monoester derivative **7** shifted from 4.34 to 5.38 ppm with a slight deviation on the chemical shift of H-4 (δ_H 4.16 in **7**, δ_H 4.11 in **1**). Meanwhile, the chemical shift of H-4 in 4-monoester derivative **8** shifted from 4.11 to 5.48 ppm with no difference in the chemical shift of H-7 (δ_H 4.33 in **8**, δ_H 4.33 in **1**). The chemical shifts of H-4 and H-7 in 4,7-diester derivative **9** shifted from 4.11 to 5.56 ppm and 4.34 to 5.41 ppm, respectively. On this basis, the structures of all the derivatives were confirmed.

2.2. Biological Evaluation

2.2.1. Cytotoxic Activity

The cytotoxicity of the natural product **1** together with its derivatives **2–16** were evaluated against human chronic myelogenous leukemia cell line K562 with doxorubicin as a positive control. The results showed that the mono-substituted derivatives displayed moderate to strong cytotoxicity against K562 cells with IC_{50} values ranging from 0.84 to 2.49 μM (Table 1). Strikingly, the inhibitory effects of **4**, **5**, and **7** were superior to that of other compounds (**2**, **6**, **8**, **10**, **11**, **13**, and **14**) with the IC_{50} values of 0.91, 0.91, and 0.84 μM, respectively. Generally, the activity of 4-mono- or 7-monoester derivatives evidenced no obvious distinction. Decreased cytotoxicity was observed on derivatives **3**, **9**, **12**, and **15** with di-substitution of both -OH groups at positions C4 and C7, indicating that the -OH groups played an important role in cytotoxic property. Moreover, in comparison to **2**, a stronger activity was observed on **5**, **7**, **10**, and **13**, which indicated that the introduction of fluorine or chlorine atoms contributed to the cytotoxicity to some extent, but it was not affected by the number and position of halogen atoms. Significantly, derivative **7** with the structure featuring a 2-chloro-4,5-difluoro-substituted benzene ring greatly suppressed K562 cells growth with an IC_{50} value of 0.84 μM, which was better than that of other compounds and slightly lower than that of **1** (IC_{50} ratio **7**/**1** = 3.5, in the same order of magnitude). Given that the aqueous solubility of the compound may be more important to be considered in terms of drug testing, as well as drug administration, the solubility measurement of **7** was also indicated. Strikingly, **7** possessed improved water solubility (220 μg/mL), which was more than 3-fold higher than that of **1** (72 μg/mL). Therefore, it represented a potential promising lead compound and encouraged us to further investigate the possible cellular mechanisms of **7**.

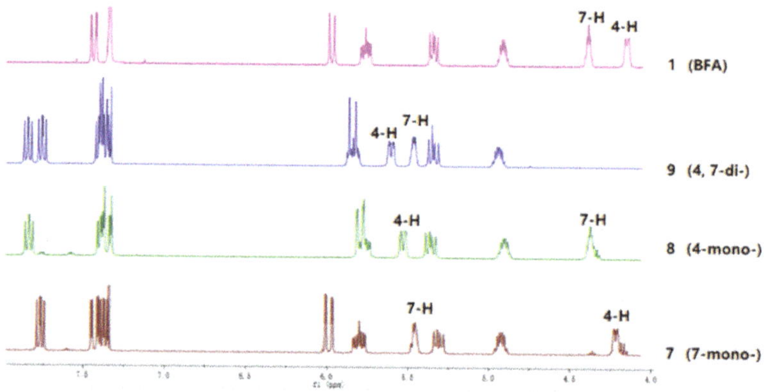

Figure 2. The partial stacking ^{1}H NMR spectra of **1** and its derivatives **7**–**9**.

2.2.2. Compound 7 Inhibited the Proliferation of K562 Cells

To elucidate the inhibitory efficacy of **7**, the cell viability was detected using an MTT assay. Cultured K562 cells were treated with **7** for 24, 48, and 72 h, and the data showed that the **7**-treated group markedly decreased the cell viability in a concentration- and time-dependent manner, with IC_{50} values of 6.69 and 0.84 μM at 48 and 72 h, respectively (Figure 3A). Meanwhile, the long-term effects of **7** on K562 cells proliferation were determined with a colony formation assay in soft agar, an in vitro indicator of malignancy. As shown in Figure 3B,C, treatment of K562 cells with **7** (0–2 μM) for 12 days dose-dependently reduced the formation of colonies, indicating the antileukemia activity of **7**. Collectively, these results indicated that **7** inhibited the proliferation of K562 cells in vitro.

2.2.3. Compound 7 Induced G0/G1 Phase Cell Cycle Arrest in K562 Cells

To explore the underlying mechanisms leading to growth inhibition further, we analyzed the effect of **7** on the cell cycle distribution of K562 cells. The results showed that **7** induced moderate G0/G1 phase arrest in K562 cells at the concentration of 4 μM. In the control group, the cells in G0/G1 phase represented 41.5%, and it increased to 54.3% in the **7**-treated group. Correspondingly, the cells in the S phase were decreased after being treated by **7** (Figure 4A,B). It is worth mentioning that was totally different from BFA inducing G2/M phase cell cycle arrest in K562 cells [34]. Collectively, cell cycle arrest in G0/G1 phase may at least in part account for **7**-induced proliferation inhibition in K562 cells.

Table 1. Cytotoxic activity of **1** and its derivatives **2–16**.

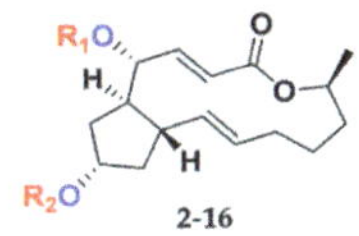

2-16

Compounds		IC50 (μM) [a]	Compounds		IC50 (μM) [a]
Structure	Substituents	K562	Structure	Substituents	K562
brefeldin A	**1** R1 = R2 = H	0.24	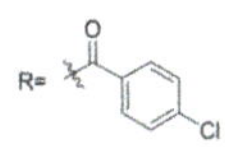	**10** R1 = H, R2 = R	1.07
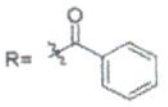	**2** R1 = H, R2 = R	2.49		**11** R1 = R, R2 = H	1.33
	3 R1 = R2 = R	4.71		**12** R1 = R2 = R	>10
	4 R1 = R, R2 = H	0.91	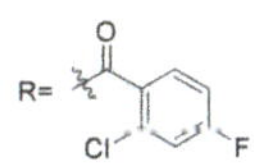	**13** R1 = H, R2 = R	1.11
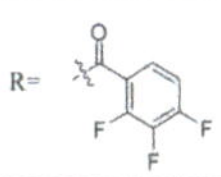	**5** R1 = H, R2 = R	0.91		**14** R1 = R, R2 = H	1.76
	6 R1 = R, R2 = H	1.22		**15** R1 = R2 = R	>10
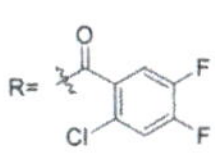	**7** R1 = H, R2 = R	0.84	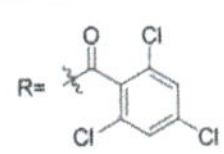	**16** R1 = H, R2 = R	>10
	8 R1 = R, R2 = H	2.06	Doxorubicin		0.06
	9 R1 = R2 = R	>10			

Note: [a] Results were the average of three independent experiments, each performed in duplicate. Standard deviations were less than ± 10%.

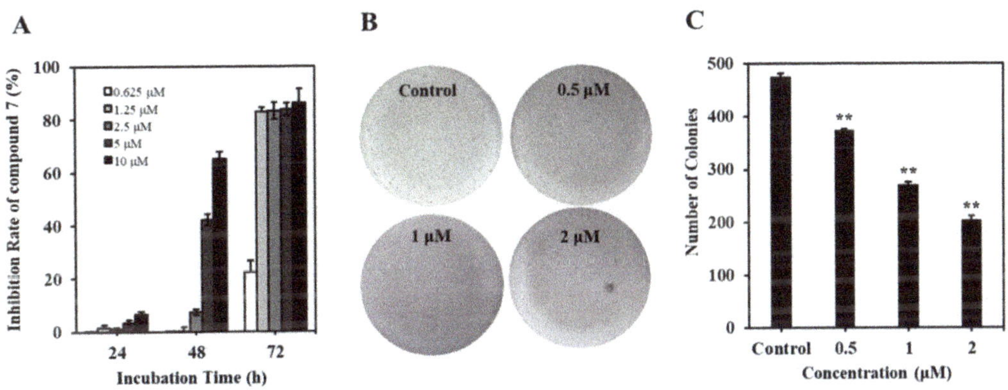

Figure 3. Compound **7** inhibited the proliferation of K562 cells. (**A**) Proliferation inhibition rates (%) of **7** against K562 cells. K562 cells were treated with **7** (0–10 μM) for 24–72 h. Cell viability was subjected to MTT assay. (**B**) Effect of **7** on soft agar colony formation of K562 cells. K562 cells were treated with 0–2 μM of **7** for indicated time. Cell proliferation was determined by colony formation. (**C**) Quantification of the colonies in soft agar. Values are expressed as mean ± SD of three independent experiments. ** $p < 0.01$, versus control.

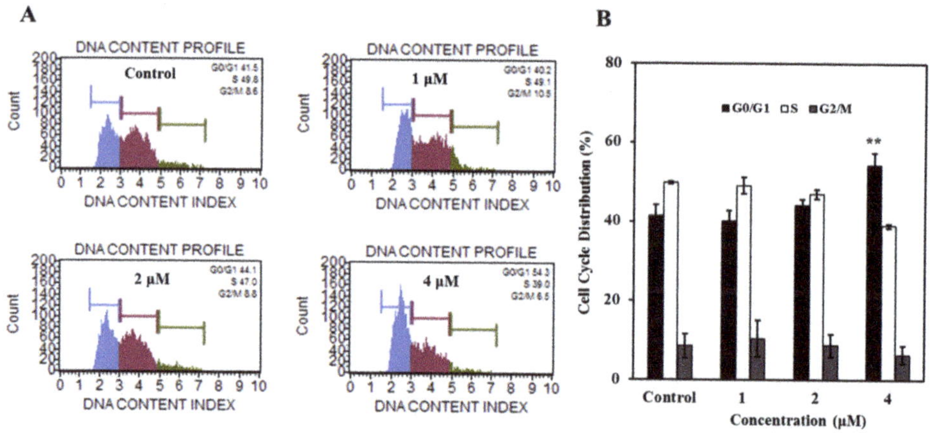

Figure 4. Compound **7** arrested cell cycle at G0/G1 phase. (**A**) Effect of compound **7** on cell cycle distribution. K562 cells after 36 h treatment with 0–4 µM of **7** were collected, washed, fixed, strained, and measured using Muse Cells Analyzer. (**B**) The histogram represented the cell cycle distributions in samples treated with or without **7**. Data are presented as mean ± SD of three independent experiments, ** $p < 0.01$, compared to the control.

2.2.4. Compound 7 Induced Caspase-Dependent Apoptosis in K562 Cells

To determine whether the proliferative inhibition induced by **7** was attributed to apoptosis, K562 cells were treated with **7** at different concentrations for 24 h, followed by Annexin V-PE/7-AAD staining measured with flow cytometry. Compound **7** induced dose-dependent apoptosis with the apoptotic cells increased from 4.14% (in the control group) to 24.31% at the concentration of 4 µM (Figure 5A,B). The proapoptotic effect of **7** was also evidenced by the elevated apoptosis markers C-Cas 3, C-Cas 9, and C-PARP (Figure 5C,D). To further confirm whether caspases activation was involved in **7**-induced cell apoptosis, pan-caspase inhibitor Z-VAD-fmk was used to observe the attenuation of apoptotic cells. Consist with our hypothesis, **7**-stimulated apoptosis was attenuated significantly in the presence of Z-VAD-fmk (Figure 5E). These results demonstrated that compound **7** induced caspase-dependent apoptosis in K562 cells.

2.2.5. Compound 7 Inactivated BCR-ABL and Affected Its Downstream Signaling Pathways in K562 Cells

With the aim of obtaining insights into the potential mechanisms underlying **7**-induced inhibition of cell proliferation in K562 cells, the activation of BCR-ABL was first examined since CML cells were highly dependent on the presence of BCR-ABL [35]. The results suggested that **7** downregulated the total and phosphorylation levels of BCR-ABL (Figure 6A), which consisted of BFA reported as a functional inhibitor and degrader of BCR-ABL in our previous work [34]. The alternation of the key downstream signaling pathways of BCR-ABL was further explored, including AKT/mTOR/S6K1 and MAPK/ERK pathways, which were also important intracellular signaling pathways in tumorigenesis [36]. BFA (**1**) was also found to decrease the downstream signaling pathways of BCR-ABL, such as p-Akt and p-STAT5, while increased p-ERK in K562 cells [34]. AKT/mTOR/S6K1 pathway is a critical way for enhanced survival of BCR-ABL in leukemia cells, and many anticancer agents exert their anticancer effect by blocking this signal pathway and consequently enhancing apoptosis [37–39]. Therefore, the inactivation of key molecules in this pathway could be effective in CML treatment. For example, PI3K inhibitor LY294002 sensitized CML cells to nilotinib and increased apoptosis [40]. PI3K and mTOR inhibitor NVP-BEZ235 in combination with imatinib or nilotinib induced significant proliferation inhibition and apoptosis in BCR-ABL-positive cell lines [41]. The Western blot analysis indicated that **7** significantly inhibited the phosphorylation of AKT, thus leading to the downstream inhibition of the signaling molecules mTOR and p70S6K (Figure 6B). However, **7** showed no significant effect against the ERK1/2 signaling pathway (Figure 6C). Combined with the differences with **1** in cell cycle arrest and signal regulation, this implied that **7** was not a simple derivative of **1** and may have its own unique mode of action. These results suggested that **7** exhibited its antileukemia effect via at least partially inhibiting the activation of BCR-ABL and subsequently inactivating the downstream AKT/mTOR/S6K1 signaling pathway in K562 cells.

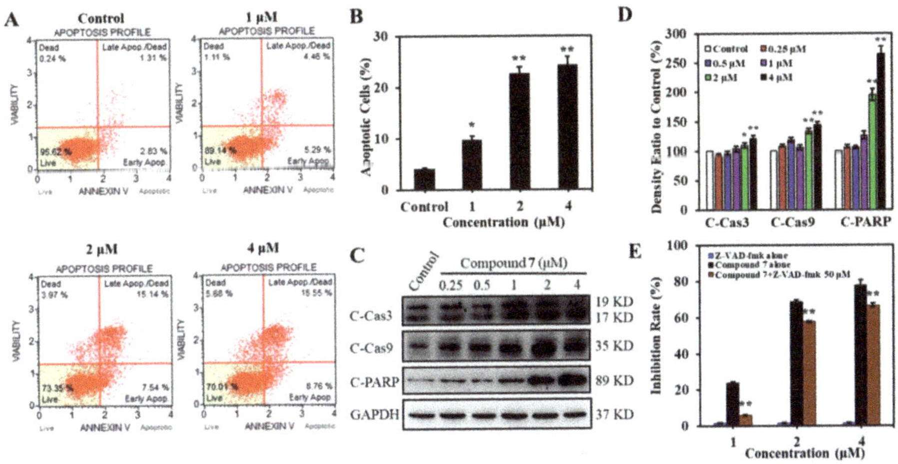

Figure 5. Compound **7** induced apoptosis in K562 cells. (**A**) Annexin V-PE/7-AAD staining in K562 cells incubated with 0–4 μM of **7** for 24 h was measured by Muse Cell Analyzer. (**B**) The bar graph depicted the percentage of apoptotic cells induced by **7**. Data are presented as mean ± SD for three independent experiments. * $p < 0.05$, ** $p < 0.01$, versus control. (**C**) Effect of **7** on apoptosis-related proteins. K562 cells were treated with vehicle or **7** at 0–4 μM for 36 h. Western blotting was performed to analyze the expression of C-Cas 3, C-Cas 9, and C-PARP. GAPDH was immunoblotted as a loading control. (**D**) Histograms show the relative abundance of the aimed bands to the control group. Data are presented as mean ± SD for three independent experiments. * $p < 0.05$, ** $p < 0.01$, versus control. (**E**) Pan caspase inhibitor Z-VAD-fmk significantly attenuated **7**-induced cell death. K562 cells were pretreated with or without Z-VAD-fmk for 1 h followed by incubation with various concentrations of **7** for 48 h, and then cells were subjected to MTT assay. Data are expressed as mean ± SD (n = 3). ** $p < 0.01$, versus **7** alone.

2.3. Molecular Modeling and Ligand Docking of Compound 7 into the Binding Site of 1

Given insights into the observation published by Renault et al. (PDB ID: 1R8Q) that the exquisite structural and chemical fit of **1** to the ARF–GDP-GEF interface accounted for its biological specificity [17], the structure of **7** was also investigated by molecular modeling to determine how well it would be tolerated in this pocket and whether it would fulfill the binding interactions necessary for inhibiting the GDP/GTP nucleotide exchange. Docking experiments were carried out with the X-ray crystal structure of the ARF1–GDP–Mg^{2+}–BFA–ARNO complex [17] using the software Molecular Operating Environment (MOE). Thus, **7** was modeled into the binding site between ARF1 and ARNO, overlapping with the structure of **1**, which was then deleted (Figure 7A). The result showed that compound **7** was well tolerated in the active site of **1** (Figure 7B,C) and achieved a little higher docking score than **1**, indicating a good geometric fit in the binding pocket.

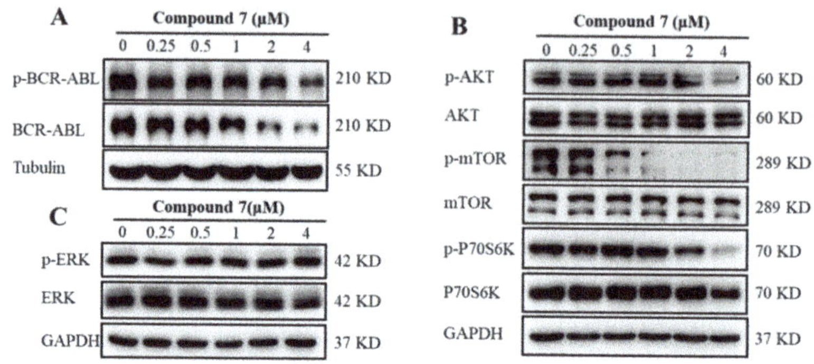

Figure 6. Compound **7** inhibited the activation of AKT/mTOR signaling pathway. (**A**) **7** induced the total and phosphorylated BCR-ABL inhibition. K562 cells were treated with indicated concentrations of **7** for 36 h, and the protein levels of BCR-ABL and p-BCR-ABL were subjected to Western blotting. (**B**) AKT/mTOR/S6K1 pathways were inactivated by **7**. Cells were treated as described before; then, the total and phosphorylated expression of AKT, mTOR, and p70S6K were evaluated by Western blotting. (**C**) Effect of **7** on ERK activation. K562 cells were treated as described above, and the protein levels of ERK and p-ERK were detected by Western blotting.

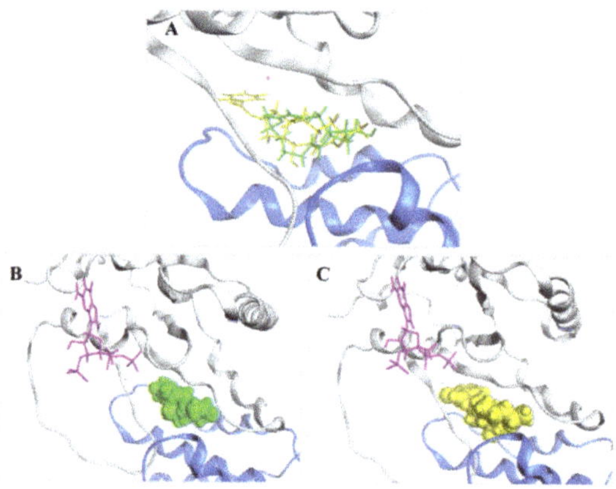

Figure 7. (**A**) Overlay of the docked pose of BFA (**1**, green) and BFA 7-*O*-2-chloro-4,5-difluorobenzoate (**7**, yellow) in the ARF1–GDP–GEF interface. (**B**) Crystal structure of **1** in the ARF1–GDP–GEF interface. (**C**) Model of **7** in the ARF1–GDP–GEF interface. Guanosine-3′-monophosphate-5′-diphosphate (GDP), purple; Mg^{2+} ion, pink; ARF1, gray; GEF, blue.

3. Materials and Methods

3.1. General Experimental Procedures

NMR spectra were recorded on a JEOL JEM-ECP NMR spectrometer. Chemical shifts δ are reported in ppm, using TMS as internal standard, and coupling constants (J) are in Hz. HRESIMS and ESIMS spectra were obtained from a Micromass Q-TOF spectrometer. Single-crystal data were measured on an Agilent Gemini Ultra diffractometer (Cu Kα radiation). UPLC-MS was performed on Waters UPLC® system (Waters Ltd., Milford, MA, USA) using a C18 column [(Waters Ltd.) ACQUITY UPLC® BEH C18, 2.1 × 50 mm, 1.7 μm; 0.5 mL/min] and ACQUITY QDa ESIMS scan from 150 to 1000 Da. Silica gel (Qing Dao Hai Yang Chemical Group Co., Qingdao, China; 200–300 mesh) and Sephadex LH-20 (Amersham Biosciences, Amersham, UK) were used for column chromatography (CC). TLC silica gel plates (Yan Tai Zi Fu Chemical Group Co., Yantai, China; G60, F-254) were used for thin-layer chromatography. Semi-preparative HPLC was operated on a Waters 1525 system using a semi-preparative C18 (Kromasil, 5 μm, 10 × 250 mm) column equipped with a Waters 2996 photodiode array detector, at a flow rate of 2.0 mL/min.

3.2. Fungal Material

The fungal strain *Penicillium* sp. (HS-N-29) was isolated from a piece of fresh tissue from the inner part of the medicinal mangrove *Acanthus ilicifolius* collected from the South China Sea. The strain was identified according to a molecular biological protocol by DNA amplification and sequencing of the ITS region as described in the literature [42]. The fungal strain was identified as *Penicillium* sp. with the accession number MW178203.

3.3. Fermentation, Extraction, and Isolation

The fungal strain was cultivated in 50 L of PDB medium (200.0 g of potato, 20.0 g of glucose in 1 L of seawater, in 500 mL Erlenmeyer flasks, each containing 250 mL of culture broth) at 28 °C with shaking for 2 weeks. The fungal culture was filtered and extracted three times with EtOAc. The EtOAc extract was combined and concentrated under vacuum to afford a dry crude extract (55.0 g). This extract was fractionated into five fractions (Fr.1–Fr.5) by silica gel VLC with a stepwise gradient of petroleum ether-EtOAc. Subsequently, Fr.3 (25.0 g) was separated into four subfractions (Fr.3-1–Fr.3-4) by silica gel CC (200–300 mesh) with a step gradient of petroleum ether-EtOAc from 3:1 to 0:1 (*v*/*v*). Fr.3-2 was further purified by semipreparative HPLC (70% MeCN–H_2O) and then recrystallized to produce **1** (2.3 g, Figures S1–S3).

3.4. General Synthetic Methods for Compounds **2–16**

Benzoic acid-derived reagent (1–2 equivalent) was added to a solution of **1** (50.0 mg, 0.18 mmol), DMAP (21.8 mg, 0.18 mmol), and EDCl (110.7 mg, 0.71 mmol) in 15 mL dry dichloromethane (DCM). The reaction mixture was stirred at 45 °C, and the progress of the reaction was monitored by silica gel TLC and UPLC-MS. After 1–3 h, the reaction mixture was quenched with water and diluted with DCM. The organic layer was separated, and the solvent was removed under reduced pressure. The residue was purified by silica gel CC followed by semi-preparative HPLC to yield unreacted **1** and derivatives **2–16** (Figures S4–S48).

Brefeldin A 7-*O*-benzoate (2): Known compound. Colorless oil; yield 11%; ^{1}H NMR (400 MHz, $CDCl_3$) δ 8.03–7.98 (2H, overlapped), 7.56 (1H, m), 7.47–7.43 (2H, overlapped), 7.37 (1H, dd, J = 15.7, 3.1 Hz), 5.94 (1H, dd, J = 15.7, 1.9 Hz), 5.73 (1H, m), 5.40 (1H, m), 5.26 (1H, dd, J = 15.2, 9.0 Hz), 4.86 (1H, m), 4.17 (1H, m), 2.53–2.33 (3H, overlapped), 2.06–1.96 (2H, overlapped), 1.92 (1H, m), 1.88–1.80 (2H, overlapped), 1.77–1.70 (2H, overlapped), 1.53 (1H, m), 1.26 (3H, d, J = 6.2 Hz), 0.96 (1H, m); ^{13}C NMR (100 MHz, $CDCl_3$) δ 166.3 (C = O), 166.3 (C = O), 151.6 (CH), 136.1 (CH), 133.1 (CH), 131.1 (CH), 130.6 (C), 129.7 (CH × 2), 128.5 (CH × 2), 117.9 (CH), 76.1 (CH), 76.0 (CH), 71.9 (CH), 52.6 (CH), 44.1 (CH), 40.3 (CH_2), 38.9 (CH_2), 34.2 (CH_2), 32.0 (CH_2), 26.8 (CH_2), 21.0 (CH_3). ESIMS m/z 407.4 $[M + Na]^+$.

Brefeldin A 4,7-*O*-dibenzoate (3): Known compound. Colorless oil; yield 43%; ^{1}H NMR (500 MHz, $CDCl_3$) δ 8.09–8.00 (4H, overlapped), 7.61–7.54 (2H, overlapped), 7.48–7.42 (4H, overlapped), 7.38 (1H, dd, J = 15.6, 3.4 Hz), 5.85–5.75 (2H, overlapped), 5.58 (1H, ddd, J = 10.4, 3.4, 1.9 Hz), 5.42 (1H, m), 5.34 (1H, dd, J = 15.2, 9.5 Hz), 4.87 (1H, m), 2.64 (1H, m), 2.48 (1H, m), 2.38 (1H, m), 2.28 (1H, m), 2.03 (1H, m), 1.92–1.84 (3H, overlapped), 1.81 (1H, m), 1.75 (1H, m), 1.55 (1H, m), 1.25 (3H, d, J = 6.1 Hz), 0.97 (1H, m); ^{13}C NMR (100 MHz, $CDCl_3$) δ 166.1 (C = O), 165.8 (C = O), 165.5 (C = O), 147.3 (CH), 135.9 (CH), 133.6 (CH), 133.1 (CH), 131.4 (CH), 130.6 (C), 129.9 (CH × 2), 129.7 (CH × 2), 129.6 (C), 128.7 (CH × 2), 128.6 (CH × 2), 118.7 (CH), 77.0 (CH), 76.2 (CH), 72.0 (CH), 50.5 (CH), 44.4 (CH), 40.3 (CH_2), 38.8 (CH_2), 34.2 (CH_2), 32.0 (CH_2), 26.7 (CH_2), 20.9 (CH_3). HRESIMS m/z 489.2263 $[M + H]^+$ (calcd. for $C_{30}H_{33}O_6^+$, 489.2272).

Brefeldin A 4-*O*-benzoate (4): Colorless oil; yield 33%; ^{1}H NMR (400 MHz, $CDCl_3$) δ 8.09–8.04 (2H, overlapped), 7.59 (1H, m), 7.49–7.42 (2H, overlapped), 7.35 (1H, dd, J = 15.7,

3.2 Hz), 5.82–5.68 (2H, overlapped), 5.50 (1H, ddd, J = 10.5, 3.3, 1.8 Hz), 5.34 (1H, dd, J = 15.2, 9.5 Hz), 4.84 (1H, m), 4.33 (1H, m), 2.50 (1H, m), 2.30 (1H, m), 2.24 (1H, m), 2.09–1.94 (2H, overlapped), 1.88–1.79 (2H, overlapped), 1.76–1.65 (2H, overlapped), 1.61–1.47 (2H, overlapped), 1.23 (3H, d, J = 6.2 Hz), 0.94 (1H, m); ^{13}C NMR (100 MHz, $CDCl_3$) δ 165.8 (C = O), 165.6 (C = O), 147.4 (CH), 136.6 (CH), 133.5 (CH), 130.8 (CH), 129.8 (CH × 2), 129.7(C), 128.7 (CH × 2), 118.4 (CH), 77.0 (CH), 72.6 (CH), 72.0 (CH), 49.9 (CH), 44.5 (CH), 43.3 (CH_2), 41.2 (CH_2), 34.2 (CH_2), 31.9 (CH_2), 26.8 (CH_2), 20.9 (CH_3). HRESIMS m/z 385.2004 [M + H]$^+$ (calcd. for $C_{23}H_{29}O_5{}^+$, 385.2010).

Brefeldin A 7-*O*-(2,3,4)-trifluorobenzoate (5): Colorless oil; yield 10%; ^{1}H NMR (500 MHz, $CDCl_3$) δ 7.70 (1H, m), 7.36 (1H, dd, J = 15.7, 3.2 Hz), 7.04 (1H, m), 5.92 (1H, dd, J = 15.8, 2.0 Hz), 5.73 (1H, m), 5.43 (1H, m), 5.27 (1H, dd, J = 15.2, 9.2 Hz), 4.87 (1H, m), 4.17 (1H, m), 2.51–2.35 (3H, overlapped), 2.06–1.95 (2H, overlapped), 1.94–1.80 (3H, overlapped), 1.79–1.72 (2H, overlapped), 1.53 (1H, m), 1.26 (3H, d, J = 6.3 Hz), 0.95 (1H, m); ^{13}C NMR (125 MHz, $CDCl_3$) δ 166.2 (C = O), 162.6 (C = O), 151.4 (CH), 135.9 (CH), 131.3 (CH), 126.4 (C), 126.4 (C), 126.3 (C), 126.3 (C), 118.0 (CH), 112.3 (CH), 112.2 (CH), 77.2 (CH), 76.0 (CH), 71.9 (CH), 52.5 (CH), 44.1 (CH), 40.2 (CH), 39.0 (CH_2), 34.3 (CH_2), 32.0 (CH_2), 26.8 (CH_2), 21.0 (CH_3). HRESIMS m/z 439.1726 [M + H]$^+$ (calcd. for $C_{23}H_{26}F_3O_5{}^+$, 439.1727).

Brefeldin A 4-*O*-(2,3,4)-trifluorobenzoate (6): Colorless oil; yield 28%; ^{1}H NMR (500 MHz, $CDCl_3$) δ 7.75 (1H, m), 7.31 (1H, dd, J = 15.7, 3.4 Hz), 7.07 (1H, m), 5.80–5.69 (2H, overlapped), 5.51 (1H, ddd, J = 10.6, 3.5, 1.9 Hz), 5.34 (1H, dd, J = 15.2, 9.6 Hz), 4.86 (1H, m), 4.35 (1H, m), 2.49 (1H, m), 2.38–2.22 (2H, overlapped), 2.08–1.96 (2H, overlapped), 1.89–1.82 (2H, overlapped), 1.77–1.67 (2H, overlapped), 1.58–1.50 (2H, overlapped), 1.25 (3H, d, J = 6.2 Hz), 0.95 (1H, m); ^{13}C NMR (125 MHz, $CDCl_3$) δ 165.7 (C = O), 162.0 (C = O), 146.6 (CH), 136.4 (CH), 130.9 (CH), 126.5 (C), 126.5 (C), 126.5 (C), 126.4 (C), 118.9 (CH), 112.5 (CH), 112.4 (CH), 78.0 (CH), 72.6 (CH), 72.1 (CH), 49.8 (CH), 44.5 (CH), 43.3 (CH_2), 41.3 (CH_2), 34.2 (CH_2), 32.0 (CH_2), 26.7 (CH_2), 20.9 (CH_3). HRESIMS m/z 439.1723 [M + H]$^+$ (calcd. for $C_{23}H_{26}F_3O_5{}^+$, 439.1727).

Brefeldin A 7-*O*-2-chloro-4,5-difluorobenzoate (7): Colorless oil; yield 15%; ^{1}H NMR (400 MHz, $CDCl_3$) δ 7.69 (1H, dd, J = 10.4, 8.4 Hz), 7.34 (1H, dd, J = 15.7, 3.2 Hz), 7.29 (1H, dd, J = 9.8, 6.9 Hz), 5.92 (1H, dd, J = 15.7, 1.9 Hz), 5.73 (1H, m), 5.38 (1H, m), 5.24 (1H, dd, J = 15.2, 8.8 Hz), 4.85 (1H, m), 4.15 (1H, ddd, J = 9.2, 3.1, 1.9 Hz), 2.53–2.31 (3H, overlapped), 2.03–1.91 (3H, overlapped), 1.90–1.80 (2H, overlapped), 1.78–1.67 (2H, overlapped), 1.53 (1H, m), 1.25 (3H, d, J = 6.3 Hz), 0.86 (1H, m); ^{13}C NMR (100 MHz, $CDCl_3$) δ 166.3 (C = O), 163.5 (C = O), 151.5 (CH), 135.8 (CH), 131.4 (CH), 120.7 (C), 120.7 (C), 120.6 (CH), 120.5 (C), 120.5 (C), 120.4 (CH), 118.0 (CH), 77.4 (CH), 75.9 (CH), 71.9 (CH), 52.3 (CH), 44.1 (CH), 40.2 (CH_2), 38.9 (CH_2), 34.2 (CH_2), 31.9 (CH_2), 26.7 (CH_2), 20.9 (CH_3). HRESIMS m/z 455.1429 [M + H]$^+$ (calcd. for $C_{23}H_{26}ClF_2O_5{}^+$, 455.1431).

Brefeldin A 4-*O*-2-chloro-4,5-difluorobenzoate (8): Colorless oil; yield 30%; ^{1}H NMR (400 MHz, $CDCl_3$) δ 7.77 (1H, dd, J = 10.3, 8.3 Hz), 7.33 (1H, m), 7.28 (1H, d, J = 12.4 Hz), 5.82–5.63 (2H, overlapped), 5.48 (1H, ddd, J = 10.5, 3.5, 1.8 Hz), 5.31 (1H, dd, J = 15.2, 9.5 Hz), 4.85 (1H, m), 4.32 (1H, m), 2.47 (1H, m), 2.33 (1H, m), 2.22 (1H, m), 2.06–1.94 (2H, overlapped), 1.91–1.80 (2H, overlapped), 1.75–1.65 (2H, overlapped), 1.57–1.47 (2H, overlapped), 1.23 (3H, d, J = 6.3 Hz), 0.93 (1H, m); ^{13}C NMR (100 MHz, $CDCl_3$) δ 165.6 (C = O), 162.6 (C = O), 146.5 (CH), 136.3 (CH), 130.9 (CH), 120.9 (C), 120.8 (C), 120.8 (CH), 120.7 (C), 120.6 (C), 120.6 (CH), 118.8 (CH), 78.3 (CH), 72.4 (CH), 72.1 (CH), 49.6 (CH), 44.5 (CH), 43.3 (CH_2), 41.2 (CH_2), 34.1 (CH_2), 31.9 (CH_2), 26.7 (CH_2), 20.9 (CH_3). HRESIMS m/z 455.1426 [M + H]$^+$ (calcd. for $C_{23}H_{26}ClF_2O_5{}^+$, 455.1431).

Brefeldin A 4,7-*O*-di-2-chloro-4,5-difluorobenzoate (9): Colorless oil; yield 35%; ^{1}H NMR (400 MHz, $CDCl_3$) δ 7.78 (1H, dd, J = 10.3, 8.3 Hz), 7.69 (1H, dd, J = 10.3, 8.3 Hz), 7.37–7.26 (3H, overlapped), 5.86–5.70 (2H, overlapped), 5.55 (1H, ddd, J = 10.1, 3.6, 1.8 Hz), 5.40 (1H, m), 5.29 (1H, dd, J = 15.4, 9.2 Hz), 4.88 (1H, m), 2.60 (1H, m), 2.50 (1H, m), 2.41–2.24 (2H, overlapped), 2.03 (1H, m), 1.96–1.70 (5H, overlapped), 1.54 (1H, m), 1.25 (3H, d, J = 6.2 Hz), 0.96 (1H, m); ^{13}C NMR (100 MHz, $CDCl_3$) δ 165.5 (C = O), 163.4 (C = O), 162.6 (C = O), 146.0 (CH), 135.3 (CH), 131.9 (CH), 121.0 (C), 121.0 (C), 120.9 (CH), 120.8 (C),

120.8 (C), 120.7 (C), 120.7 (C), 120.7 (CH), 120.6 (CH), 120.5 (C), 120.5 (C), 120.4 (CH), 119.3 (CH), 78.1 (CH), 77.3 (CH), 72.1 (CH), 50.0 (CH), 44.3 (CH), 40.2 (CH_2), 38.8 (CH_2), 34.2 (CH_2), 31.9 (CH_2), 26.6 (CH_2), 20.9 (CH_3). HRESIMS m/z 629.1117 $[M + H]^+$ (calcd. for $C_{30}H_{27}Cl_2F_4O_6^+$, 629.1115).

Brefeldin A 7-*O*-(4)-chlorobenzoate (10): Colorless oil; yield 10%; ^{1}H NMR (600 MHz, $CDCl_3$) δ 7.96–7.92 (2H, overlapped), 7.43–7.40 (2H, overlapped), 7.37 (1H, dd, J = 15.6, 3.0 Hz), 5.93 (1H, d, J = 15.5 Hz), 5.74 (1H, m), 5.39 (1H, m), 5.24 (1H, dd, J = 15.2, 9.2 Hz), 4.87 (1H, m), 4.18 (1H, d, J = 9.6 Hz), 2.51–2.33 (3H, overlapped), 2.05–1.96 (2H, overlapped), 1.91 (1H, m), 1.88–1.81 (2H, overlapped), 1.78–1.70 (2H, overlapped), 1.53 (1H, m), 1.27 (3H, d, J = 6.4 Hz), 0.96 (1H, m); ^{13}C NMR (150 MHz, $CDCl_3$) δ 166.2 (C = O), 165.4 (C = O), 151.4 (CH), 139.6 (C), 136.0 (CH), 131.3 (CH), 131.1 (CH × 2), 129.0 (C), 128.9 (CH × 2), 118.0 (CH), 76.4 (CH), 76.0 (CH), 71.9 (CH), 52.5 (CH), 44.1 (CH), 40.3 (CH_2), 38.9 (CH_2), 34.3 (CH_2), 32.0 (CH_2), 26.8 (CH_2), 21.0 (CH_3). HRESIMS m/z 419.1620 $[M + H]^+$ (calcd. for $C_{23}H_{28}ClO_5^+$, 419.1620).

Brefeldin A 4-*O*-(4)-chlorobenzoate (11): Colorless oil; yield 30%; ^{1}H NMR (600 MHz, $CDCl_3$) δ 8.02–7.95 (2H, overlapped), 7.45–7.40 (2H, overlapped), 7.32 (1H, dd, J = 15.7, 3.3 Hz), 5.77–5.67 (2H, overlapped), 5.48 (1H, ddd, J = 10.5, 3.3, 1.8 Hz), 5.32 (1H, dd, J = 15.2, 9.6 Hz), 4.84 (1H, m), 4.30 (1H, m), 2.47 (1H, m), 2.31 (1H, m), 2.23 (1H, m), 2.05–1.92 (2H, overlapped), 1.88–1.81 (2H, overlapped), 1.71 (1H, m), 1.66 (1H, m), 1.56–1.47 (2H, overlapped), 1.22 (3H, d, J = 6.2 Hz), 0.92 (1H, m); ^{13}C NMR (150 MHz, $CDCl_3$) δ 165.8 (C = O), 164.7 (C = O), 147.2 (CH), 140.0 (C), 136.5 (CH), 131.2 (CH × 2), 130.8 (CH), 129.0 (CH × 2), 128.1 (C), 118.4 (CH), 77.3 (CH), 72.4 (CH), 72.1 (CH), 49.8 (CH), 44.4 (CH), 43.3 (CH_2), 41.1 (CH_2), 34.1 (CH_2), 31.9 (CH_2), 26.7 (CH_2), 20.9 (CH_3). HRESIMS m/z 419.1626 $[M + H]^+$ (calcd. for $C_{23}H_{28}ClO_5^+$, 419.1620).

Brefeldin A 4,7-*O*-di-(4)-chlorobenzoate (12): Colorless oil; yield 36%; ^{1}H NMR (600 MHz, $CDCl_3$) δ 8.03–7.88 (4H, overlapped), 7.46–7.36 (4H, overlapped), 7.34 (1H, dd, J = 15.7, 3.3 Hz), 5.84–5.72 (2H, overlapped), 5.55 (1H, ddd, J = 10.4, 3.4, 1.8 Hz), 5.37 (1H, m), 5.28 (1H, dd, J = 15.2, 9.6 Hz), 4.84 (1H, m), 2.60 (1H, m), 2.44 (1H, m), 2.32 (1H, m), 2.22 (1H, m), 2.01 (1H, m), 1.92–1.80 (3H, overlapped), 1.81–1.68 (2H, overlapped), 1.52 (1H, m), 1.22 (3H, d, J = 6.1 Hz), 0.88 (1H, m); ^{13}C NMR (125 MHz, $CDCl_3$) δ 165.5 (C = O), 165.1 (C = O), 164.5 (C = O), 146.8 (CH), 139.9 (C), 139.4 (C), 135.5 (CH), 131.5 (CH), 131.1 (CH × 2), 130.9 (CH × 2), 128.9 (CH × 2), 128.8 (C), 128.7 (CH × 2), 127.9 (C), 118.6 (CH), 77.0 (CH), 76.3 (CH), 72.0 (CH), 50.1 (CH), 44.1 (CH), 40.1 (CH_2), 38.5 (CH_2), 34.1 (CH_2), 31.8 (CH_2), 26.5 (CH_2), 20.8 (CH_3). HRESIMS m/z 557.1486 $[M + H]^+$ (calcd. for $C_{30}H_{31}Cl_2O_6^+$, 557.1492).

Brefeldin A 7-*O*-2-chloro-4-fluorobenzoate (13): Colorless oil; yield 12%; ^{1}H NMR (400 MHz, $CDCl_3$) δ 7.85 (1H, dd, J = 8.8, 6.1Hz), 7.35 (1H, dd, J = 15.7, 3.2 Hz), 7.19 (1H, dd, J = 8.5, 2.5 Hz), 7.03 (1H, ddd, J = 8.8, 7.6, 2.5 Hz), 5.92 (1H, dd, J = 15.7, 2.0 Hz), 5.73 (1H, m), 5.41 (1H, m), 5.26 (1H, dd, J = 15.2, 8.9 Hz), 4.87 (1H, m), 4.17 (1H, ddd, J = 9.4, 3.2, 2.0 Hz), 2.52–2.33 (3H, overlapped), 2.04–1.80 (5H, overlapped), 1.78–1.71 (2H, overlapped), 1.52 (1H, m), 1.28–1.24 (3H, d, J = 6.3 Hz), 0.95 (1H, m); ^{13}C NMR (100 MHz, $CDCl_3$) δ 166.3 (C = O), 164.5 (C = O), 151.4 (CH), 135.9 (CH), 133.7 (C), 133.6 (C), 131.3 (CH), 118.9 (C), 118.6 (CH), 118.0 (CH), 114.4 (CH), 114.2 (CH), 76.9 (CH), 76.0 (CH), 71.9 (CH), 52.5 (CH), 44.2 (CH), 40.2 (CH_2), 38.9 (CH_2), 34.3 (CH_2), 32.0 (CH_2), 26.8 (CH_2), 21.0 (CH_3); HRESIMS m/z 437.1522 $[M + H]^+$ (calcd. for $C_{23}H_{27}ClFO_5^+$, 437.1526).

Brefeldin A 4-*O*-2-chloro-4-fluorobenzoate (14): Colorless oil; yield 30%; ^{1}H NMR (600 MHz, $CDCl_3$) δ 7.95 (1H, dd, J = 8.8, 6.1 Hz), 7.31 (1H, dd, J = 15.7, 3.4 Hz), 7.22 (1H, dd, J = 8.5, 2.5 Hz), 7.07 (1H, m), 5.81–5.70 (2H, overlapped), 5.51 (1H, ddd, J = 10.5, 3.4, 1.8 Hz), 5.32 (1H, dd, J = 15.2, 9.6 Hz), 4.87 (1H, m), 4.35 (1H, m), 2.49 (1H, m), 2.32 (1H, m), 2.24 (1H, m), 2.08–1.96 (2H, overlapped), 1.89–1.82 (2H, overlapped), 1.80–1.68 (2H, overlapped), 1.57–1.52 (2H, overlapped), 1.25 (3H, d, J = 6.3 Hz), 0.94 (1H, m); ^{13}C NMR (150 MHz, $CDCl_3$) δ 165.8 (C = O), 163.7 (C = O), 146.9 (CH), 136.4 (CH), 133.9 (C), 133.8 (C), 130.9 (CH), 119.1 (CH), 118.9 (C), 118.8 (CH), 114.5 (CH), 114.3 (CH), 77.8 (CH), 72.6

(CH), 72.1 (CH), 49.8 (CH), 44.5 (CH), 43.4 (CH_2), 41.3 (CH_2), 34.2 (CH_2), 31.9 (CH_2), 26.7 (CH_2), 20.9 (CH_3). HRESIMS *m/z* 437.1530 $[M + H]^+$ (calcd. for $C_{23}H_{27}ClFO_5^+$, 437.1526).

Brefeldin A 4,7-*O*-di-2-chloro-4-fluorobenzoate (15): Colorless oil; yield 36%; ^{1}H NMR (600 MHz, $CDCl_3$) δ 7.94 (1H, dd, J = 8.8, 6.1 Hz), 7.85 (1H, dd, J = 8.8, 6.1 Hz), 7.32 (1H, dd, J = 15.7, 3.5 Hz), 7.26–7.17 (2H, overlapped), 7.08–7.01 (2H, overlapped), 5.84–5.73 (2H, overlapped), 5.56 (1H, ddd, J = 10.1, 3.5, 1.8 Hz), 5.42 (1H, m), 5.30 (1H, m), 4.88 (1H, m), 2.60 (1H, m), 2.49 (1H, m), 2.40–2.28 (2H, overlapped), 2.02 (1H, m), 1.95–1.83 (3H, overlapped), 1.80 (1H, m), 1.74 (1H, m), 1.55 (1H, m), 1.25 (3H, d, J = 6.2 Hz), 0.97 (1H, m); ^{13}C NMR (150 MHz, $CDCl_3$) δ 165.6 (C = O), 164.5 (C = O), 163.7 (C = O), 146.5 (CH), 135.6 (CH), 133.9 (C), 133.9 (C), 133.7 (C), 133.6 (C), 131.7 (CH), 119.1 (CH $\times$ 2), 118.9 (CH), 118.9 (C), 118.7 (C), 114.5 (CH), 114.4 (CH), 114.4 (CH), 114.2 (CH), 77.7 (CH), 76.9 (CH), 72.1 (CH), 50.2 (CH), 44.4 (CH), 40.2 (CH_2), 38.9 (CH_2), 34.2 (CH_2), 31.9 (CH_2), 26.6 (CH_2), 20.9 (CH_3). HRESIMS *m/z* 593.1309 $[M + H]^+$ (calcd. for $C_{30}H_{29}Cl_2F_2O_6^+$, 593.1304).

Brefeldin A 7-*O*-(2,4,6)-trichlorobenzoate (16): Colorless oil; yield 15%; ^{1}H NMR (500 MHz, $CDCl_3$) δ 7.37–7.29 (3H, overlapped), 5.90 (1H, dd, J = 15.7, 1.9 Hz), 5.71 (1H, m), 5.46 (1H, m), 5.23 (1H, dd, J = 15.3, 8.5Hz), 4.84 (1H, m), 4.14 (1H, m), 2.46–2.37 (3H, overlapped), 2.05 (1H, d, J = 5.0 Hz), 2.01–1.90 (3H, overlapped), 1.87–1.78 (3H, overlapped), 1.73 (1H, m), 1.52 (1H, m), 1.25 (3H, d, J = 6.3 Hz), 0.92 (1H, m); ^{13}C NMR (100 MHz, $CDCl_3$) δ 166.3 (C = O), 163.8 (C = O), 151.4 (CH), 136.2 (C), 135.9 (CH), 132.6 (CH), 132.3 (C), 131.2 (CH), 128.2 (CH), 128.2 (C $\times$ 2),117.9 (CH), 78.0 (CH), 75.9 (CH), 71.9 (CH), 52.3 (CH), 44.1 (CH), 40.0 (CH_2), 38.6 (CH_2), 34.2 (CH_2), 31.9 (CH_2), 26.8 (CH_2), 21.0 (CH_3). HRESIMS *m/z* 487.0837 $[M + H]^+$ (calcd. for $C_{23}H_{26}Cl_3O_5^+$, 487.0840).

3.5. Biological Assays

3.5.1. Reagents

Antibodies against AKT, phosphorylated AKT at S473, ERK1/2, phosphorylated ERK1/2 (T202/Y204), mTOR, phosphorylated mTOR (S2481), p70S6K, phosphorylated p70S6K (T421/S424), cleaved caspase-3 (C-Cas3), cleaved caspase-9 (C-Cas9), and cleaved PARP (C-PARP) were purchased from Cell Signaling Technology (Boston, MA, USA). Antibodies against GAPDH and Tubulin were obtained from Huaan Biotechnology Co., Ltd. (Hangzhou, China). Z-VAD-fmk was obtained from Selleck Chemicals (Houston, TX, USA). Muse™ Cell Cycle Kit and Muse® Annexin V & Dead Cell Kit were purchased from Millipore (Billerica, MA, USA). Other reagents were purchased from Beyotime Biotechnology, Shanghai, China.

3.5.2. Cell Lines and Cell Culture

Human chronic myelogenous leukemia cell line K562 was purchased from Shanghai Cell Bank, Chinese Academy of Sciences, and cells were maintained in Iscove's Modified Dulbecco's Medium (GIBCO, Grand Island, NY, USA) with 10% fetal bovine serum (FBS) and 1% penicillin/streptomycin in a humidified incubator at 37 °C under 5% CO_2.

3.5.3. Cell Proliferation Assay

The 3-(4,5-dimethylthiazol-2-yl)-2,5-diphenyltetrazolium bromide (MTT) assay was performed to determine cell viability. Briefly, K562 cells were seeded in 96-well plates and treated for the indicated time with various concentrations of compound 7. Then, 20 μL of MTT reagent was added to each well and further incubated for 4 h. Next, the formazan product was dissolved with acidic isopropanol (100 μL) incubated overnight. Finally, the absorbance was measured at 570 nm using a SpectraMax® i3x multi-mode microplate reader (Molecular Devices, San Jose, CA, USA). Then, cells viability was calculated.

3.5.4. Soft Agar Colony Formation Assay

Soft agar colony formation assay was performed as described previously [43]. In brief, 6-well plate was first coated with 1.2% agarose with an equal volume of 2× Dulbecco's Modified Eagle's Medium containing 20% fetal bovine serum, then K562 cells (2000/well) were mixed with the culture medium containing 0.4% agarose and indicated concentration of compound **7**, and then the mixture immediately overlaid on the pre-coated plates. The culture medium was changed every 3 days. After incubation for 12 d at 37 °C, cells were stained with 0.005% crystal violet, and colonies consisting of 50 or more cells were counted.

3.5.5. Cell Cycle Analysis

K562 cells were seeded in 6-well plates (3×10^5 cells/well) and treated with different concentrations of compound **7** for 36 h; the control group was treated with the same diluted DMSO. Then, cells were harvested, washed with ice-cold phosphate-buffered saline (PBS), and fixed in 70% cold ethanol overnight at −20 °C. Fixed cells were then collected, washed, and stained with 200 μL of Muse™ cell cycle reagent for 30 min in the dark at room temperature. The cell cycle distribution was immediately analyzed by Muse Cell Analyzer (Millipore, Billerica, MA, USA).

3.5.6. Cell Apoptosis Analysis

Apoptosis was determined by Annexin V-PE/7-AAD staining [44]. After treatment with compound **7** for 36 h, cells were collected, centrifuged, and washed with ice-cold PBS. Then cells were resuspended in 100 μL Iscove's Modified Dulbecco's Medium with 1% FBS and stained with Muse® Annexin V & Dead Cell Kit (Millipore, Billerica, MA, USA) for 20 min in the dark at room temperature and finally analyzed by Muse Cell Analyzer (Millipore, Billerica, MA, USA).

3.5.7. Western Blotting Assay

Cells were seeded in 6-well plates (3×10^5 cells/well) and incubated with compound **7** for the indicated time. Then, cells were collected, washed, suspended, and lysed in loading buffer (0.125 M Tris-HCl, 5% 2-mMercaptoethanol, 30 mg/mL sodium dodecyl sulfate (SDS), 10% glycerol, 0.5 mg/mL bromophenol blue) for 40 min at 4 °C. Proteins were separated by electrophoresis on 6–12% SDS-polyacrylamide gels and transferred to NC membranes (Millipore, Billerica, MA, USA). The membrane was blocked in 5% skim milk for 1 h and incubated with corresponding primary antibodies overnight at 4 °C, and subsequently, the membranes were incubated with HRP-secondary antibody at room temperature for 1 h and finally detected by Tanon 5200 (Tanon, Beijing, China).

3.5.8. Statistical Analysis

The results shown in this study are represented as the mean values ± SD. Comparisons between the groups were assessed by Student's t-test, and $p < 0.05$ was defined as statistically significant.

3.6. Solubility Measurement

Ten milligrams of **1** and **7** was added into the 15 mL centrifuge tubes, then 10 mL of water was added, and the tubes were shaken on a vortexes (Shanghai Qite Analytical Instrument Co., Shanghai, China; QT-2) at 1000 rpm for 30 min at room temperature. Subsequently, the tubes were ultrasonic dissolved for a further 3 h in an ultrasonic cleaner (Kunshan Ultrasonic Instrument Co., Kunshan, China; KQ-300DE). After completion of dissolution, the suspension was centrifuged at 15 000 rpm (Thermo Fisher, Waltham, MA, USA, Sorvall Legend Micro 17) for 10 min to precipitate undissolved particles. Then, the solid and liquid phases were separated, and the undissolved solid was dried and weighed.

3.7. Molecular Modeling and Protein–Ligand Docking

The crystal structure of **1** in the interface between ARF1-GDP and its GEF protein ARNO was downloaded from the Protein Data Bank (PDB ID: 1R8Q) [13]. The structure of **7** was selected for docking, followed by structure optimization with the software MOE (Chemical Computing Group ULC, Montreal, QC, Canada). The target proteins were performed for protonation with the Protonate 3D function in MOE and expulsion of water.

The 3D structure of **7** was constructed with drawing software ChemDraw & Chem3D, and MM2 minimized in Chem3D prior to molecular docking. Then, **7** was docked in the binding pocket overlapped with **1**. Molecular docking with the Rigid Receptor parameter was conducted within MOE.

4. Conclusions

In this study, a series of derivatives of **1** were designed and synthesized, and their inhibitory effects against K562 cells were evaluated. The SARs studies revealed that the monoester derivatives exhibited stronger cytotoxic activity than those of diester derivatives. Moreover, the introduction of halogen atoms on the benzene rings showed a certain improvement in potency. The results exhibited that compound **7** showed great potential cytotoxic activity on K562 cells compared to other tested compounds, while the effect was slightly weaker than **1**. Further investigations indicated that **7** inhibited the growth of K562 cells, arrested cell cycle, and induced apoptosis. Additionally, the mechanism underlying **7**-induced cell proliferation inhibition was partially related to the inactivation of the BCR-ABL signaling pathway. The molecular models indicated that **7** was well tolerated in the interface between the ARF and ARNO proteins. In summary, the current results demonstrated that **7** has great promise against BCR-ABL positive cells and may serve as an efficacious antileukemia agent.

Supplementary Materials: The following are available online at https://www.mdpi.com/article/10.3390/md20010026/s1, Figures S1–S48: ^{1}H NMR, ^{13}C NMR, and HRESIMS/ESIMS spectra of compounds **1–16**.

Author Contributions: X.-X.L., investigation, visualization, writing—original draft, writing—review and editing; Y.-Y.J., investigation, conceptualization, writing—original draft, writing—review and editing; Y.-W.W., investigation; Y.-C.G., supervision, writing—review and editing; G.-Y.C., supervision and funding acquisition; C.-L.S., M.L. and M.-Y.W., project administration, supervision, and funding acquisition. All authors have read and agreed to the published version of the manuscript.

Funding: This research was funded by the Program of National Natural Science Foundation of China (Nos. 41776141, U1706210, 81872792, 41676127, and 41322037), the National Key Research and Development Program of China (No. 2017YFE0195000), the Program of Natural Science Foundation of Shandong Province of China (No. ZR2019BD047), the Fundamental Research Funds for the Central Universities (No. 201841004), the Marine S & T Fund of Shandong Province for Pilot National Laboratory for Marine Science and Technology (Qingdao) (No. 2018SDKJ0403-2), and the Taishan Scholars Program, China (No. tsqn20161010). The project was also funded by State Key Laboratory for Chemistry and Molecular Engineering of Medicinal Resources (Guangxi Normal University) (CMEMR2019-B05) and Key Laboratory of Tropical Medicinal Resource Chemistry of Ministry of Education, Hainan Normal University (RDZH2021003).

Institutional Review Board Statement: Not applicable.

Data Availability Statement: Data are contained within the article or Supplementary Materials.

Acknowledgments: We thank Syngenta for the fellowship to Yao-Yao Jiang.

Conflicts of Interest: The authors declare no conflict of interest.

References

1. Quintás-Cardama, A.; Cortes, J. Molecular biology of BCR-ABL1-positive chronic myeloid leukemia. *Blood* **2009**, *113*, 1619–1630. [CrossRef] [PubMed]
2. Lugo, T.; Pendergast, A.; Muller, A.; Witte, O. Tyrosine kinase activity and transformation potency of BCR-ABL oncogene products. *Science* **1990**, *247*, 1079–1082. [CrossRef] [PubMed]
3. Danial, N.; Rothman, P. JAK-STAT signaling activated by ABL oncogenes. *Oncogene* **2000**, *19*, 2523–2531. [CrossRef] [PubMed]
4. Quintás-Cardama, A.; Kantarjian, H.; Cortes, J. Imatinib and beyond-exploring the full potential of targeted therapy for CML. *Nat. Rev. Clin. Oncol.* **2009**, *6*, 535–543. [CrossRef]
5. Isfort, S.; Amsberg, G.K.-V.; Schafhausen, P.; Koschmieder, S.; Brümmendorf, T.H. Bosutinib: A novel second-generation tyrosine kinase inhibitor. *Small Mol. Oncol.* **2014**, *201*, 81–97.
6. Blay, J.; von Mehren, M. Nilotinib: A novel, selective tyrosine kinase inhibitor. *Semin. Oncol.* **2011**, *38*, S3–S9. [CrossRef]

7. Shah, N.; Tran, C.; Lee, F.; Chen, P.; Norris, D.; Sawyers, C. Overriding imatinib resistance with a novel ABL kinase inhibitor. *Science* **2004**, *305*, 399–401. [CrossRef]
8. Pan, X.; Liang, L.; Sun, Y.; Si, R.; Zhang, Q.; Wang, J.; Fu, J.; Zhang, J.; Zhang, J. Discovery of novel BCR-ABL inhibitors with flexible linker. Part 1: Confirmation optimization of phenyl-1H-indazol-3-amine as hinge binding moiety. *Eur. J. Med. Chem.* **2019**, *178*, 232–242. [CrossRef]
9. Hou, X.M.; Liang, T.M.; Guo, Z.Y.; Wang, C.Y.; Shao, C.L. Discovery, absolute assignments, and total synthesis of asperversiamides A-C and their potent activity against *Mycobacterium marinum*. *Chem. Commun.* **2019**, *55*, 1104–1107. [CrossRef]
10. Hai, Y.; Wei, M.Y.; Wang, C.Y.; Gu, Y.C.; Shao, C.L. The intriguing chemistry and biology of sulfur-containing natural products from marine microorganisms (1987–2020). *Mar. Life Sci. Technol.* **2021**, *3*, 488–518. [CrossRef]
11. Singleton, V.L.; Bohonos, N.; Ullstrup, A.J. Decumbin, a new compound from a species of *Penicillium*. *Nature* **1958**, *181*, 1072–1073. [CrossRef]
12. Trisuwan, K.; Rukachaisirikul, V.; Sukpondma, Y.; Phongpaichit, S.; Preedanon, S.; Sakayaroj, J. Lactone derivatives from the marine-derived fungus *Penicillium* sp. PSU-F44. *Chem. Pharm. Bull.* **2009**, *57*, 1100–1102. [CrossRef]
13. Hu, Z.F.; Qin, L.L.; Ding, W.J.; Liu, Y.; Ma, Z.J. New analogues of brefeldin A from sediment-derived fungus *Penicillium* sp. DT-F29. *Nat. Prod. Res.* **2016**, *30*, 2311–2315. [CrossRef]
14. Cheng, X.; Yu, L.; Wang, Q.; Ding, W.; Chen, Z.; Ma, Z. New brefeldins and penialidins from marine fungus *Penicillium* janthinellum DT-F29. *Nat. Prod. Res.* **2018**, *32*, 282–286. [CrossRef]
15. Zhang, J.M.; Jiang, Y.Y.; Huang, Q.F.; Lu, X.X.; Wang, G.H.; Shao, C.L.; Liu, M. Brefeldin A delivery nanomicelles in hepatocellular carcinoma therapy: Characterization, cytotoxic evaluation in vitro, and antitumor efficiency in vivo. *Pharmacol. Res.* **2021**, *172*, 105800–105810. [CrossRef]
16. Mossessova, E.; Corpina, R.A.; Goldberg, J. Crystal structure of ARF1·Sec7 complexed with brefeldin A and its implications for the guanine nucleotide exchange mechanism. *Mol. Cell* **2003**, *12*, 1403–1411. [CrossRef]
17. Renault, L.; Guibert, B.; Cherfils, J. Structural snapshots of the mechanism and inhibition of a guanine nucleotide exchange factor. *Nature* **2003**, *426*, 525–530. [CrossRef]
18. Fujiwara, T.; Oda, K.; Yokota, S.; Takatsuki, A.; Ikehara, Y. Brefeldin A causes disassembly of the Golgi complex and accumulation of secretory proteins in the endoplasmic reticulum. *J. Biol. Chem.* **1988**, *263*, 18545–18552. [CrossRef]
19. Lippincott-Schwartz, J.; Yuan, L.C.; Bonifacino, J.S.; Klausner, R.D. Rapid redistribution of Golgi proteins into the ER in cells treated with brefeldin A: Evidence for membrane cycling from Golgi to ER. *Cell* **1989**, *56*, 801–813. [CrossRef]
20. Driouich, A.; Zhang, G.F.; Staehelin, L.A. Effect of brefeldin A on the structure of the Golgi apparatus and on the synthesis and secretion of proteins and polysaccharides in sycamore maple (Acer pseudoplatanus) suspension-cultured cells. *Plant Physiol.* **1993**, *101*, 1363–1373. [CrossRef]
21. Rouhana, J.; Padilla, A.; Estaran, S.; Bakari, S.; Delbecq, S.; Boublik, Y.; Chopineau, J.; Pugniere, M.; Chavanieu, A. Kinetics of interaction between ADP-ribosylation factor-1 (Arf1) and the Sec7 domain of Arno guanine nucleotide exchange factor, modulation by allosteric factors, and the uncompetitive inhibitor brefeldin A. *J. Biol. Chem.* **2013**, *288*, 4659–4672. [CrossRef]
22. Prieto-Dominguez, N.; Parnell, C.; Teng, Y. Drugging the small GTPase pathways in cancer treatment: Promises and challenges. *Cells* **2019**, *8*, 255. [CrossRef]
23. Anadu, N.O.; Davisson, V.J.; Cushman, M. Synthesis and anticancer activity of Brefeldin A ester derivatives. *J. Med. Chem.* **2006**, *49*, 3897–3905. [CrossRef]
24. Kikuchi, S.; Shinpo, K.; Tsuji, S.; Yabe, I.; Niino, M.; Tashiro, K. Brefeldin A-induced neurotoxicity in cultured spinal cord neurons. *J. Neurosci. Res.* **2003**, *71*, 591–599. [CrossRef]
25. He, B.; Wang, Y.; Zheng, Y.; Chen, W.; Zhu, Q. Synthesis and cytotoxic evaluation of acylated Brefeldin A derivatives as potential anticancer agents. *Chem. Biol. Drug Des.* **2013**, *82*, 307–316. [CrossRef]
26. Zhu, J.W.; Nagasawa, H.; Nagura, F.; Mohamad, S.B.; Uto, Y.; Ohkura, K.; Hori, H. Elucidation of strict structural requirements of Brefeldin A as an inducer of differentiation and apoptosis. *Bioorg. Med. Chem.* **2000**, *8*, 455–463. [CrossRef]
27. Wu, Y.; Shen, X.; Yang, Y.-Q.; Hu, Q.; Huang, J.-H. Enantioselective total synthesis of (+)-brefeldin A and 7-*epi*-brefeldin A. *J. Org. Chem.* **2004**, *69*, 3857–3865. [CrossRef]
28. Proksa, B.; Uhrin, D.; Adamcova, J.; Fuska, J. Oxidation of brefeldin A. *Pharmazie* **1992**, *47*, 582–584. [PubMed]
29. Fox, B.M.; Vroman, J.A.; Fanwick, P.E.; Cushman, M. Preparation and evaluation of sulfide derivatives of the antibiotic brefeldin A as potential prodrug candidates with enhanced aqueous solubilities. *J. Med. Chem.* **2001**, *44*, 3915–3924. [CrossRef] [PubMed]
30. Zhu, J.W.; Hori, H.; Nojiri, H.; Tsukuda, T.; Taira, Z. Synthesis and activity of brefeldin A analogs as inducers of cancer cell differentiation and apoptosis. *Bioorg. Med. Chem. Lett.* **1997**, *7*, 139–144. [CrossRef]
31. Seehafer, K.; Rominger, F.; Helmchen, G.; Langhans, M.; Robinson, D.G.; Oezata, B.; Bruegger, B.; Strating, J.R.P.M.; van Kuppeveld, F.J.M.; Klein, C.D. Synthesis and biological properties of novel brefeldin A analogues. *J. Med. Chem.* **2013**, *56*, 5872–5884. [CrossRef]
32. Haruma, T. Antitumor Agent Containing Acyl Thiourea Compound and Antitumor Effect Potentiator for Use with Immunocheckpoint Regulator. WO Patent WO2019049956A1, 14 March 2019.
33. Van Pee, K.-H.; Ludwig-Mueller, J. Halogenated indole derivatives. *Curr. Top. Phytochem.* **2002**, *5*, 1–21.

34. Zhang, J.M.; Wang, C.F.; Wei, M.Y.; Dong, H.; Gu, Y.C.; Mo, X.M.; Shao, C.L.; Liu, M. Brefeldin A induces apoptosis, inhibits BCR-ABL activation, and triggers BCR-ABL degradation in chronic myeloid leukemia K562 cells. *Anticancer Agents Med. Chem.* 2021, *in press*. [CrossRef]
35. Chereda, B.; Melo, J.V. Natural course and biology of CML. *Ann. Hematol.* **2015**, *94*, 107–121. [CrossRef]
36. Martin, G.S. Cell signaling and cancer. *Cancer Cell* **2003**, *4*, 167–174. [CrossRef]
37. Yuan, Z.; Wang, F.; Zhao, Z.; Zhao, X.; Qiu, J.; Nie, C.; Wei, Y. BIM-mediated AKT phosphorylation is a key modulator of arsenic trioxide-induced apoptosis in cisplatin-sensitive and -resistant ovarian cancer cells. *PLoS ONE* **2011**, *6*, e20586. [CrossRef]
38. He, W.; Yu, S.; Wang, L.; He, M.; Cao, X.; Li, Y.; Xiao, H. Exendin-4 inhibits growth and augments apoptosis of ovarian cancer cells. *Mol. Cell Endocrinol.* **2016**, *436*, 240–249. [CrossRef]
39. Bertacchini, J.; Heidari, N.; Mediani, L.; Capitani, S.; Shahjahani, M.; Ahmadzadeh, A.; Saki, N. Targeting PI3K/AKT/mTOR network for treatment of leukemia. *Cell. Mol. Life Sci.* **2015**, *72*, 2337–2347. [CrossRef]
40. Airiau, K.; Mahon, F.X.; Josselin, M.; Jeanneteau, M.; Belloc, F. PI3K/mTOR pathway inhibitors sensitize chronic myeloid leukemia stem cells to nilotinib and restore the response of progenitors to nilotinib in the presence of stem cell factor. *Cell Death Dis.* **2013**, *4*, 827–835. [CrossRef]
41. Okabe, S.; Tauchi, T.; Tanaka, Y.; Kitahara, T.; Kimura, S.; Maekawa, T.; Ohyashiki, K. Efficacy of the dual PI3K and mTOR inhibitor NVP-BEZ235 in combination with nilotinib against BCR-ABL-positive leukemia cells involves the ABL kinase domain mutation. *Cancer Biol. Ther.* **2014**, *15*, 207–215. [CrossRef]
42. Wang, S.; Li, X.M.; Teuscher, F.; Li, D.L.; Diesel, A.; Ebel, R.; Proksch, P.; Wang, B.G. Chaetopyranin, a benzaldehyde derivative, and other related metabolites from *Chaetomium globosum*, an endophytic fungus derived from the marine red alga *Polysiphonia urceolata*. *J. Nat. Prod.* **2006**, *69*, 1622–1625. [CrossRef]
43. Zhi, Y.; Wu, X.; Shen, W.; Wang, Y.; Zhou, X.; He, P.; Pan, J.; Chen, Z.; Li, W.; Zhou, Z. Synthesis and pharmacological evaluation of novel epidermal growth factor receptor inhibitors against prostate tumor cells. *Oncol. Lett.* **2018**, *16*, 6522–6530. [CrossRef]
44. Lu, X.; Geng, J.; Zhang, J.; Miao, J.; Liu, M. Xanthohumol, a prenylated flavonoid from hops, induces caspase-dependent degradation of oncoprotein BCR-ABL in K56.62 cells. *Antioxidants* **2019**, *8*, 402. [CrossRef]

marine drugs

Article

5-*O*-(*N*-Boc-L-Alanine)-Renieramycin T Induces Cancer Stem Cell Apoptosis via Targeting Akt Signaling

Darinthip Suksamai [1,2], Satapat Racha [3], Nicharat Sriratanasak [1,4], Chatchai Chaotham [1,5], Kanokpol Aphicho [6], Aye Chan Khine Lin [2,6], Chaisak Chansriniyom [6,7], Khanit Suwanborirux [6,7], Supakarn Chamni [6,7] and Pithi Chanvorachote [1,4,*]

1 Center of Excellence in Cancer Cell and Molecular Biology, Faculty of Pharmaceutical Sciences, Chulalongkorn University, Bangkok 10330, Thailand; 6272002733@student.chula.ac.th (D.S.); nicharat.s@alumni.chula.ac.th (N.S.); chatchai.c@chula.ac.th (C.C.)
2 Graduate Program of Pharmaceutical Science and Technology, Faculty of Pharmaceutical Science, Chulalongkorn University, Bangkok 10330, Thailand; 6373015133@student.chula.ac.th
3 Interdisciplinary Program in Pharmacology, Graduate School, Chulalongkorn University, Bangkok 10330, Thailand; 6481007020@student.chula.ac.th
4 Department of Pharmacology and Physiology, Faculty of Pharmaceutical Sciences, Chulalongkorn University, Bangkok 10330, Thailand
5 Department of Biochemistry and Microbiology, Faculty of Pharmaceutical Sciences, Chulalongkorn University, Bangkok 10330, Thailand
6 Natural Products and Nanoparticles Research Unit (NP2), Chulalongkorn University, Bangkok 10330, Thailand; kanokpol.a@alumni.chula.ac.th (K.A.); chaisak.c@pharm.chula.ac.th (C.C.); khanit.s@chula.ac.th (K.S.); supakarn.c@pharm.chula.ac.th (S.C.)
7 Department of Pharmacognosy and Pharmaceutical Botany, Faculty of Pharmaceutical Sciences, Chulalongkorn University, Bangkok 10330, Thailand
* Correspondence: pithi.c@chula.ac.th; Tel.: +662-218-8344

Citation: Suksamai, D.; Racha, S.; Sriratanasak, N.; Chaotham, C.; Aphicho, K.; Lin, A.C.K.; Chansriniyom, C.; Suwanborirux, K.; Chamni, S.; Chanvorachote, P. 5-*O*-(*N*-Boc-L-Alanine)-Renieramycin T Induces Cancer Stem Cell Apoptosis via Targeting Akt Signaling. *Mar. Drugs* **2022**, *20*, 235. https://doi.org/10.3390/md20040235

Academic Editors: Celso Alves and Marc Diederich

Received: 7 February 2022
Accepted: 27 March 2022
Published: 29 March 2022

Publisher's Note: MDPI stays neutral with regard to jurisdictional claims in published maps and institutional affiliations.

Copyright: © 2022 by the authors. Licensee MDPI, Basel, Switzerland. This article is an open access article distributed under the terms and conditions of the Creative Commons Attribution (CC BY) license (https://creativecommons.org/licenses/by/4.0/).

Abstract: Cancer stem cells (CSCs) drive aggressiveness and metastasis by utilizing stem cell-related signals. In this study, 5-*O*-(*N*-Boc-L-alanine)-renieramycin T (OBA-RT) was demonstrated to suppress CSC signals and induce apoptosis. OBA-RT exerted cytotoxic effects with a half-maximal inhibitory concentration of approximately 7 μM and mediated apoptosis as detected by annexin V/propidium iodide using flow cytometry and nuclear staining assays. Mechanistically, OBA-RT exerted dual roles, activating p53-dependent apoptosis and concomitantly suppressing CSC signals. A p53-dependent pathway was indicated by the induction of p53 and the depletion of anti-apoptotic Myeloid leukemia 1 (Mcl-1) and B-cell lymphoma 2 (Bcl-2) proteins. Cleaved poly (ADP-ribose) polymerase (Cleaved-PARP) was detected in OBA-RT-treated cells. Interestingly, OBA-RT exerted strong CSC-suppressing activity, reducing the ability to form tumor spheroids. In addition, OBA-RT could induce apoptosis in CSC-rich populations and tumor spheroid collapse. CSC markers, including prominin-1 (CD133), Octamer-binding transcription factor 4 (Oct4), and Nanog Homeobox (Nanog), were notably decreased after OBA-RT treatment. Upstream CSCs regulating active Akt and c-Myc were significantly decreased; indicating that Akt may be a potential target of action. Computational molecular modeling revealed a high-affinity interaction between OBA-RT and an Akt molecule. This study has revealed a novel CSC inhibitory effect of OBA-RT via Akt inhibition, which may improve cancer therapy.

Keywords: 5-*O*-(*N*-Boc-L-alanine)-renieramycin T; *Xestospongia* sp.; marine sponge; lung cancer; anti-cancer; cancer stem cells; apoptosis; Akt; c-Myc

1. Introduction

Lung cancer is an important human cancer. At present, several strategies are used for lung cancer treatment, including surgery, chemotherapy, radiotherapy, and targeted therapy; however, drug resistance and the spread of the cells to form metastases frequently result in poor prognosis and treatment failure. Advances in molecular and clinical research have highlighted the role of a cancer cell population, namely cancer stem cells (CSCs), and the concept of CSCs has dramatically altered the understanding view of cancer cell biology, pathogenesis, and the clinical response [1]. Therefore, the current drug discovery theme has focused on the undifferentiated cancer cell population, as the available therapy primarily eradicates the non-CSC population in the tumor, thereby sparing drug-resistant CSCs [2]. High tumorigenic potentials augment cellular survival and drug-resistant mechanisms, and the metastatic abilities of lung CSCs depend on the specific stem cell-related signaling pathways [3].

Myc is a family of proto-oncoproteins that regulate cell growth, survival, and proliferation [4]. In lung cancer, c-Myc is recognized as a key factor facilitating cell growth, drug resistance, and dissemination. In addition, its dominant role in controlling CSC properties supports the concept that targeting c-Myc could be a potential method for lung cancer therapy [5]. A number of studies and observations show the co-incidence of c-Myc and activated PI3K/Akt in transformed cells. Moreover, the PI3K/Akt/c-Myc signaling axis could promote CSC properties in cancers [6].

The deregulation of Akt is associated with several features of cancers, and Akt-targeting compounds can improve cancer therapies. In addition, a number of Akt inhibitors have been investigated for lung cancer treatment [7]. Natural tetrahydroisoquinoline of marine origin and their analogs, such as ecteinascidins from tunicates, exhibit potent cytotoxicity against several types of cancer cells, and they have been approved for clinical use in the treatment of cancers, including advanced soft-tissue sarcoma and ovarian cancer in the case of ecteinascidin 743 (trabectedin) [8] and metastatic small cell lung cancer in the case of the semisynthetic analog, namely lurbinectedin [9].

However, the mechanism of action of ecteinascidins is not fully understood. Ecteinascidins can exert anticancer activities via binding with DNA and DNA-binding proteins and mediating cell apoptosis [10]. Ecteinascidins target Akt as it can dramatically decrease phosphorylated Akt (s473-AKT or p-Akt) [11] and reduce the expression level of several anti-apoptotic proteins, such as Bcl-2 and Mcl-1 [12]. A recent pre-clinical study in the xenograft mice model of uterine cervical cancer revealed that lurbinectedin effectively eliminates CSCs [9]. Renieramycins, which are bis(tetrahydroisoquinoline)quinone alkaloids found in sea sponges and nudibranchs, are members of the same soframycin family as tris(tetrahydroisoquinoline) ecteinascidins [13] and have also demonstrated potent anticancer activities [14], particularly renieramycin M (RM), which is the major bis(tetrahydroisoquinolinequinone) constituent isolated from potassium cyanide-pretreated *Xestospongia* sp. collected in Thailand [15] and the Philippines [16]. RM can sensitize resistance to anoikis via decreasing cellular levels of survival and apoptotic proteins (including p-Akt, p-ERK, Bcl-2, and Mcl-1) [15] and attenuate CSC-like phenotypes [17] in H460 cells. Similar to derivatizations of ecteinascidins [18], late-stage modifications on either the A- or E-ring quinone of RM have been found to alter the mode of action and cellular targeting pattern, which can lead to enhanced selectivity and activity. A series of 5-*O*-Boc-amino ester derivatives of RM is synthesized and successfully used in a structural cytotoxicity relationship study [19], indicating that Boc-protected amino acid moieties serve as empirical groups in the introduction of additional compound–target intermolecular interaction networks and modifying their physicochemical properties. The cinnamoyl ester derivative of RM has superior cytotoxicity compared with the parent compound [20], and it can suppress CSCs potentially by inhibiting Akt [21]. Renieramycin T (RT), a hybrid renieramycin–ecteinascidin analog derived from RM with a methylhydroxybenzodioxole unit resembling ecteinascidin [22], could promote p53-dependent apoptosis via near-to-complete depletion of Mcl-1 and partly decrease the cellular level of Bcl-2, whereas RT did not affect Akt [23]. A trabectedin-mimic derivative of RT, 5-*O*-acetyl-renieramycin T (*O*-acetyl RT), could significantly deplete Akt and reverse CSC-associated cisplatin resistance in non-small-cell lung carcinoma (NSCLC) [24]. Protections at the phenolic alcohol at C-5 can enhance the cytotoxicity of RT derivatives [25]. Based on previous developments, we synthesized the 5-*O*-(*N*-Boc-L-alanine)-renieramycin T (OBA-RT) from RM and investigated the induction of cancer cell apoptosis and the CSC-suppressing effect. Using molecular pharmacological and computational modeling approaches, we reported the potential CSC-targeting activities of this new compound, which could improve anticancer therapy.

2. Results

2.1. Semi-Synthesis of 5-O-(N-Boc-L-Alanine)-Renieramycin T (OBA-RT)

OBA-RT was semi-synthesized from RM through a two-step reaction comprising the facile light-mediated conversion of RM into RT [26] and the *N*-Boc-L-alanine conjugation to RT by esterification (Figure 1). RM was irradiated with LED blue light and was subjected to photoredox transformation of methoxybenzoquinone into hydroxybenzo [1,3] dioxole, yielding RT with a 1,3-dioxole ring at C-7 and C-8, and a hydroxy group at C-5, which enabled the subsequent conjugation with *N*-Boc-L-alanine. The Steglich esterification of RT with *N*-Boc-L-alanine was performed using 1-ethyl-3-(3-dimethylaminopropyl)carbodiimide (EDCI)/4-dimethylaminopyridine (DMAP) as coupling reagents. In addition to high-resolution mass spectrometry and IR spectroscopy, the chromatographically purified OBA-RT was subjected to ^{1}H and ^{13}C NMR spectroscopy, which indicated the identity of the compound (see Supplementary Information for NMR spectra Figures S1–S5). The characteristic proton chemical shifts of the *N*-Boc-L-alanine motif included a broad doublet of a carbamate hydrogen (3′-NH) at 5.01 ppm, a triplet of the α-proton of alanine (2′-H) at 4.58 ppm, a doublet of methyl protons of alanine (7′-CH_3) at 1.70 ppm, and the 9H-equivalent singlet of the tert-butyl group (6′-CH_3) at 1.46 ppm. The characteristic pair of doublets of methylenedioxy protons at 5.97 ppm corresponded to the tetrahydroisoquinoline benzodioxole of renieramycin T. Regarding ^{13}C-NMR spectrum, the *N*-Boc-L-alanine carbonyl of carbamate at C4′, ester carbonyl at C1′, α-carbon of alanine (C2′), methyl carbon of alanine (C7′) and methylenedioxy carbon peaks appeared at 158.3, 171.2, 49.3, 18.6, and 101.8 ppm, respectively.

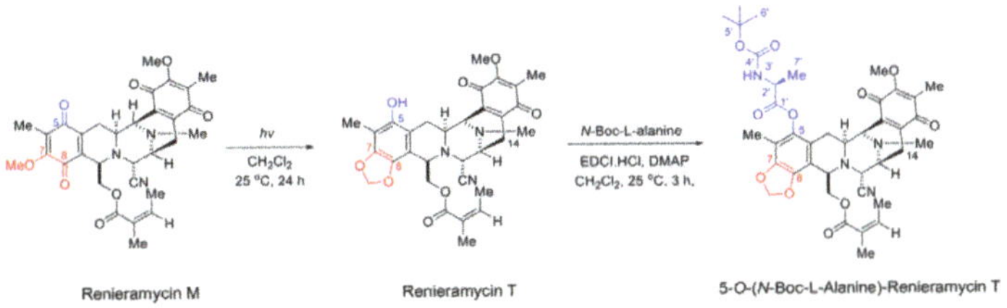

Figure 1. Semi-synthesis of 5-*O*-(*N*-Boc-L-alanine)-renieramycin T (OBA-RT). Photoconversion of renieramycin M to renieramycin T generated a phenolic alcohol at C-5 as a conjugation handle for Steglich esterification with *N*-Boc-L-alanine via EDCI/DMAP coupling, yielding OBA-RT.

2.2. Cytotoxicity and Apoptosis-Inducing Effect of OBA-RT

We determined the cytotoxic profile of OBA-RT in NSCLC A549 cells to elucidate the anticancer potential of OBA-RT. After treating the cells with various concentrations of OBA-RT (0–25 μM) for 24 h, cell viability was evaluated by using the 3-(4,5-dimethylthiazolyl-2)-2,5-diphenyltetrazolium bromide assay. The results showed that OBA-RT significantly reduced the viability of A549 cells (Figure 2a) with a half-maximal inhibitory concentration (IC_{50}) value of 7.30 ± 0.07 μM (Figure 2b). The cytotoxic effects of OBA-RT were considered non-toxic at concentrations of ≤0.05 μM in A549 cells.

We confirmed the effect of OBA-RT in causing decreased cell survival by investigating the surviving cells after treatment by colony formation assay. Surviving A549 cells after treatment with OBA-RT (5, 10, and 25 μM) for 24 h were counted and seeded for the colony formation assay without further treatment. Crystal violet-stained colonies, showing the reproduction of a new cancer colony from a single cell, are shown in Figure 2c,d. The results showed that the resistant cells receiving OBA-RT at 5 to 25 μM could not form colonies (Figure 2c,d).

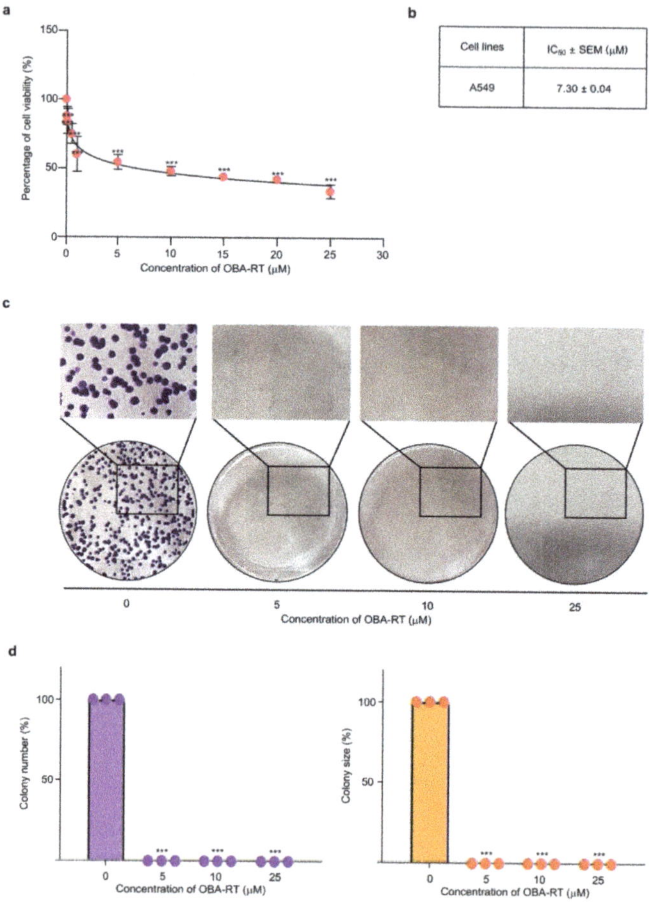

Figure 2. OBA-RT reduces the viability of non-small-cell lung cancer (NSCLC) cells. (**a**) A549 cells were treated with various concentrations of OBA-RT (0–25 μM) for 24 h. Cell viability was determined by MTT assay. (**b**) The half-maximal inhibitory concentration (IC_{50}) at 24 h was calculated. (**c**,**d**) The effect of OBA-RT on colony formation of A549 cells was observed using a colony formation assay. Colonies were stained by crystal violet. Data are represented as the mean ± SEM (n = 3). *** $p < 0.0001$ compared with untreated control cells.

2.3. OBA-RT Induced Apoptosis through p53 Activation

In determining the mode of cell death induced by OBA-RT, A549 cells were treated with OBA-RT (0–25 μM) for 24 h, and the apoptosis and necrosis cells were quantified using the Hoechst 33342/propidium iodide (PI) double staining assay. Hoechst 33342 staining was used to evaluate the nuclear morphology of apoptotic cells, showing condensed or fragmented nuclei, whereas PI stains the nucleus of necrotic cells. The results indicate that OBA-RT could increase apoptosis in a dose-dependent manner, whereas necrotic cells were minimally detected in response to all treatments. Therefore, OBA-RT primarily induced apoptotic cell death in our experimental setting (Figure 3a,b). Other apoptotic cell features, including the presence of extracellular phosphatidylserine, were determined to confirm the apoptosis-inducing effect of OBA-RT. Flow cytometric analysis of annexin V/PI staining of the OBA-RT-treated cells showed that OBA-RT could increase the number of annexin V-positive apoptotic cells (Figure 3c). As shown in Figure 3d, the percentage of early apoptotic cells was 27.28%, 43.72%, and 59.66% in A549 cells treated with OBA-RT at concentrations of 5, 10, and 25 μM, respectively.

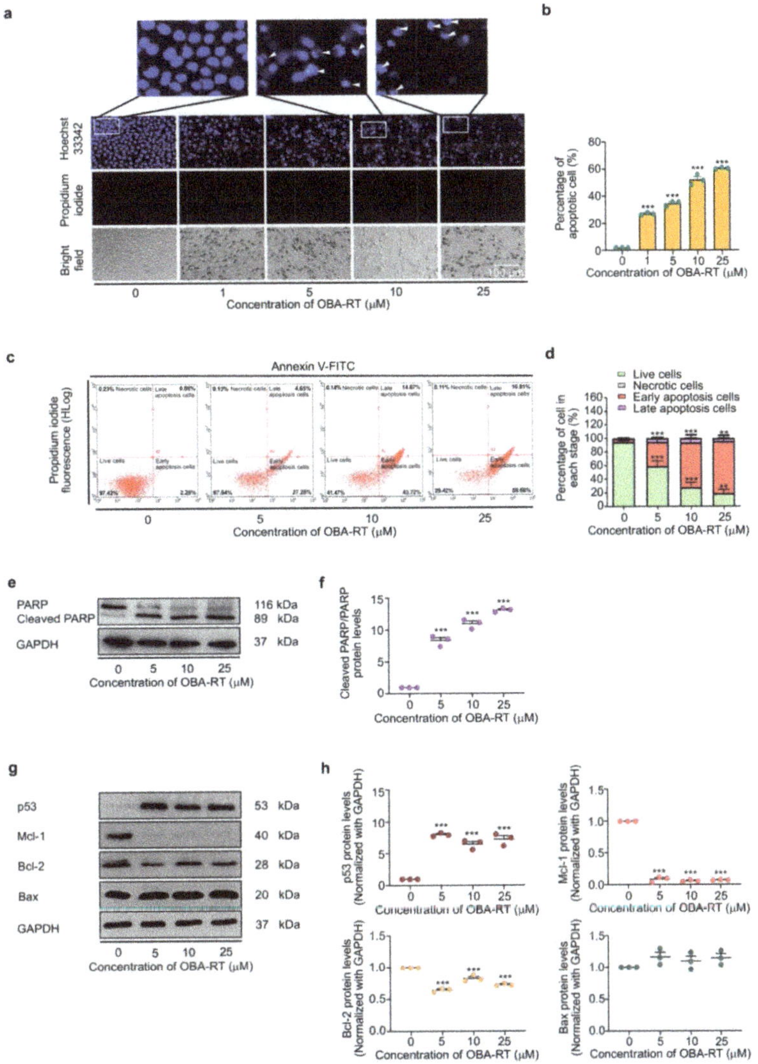

Figure 3. OBA-RT induces apoptosis in a p53-dependent manner. (**a**,**b**) The nuclei of A549 cells treated with OBA-RT were stained with Hoechst 33342/propidium iodide (PI) and calculated as a percentage compared with untreated control cells. The fragmented nuclei in apoptotic cells were indicted by arrowheads. (**c**) Apoptotic and necrotic cell death was determined using the annexin V/PI staining assay. (**d**) Percentages of cells at each stage were calculated. (**e**) OBA-RT at a concentration of 0-25 μM for 24 h induces cleavage of PARP, as examined by Western blot analysis. (**f**) Relative protein levels were quantified by densitometry. (**g**) The expression levels of apoptosis-associated proteins Bcl-2, Mcl-1, Bax, and p53 in A549 cells treated with OBA-RT (0–25 μM) for 24 h were examined by Western blot analysis. To confirm equal loading of the protein samples, the blots were reprobed with the GAPDH antibody. (**h**) Relative protein levels were quantified by densitometry. Data are presented as mean ± SEM (n = 3). *** $p < 0.0001$ compared with untreated control cells.

In addition, the specific apoptotic marker protein, namely poly (ADP-ribose) polymerase (PARP), and its cleaved form were detected in the treated cells. For mechanistic analysis, we monitored the alteration of apoptosis regulatory proteins, which belong to the Bcl-2 family and its upstream regulator p53 proteins. Protein determination was performed by Western blotting. Lung cancer cells were treated with OBA-RT (0–25 μM) for 24 h. Western blotting revealed that in response to OBA-RT treatment, the cleaved form of PARP was significantly increased compared with the untreated control cells, as shown in Figure 3e,f. For apoptosis induction, the major regulators of p53-dependent apoptosis, such as p53, anti-apoptotic proteins (Mcl-1 and Bcl-2), and pro-apoptotic proteins (Bax), were investigated in OBA-RT-treated cells. The results revealed that p53 was dramatically increased in response to compound treatment. Moreover, anti-apoptotic Bcl-2 and Mcl-1 were decreased, whereas pro-apoptotic Bax was found to be slightly altered (Figure 3g,h).

2.4. OBA-RT Suppresses CSC Spheroid Formation

CSCs have become an important target for the determination of novel anticancer drugs. The ability of cancer cells to form tumor spheroids has been referred to as augmented CSC potential. Next, we tested whether OBA-RT possessed CSC-suppressing activity. A549 cells were treated with OBA-RT at concentrations of 0-25 μM for 24 h, and the cells were subjected to a spheroid formation assay. The results showed that the cells treated with OBA-RT (5–25 μM) exhibited a reduced ability to form tumor spheroids in a concentration-dependent manner (Figure 4a–c). To further confirm the CSC-killing population, the apoptotic induction of OBA-RT in the CSC population of A549 cells was elucidated. A CSC-rich population was established in the lung cancer cells. The CSC spheroids were seeded in 96-well plates by ultralow attachment at a density of one spheroid per well. The spheroids were treated with OBA-RT (0–25 μM) for 24 h. In addition, the untreated spheroids exhibited normal survival features, and the OBA-RT-treated spheroids detached and dissociated (Figure 4d). Hoechst 33342 staining of the treated spheroids further revealed the apoptotic character of DNA fragmentation and/or DNA condensation in the OBA-RT-treated spheroids (Figure 4d–f). Collectively, OBA-RT possessed anti-CSC phenotypes that could induce CSC apoptosis.

2.5. OBA-RT Suppresses CSC Signals in A549 Cells

We determined CD133, a well-known CSC marker in response to compound treatment, to confirm the CSC-suppressing effect of OBA-RT. The cells were similarly treated with 0–25 μM OBA-RT for 24 h. The level of CD133 was then analyzed by immunofluorescence detected by a specific CD133 antibody. Figure 5a,b show that CD133 fluorescence intensity at concentrations of 5–25 μM significantly decreased when compared with the non-treatment control.

Inhibiting CSC-maintaining cellular signals is a potential way to reduce and improve clinical outcome in CSC-driven cancers, including lung cancer. The stemness properties of cancer are regulated by several pathways, and the Akt pathway can regulate pluripotent transcription factors, namely Nanog and Oct4. Considering that OBA-RT could suppress the CSC phenotypes in lung cancer cells, we further tested whether this compound could effectively inhibit the CSC upstream signals via Akt inhibition and deplete the transcription factors of stem cells. The A549 cells were treated with various concentrations of OBA-RT (0–25 μM) for 24 h. In addition, CSC transcription factors, namely Oct4 and Nanog, and CSC regulatory proteins, namely Akt, p-Akt, and c-Myc proteins, were analyzed by Western blotting analysis. The results revealed that Nanog, Oct4, and c-Myc were significantly decreased after OBA-RT treatment at concentrations of 5 and 25 μM. Akt signaling was highlighted as a therapeutic target for CSC-driven and malignant cancers; thus, the protein expression ratio of phosphorylated Akt/Akt was evaluated. After treatment of OBA-RT (5–25 μM) for 24 h, the p-Akt/Akt ratio was dramatically diminished when compared with the non-treatment control (Figure 5c,d).

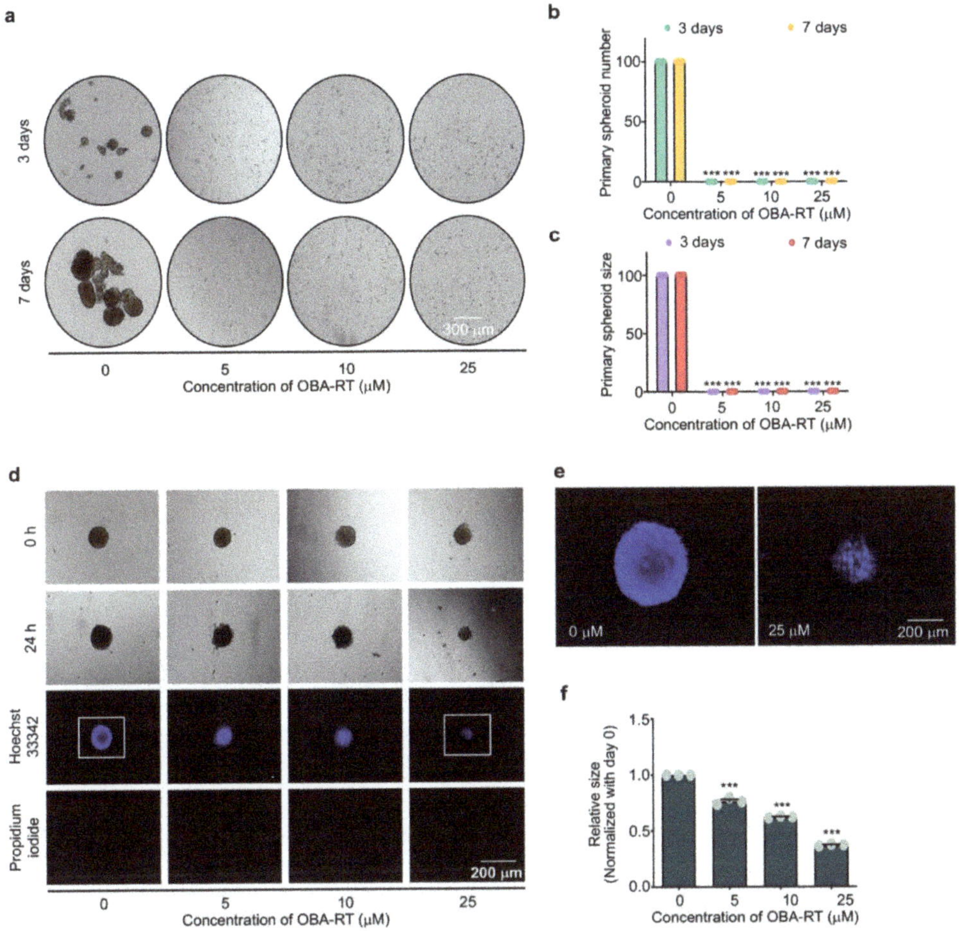

Figure 4. OBA-RT suppresses cancer stem cell (CSC) phenotypes in A549 human non-small-cell lung cancer cells. To assess the spheroid formation activity, (**a**) Cells were pre-treated with OBA-RT for 24 h and allowed to form primary spheroids for 7 days. The numbers (**b**) and sizes (**c**) of primary spheroids were calculated. (**d**) To further confirm the CSC-killing activity of OBA-RT, the CSC-rich populations in 3D culture were established by forming primary spheroids for 7 days. The primary spheroids were suspended into single cells to form CSC-rich spheroids for 14 days in ultralow-attachment 96-well plates. The CSC-rich spheroids were then treated with OBA-RT at concentrations of 0–25 μM for 24 h. (**e**) The apoptotic cells were determined by Hoechst 33342 staining. (**f**) Relative size of CSC spheroids was quantified. Data are presented as mean ± SEM ($n = 3$). *** $p < 0.0001$ compared with untreated control cells.

2.6. Molecular Docking Simulations Indicated the OBA-RT Interactions with the Allosteric Pocket of Akt-1 Protein

We performed a molecular docking simulation of OBA-RT with Akt (PDB code: 5KCV) to evaluate the possibility of a direct interaction between OBA-RT and Akt. In verifying the docking protocol, we redocked miransertib into its original binding site on Akt using Autodock Vina. The root mean square deviation (RMSD) of the redocked ligand was a small RMSD value (0.484 Å). The results (Figure 6d) indicated that the docking protocol was correct (RMSD < 2 Å) [27]. The binding energies of OBA-RT and co-crystal ligand miransertib have been reported in Table 1. OBA-RT could bind with Akt-1 with binding energy of −8.1 kcal/mol. As shown in Figure 6, OBA-RT forms two hydrogen bonds with Thr82 and Glu203 and forms hydrophobic interactions with Asn53, Asn54, Ser56, Ala58, Gln79, Trp80, Leu202, Ser205, Leu264, Lys268, Val270, and Asp292.

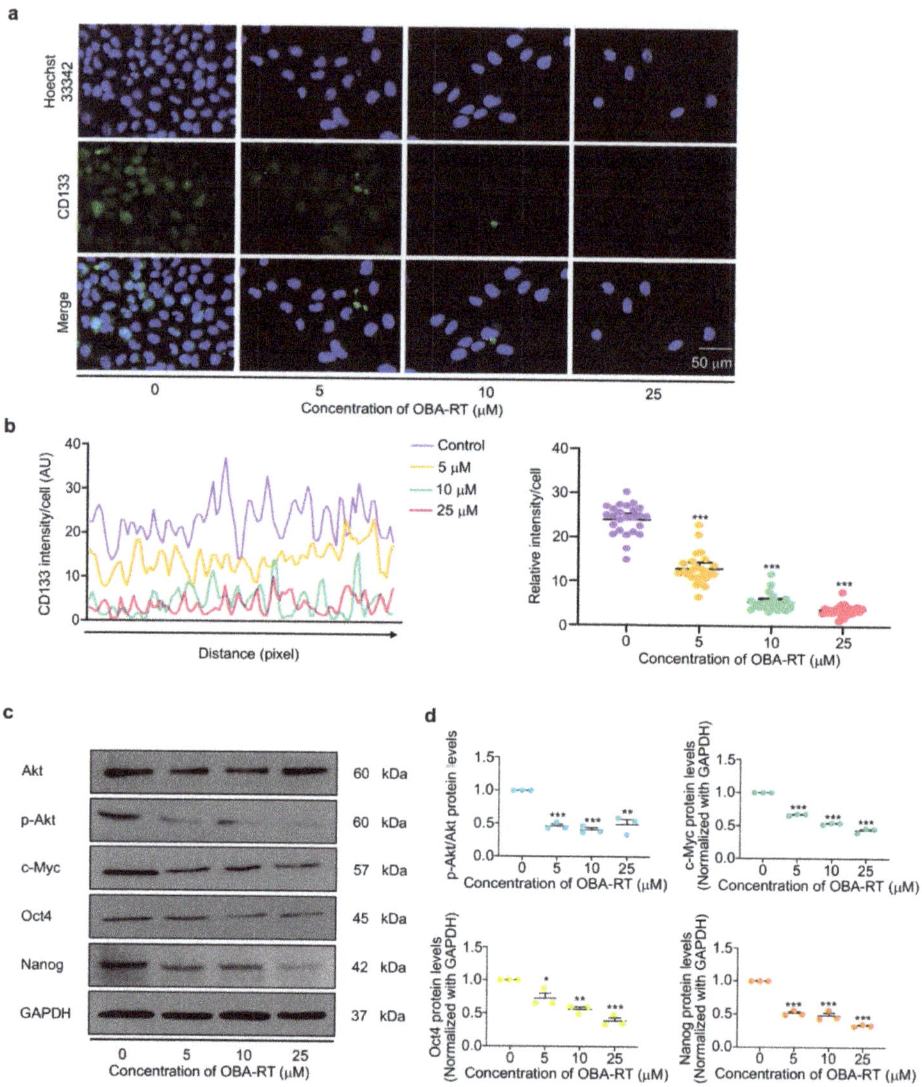

Figure 5. (**a**) OBA-RT inhibits Akt and suppresses CSCs. A549 cells were treated with OBA-RT for 24 h. The cells were co-stained with CD133 antibodies and Hoechst 33342. The expression of CD133 was examined by immunofluorescence (IF). (**b**) The fluorescence intensity was analyzed by ImageJ software. (**c**) The expression of activated Akt (p-Akt), total Akt, and the expression levels of stemness-related proteins Oct4, Nanog, and c-Myc in A549 cells treated with OBA-RT (0–25 uM) for 24 h were examined by Western blot analysis. To confirm equal loading of the protein samples, the blots were reprobed with the GAPDH antibody. (**d**) Relative protein levels were quantified by densitometry. Data are presented as mean ± SEM (n = 3). * $0.01 \leq p < 0.05$, ** $p < 0.01$, *** $p < 0.0001$ compared with untreated control cells.

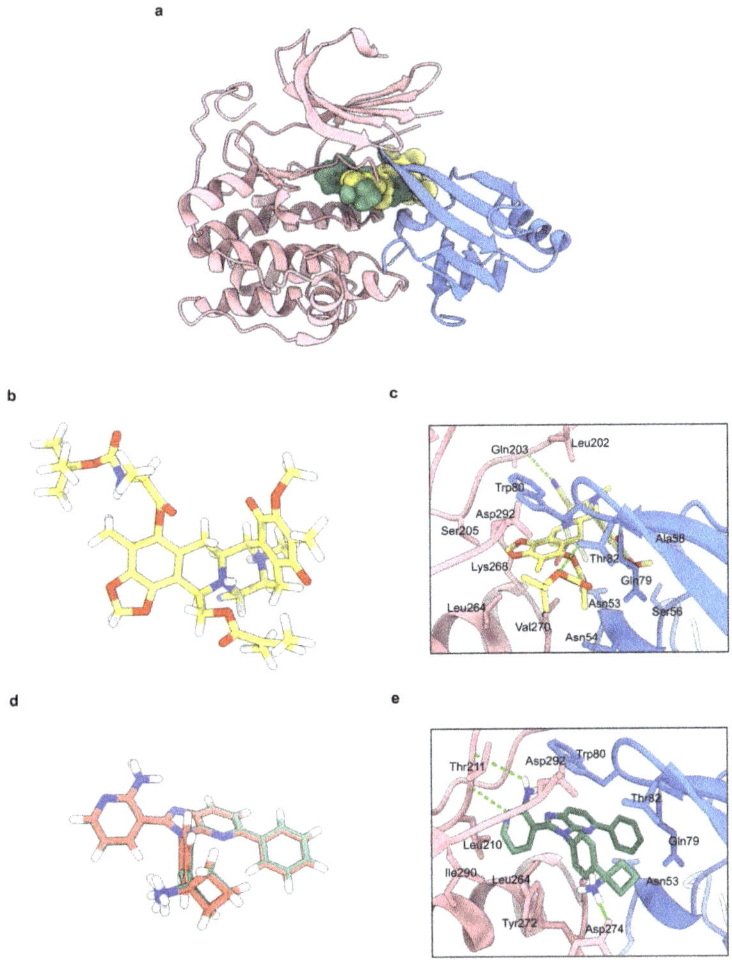

Figure 6. (**a**) Co-crystal structure of Akt-1 in complex with OBA-RT and miransertib (PDB code: 5KCV). The kinase domain is shown in pink, PH domain in blue, OBA-RT in yellow, and miransertib in green. (**b**) 3D chemical structure of OBA-RT. (**c**) The binding mode of OBA-RT to the allosteric pocket of Akt-1. One of two major hydrogen bonds was formed between the carbamate ether oxygen of Boc-L-alanine moiety and Thr82 while the butyl group was contributed to hydrophobic interactions with Leu264, Leu268, and Val270. (**d**) Redocking of miransertib in Akt-1 (PDB code: 5KCV); overlap of the co-crystal ligand miransertib (red) and redocking (green). (**e**) The binding mode of miransertib to the allosteric pocket of Akt-1. Hydrogen bonds are displayed as green dashed lines.

Table 1. Binding energy in kcal/mol of OBA-RT compared to co-crystal ligand miransertib.

Compounds	Binding Energy (kcal/mol)	Hydrogen Bond Interactions	Hydrophobic Interactions
Miransertib (Co-crystal ligand)	−12.8	Thr211, Tyr272	Asn53, Gln79, Trp80, Thr82, Leu210, Leu264, Val270, Tyr272, Asp274, Ile290
OBA-RT	−8.1	Thr82, Glu203	Asn53, Asn54, Ser56, Ala58, Gln79, Trp80, Leu202, Ser205, Leu264, Lys268, Val270, Asp292

3. Discussion

We reported a facile and concise semi-synthesis of OBA-RT (Figure 1) from RM isolated from the blue sponge *Xestospongia* sp. using benzoquinone/naphthoquinone-type photoredox chemistry [28] and Steglich esterification. In addition, phototransformation might account for the abiotic formation of hydroxybenzodioxole in naturally occurring saframycin-type tetrahydroisoquinolinequinones as an alternative enzymatic oxidative cyclization for the biosynthesis [28]. This photosynthetic approach for C–H activation at C-5 would be useful for other tetrahydroisoquinolinequinones, such as jorunnamycins, although the extent of utility and compatibility with other substitutions require further investigation. Compared with the three-step hydrogenation/esterification/oxidation scheme [19], this synthesis strategy should be amenable for any 5-*O*-conjugation of RT and related compounds. For example, the synthesis of a series of amino acid RT conjugates to allow the study of the structure–activity relationship could be performed using this two-step scheme. Moreover, it could enable creative functionalization, such as antibody–drug conjugations, fluorescence dye ligation for microscopy, and activity-based or photoaffinity probes for a target engagement study based on proteomics.

In this study, our data indicated that OBA-RT has a cytotoxic effect on human A549 cells with an IC_{50} value of 7.30 ± 0.07 μM and displays molecular pharmacological properties in cancer cells similar to previously reported structurally related compounds (Figure 2a,b). Our study revealed that OBA-RT treatment could significantly inhibit cell viability (Figure 2c–d) by inducing apoptotic cell death (Figure 3a–d).

One important apoptotic pathway is the p53-dependent pathway. The tumor suppressor p53 protein plays an important role in regulating DNA repair, cell cycle arrest, and apoptotic cell death. In response to DNA damage, p53 was activated via Ataxia telangiectasia-mutated kinases [29]. The activation of p53 resulted in the alteration of the cellular balance of Bcl-2 family proteins, thereby increasing the pro-apoptotic members and decreasing the anti-apoptotic proteins. This alteration causes the release of the mitochondrial contents to the cytoplasm, and such contents motivate the function of caspases leading to apoptotic cell death. However, inducing apoptosis is not sufficient to eliminate cancer. In this research, the results show that OBA-RT has a mechanism of action similar to that of RT by inducing the p53-dependent signaling pathway and suppressing Mcl-1, which is an anti-apoptotic marker (Figure 3g,h). Interestingly, the protein analysis shows a predominant effect of the cellular protein levels of Mcl-1. Mcl-1 is an anti-apoptotic protein that has gained increasing interest in lung cancer cell biology because it is highly expressed in lung cancer [30]. Furthermore, Mcl-1 is important for the survival of lung cancer cells.

Particular populations of cancer cells, namely CSCs, have been reported as key driving factors for malignancy in several cancers. The conventional cancer therapy can only eliminate cancer cells and not CSCs. The CSCs can escape, resulting in the relapse of the disease in the future [2]. Indeed, different anti-CSC strategies have been assessed by inhibiting many intracellular signaling pathways, such as Wnt/TCF, signal transducer and activator of transcription 3, namely NF-κB and Akt. Akt signaling can be considered as a key regulator for cancers and CSC phenotypes. Notably, Akt signaling plays a critical role in regulating CSC maintenance and properties [31]. Previous studies have revealed that Akt is directly linked to the master pluripotency factor Oct4 [32] and regulating transcription factors Nanog and Sox2, and reversed therapy resistance [33]. A series of reports has shown that Akt inhibition may lead to CSC suppression. For example, Rhodes revealed that GSK690693 is a novel Akt kinase inhibitor that has recently entered phase I clinical trials. GSK690693 inhibited proliferation and induced apoptosis in a subset of tumor cells with potency consistent with the intracellular inhibition of Akt kinase activity that showed reductions in phosphorylated Akt substrates in vivo [34]. In 2019, Chantarawong reported that *O*-acetyl RT can suppress CSCs in lung cancer by depleting the AKT signal [24]. Interestingly, *O*-acetyl RT has a chemical structure similar to OBA-RT. Hongwiangchan also reported that CIN-RM suppressed CSCs by inhibiting the AKT signaling pathway, resulting in the downregulation of stem cell transcription factors, including Nanog, Oct4, and Sox2 [21]. Nanog and Oct4 are the key transcription factors that control self-renewal and the pluripotency of CSCs, and are prognostic biomarkers in lung CSCs under regulation of the Akt signaling pathway [35].

The inhibition of Akt at an essential binding site for protein activity is a powerful strategy. At present, several critical binding sites have been focused on. Consequently, allosteric Akt inhibitors have been highly emphasized because of their role in blocking the kinase activity of Akt and interfering a pleckstrin homology (PH)-domain membrane- mediated recruitment [36]. This inhibition prevents Akt kinase activation and phosphorylation. In this study, considering the allosteric mechanism of OBA-RT, we performed molecular docking simulations using the binding interaction pattern of OBA-RT with the allosteric pocket of Akt-1. The molecular docking result revealed that OBA-RT could bind with Akt-1 with a binding energy of −8.1 kcal/mol, which is suitable for a potential interaction with Akt. The binding interaction pattern of OBA-RT with the allosteric pocket of Akt-1 is illustrated in Figure 6. The allosteric pocket of Akt-1 was located between the kinase domain and N-terminal PH domain [37]. OBA-RT forms a hydrogen bond with Gln203 and hydrophobic interactions with Leu202, Ser205, Leu264, Lys268, Val270, and Asp292 in the kinase domain. Moreover, it forms a hydrogen bond with Thr82 and hydrophobic interactions with Asn53, Asn54, Ser56, Ala58, Gln79, and Trp80 in the PH domain. Trp80 has been reported as an important residue for the allosteric Akt-1 inhibitor [38]. The Boc-L-alanine extension contributed significantly to the overall affinity of OBA-RT to Akt; that is, the hydrogen bond formed between the carbamate ether oxygen and the hydroxyl group of Thr82 and the hydrophobic interaction formed between the terminal tert-butyl group and Leu264, Lys268, and Val270. In addition, OBA-RT showed a similar binding pattern compared with miransertib, an oral allosteric Akt-1 inhibitor, by hydrophobic interaction with Trp80. Thus, the analyses suggest that OBA-RT could interact with Akt-1 via an allosteric mechanism, which demonstrates the ability of OBA-RT to inhibit Akt-1, following the previous experimental results. This result could support the conclusion that OBA-RT could be a potential anticancer agent by targeting Akt activation through an allosteric mechanism. Based on our computational analysis, OBA-RT-resistant cell lines with Akt variants harboring mutations in a key residue predicted to directly bind to OBA-RT can be generated for experimental validation. In vitro biophysical analyses for the determination of binding parameters between Akt and OBA-RT, such as isothermal titration calorimetry and thermal shift assay, might be conducted to verify the target engagement. By functionalizing OBA-RT with biotin or a bio-orthogonal group to be used in pull-down assays, chemoproteomics could be used to identify the complete set of cellular targets beyond Akt.

The cellular target profiling provided in this work contributes to a new perspective on tetrahydroisoquinoline antitumor antibiotics and may inform further systematic medicinal chemistry development of compounds in this class with defined molecular pharmacology details for next-generation therapy for intractable cancers.

4. Materials and Methods

4.1. Reagents and Antibodies

Dulbecco's Modified Eagle's Medium (DMEM) medium, fetal bovine serum (FBS), penicillin/streptomycin, L-glutamine, phosphate-buffered saline (PBS), and trypsin-EDTA were obtained from Gibco (Grand Island, NY, USA). 3-(4,5-dimethylthiazol-2-yl)-2,5-Diphenyltetrazoliumbromide (MTT), dimethyl sulfoxide (DMSO), Hoechst 33342, propidium iodide (PI), and bovine serum albumin (BSA) were obtained from Sigma-Aldrich, Co. (St. Louis, MO, USA). The following primary antibodies, PARP (#9532), p53 (#9282), Mcl-1 (#94296), Bcl-2 (#4223), BAX (#5023), Akt (#9272), phosphorylated Akt (#4060), Nanog (#4903), Oct4 (#2840), c-Myc (#5605), and GADPH (#5174) were obtained from Cell Signaling Technology (Danvers, MA, USA). CD133 (#CA1217) was obtained from Cell Applications (San Diego, CA, USA). The respective secondary antibodies, anti-rabbit IgG (#7074) and anti-mouse (#7076), were obtained from Cell Signaling Technology (Danvers, MA, USA).

4.2. Semi-Synthesis of 5-O-(N-Boc-L-Alanine)-Renieramycin T (OBA-RT)

Renieramycin M was isolated from the Thai blue sponge *Xestospongia* sp. collected at Si-chang Island, in the Gulf of Thailand, with assistance from the Aquatic Recourses Research Institute, Chulalongkorn University, and permission from the Department of Fisheries, Ministry of Agriculture and Cooperatives, Thailand (0510.2/8234, Date 28 October 2019). The fresh blue sponge was mashed, pre-treated with potassium cyanide (10 mM) in phosphate buffer at pH 7, macerated in methanol, concentrated, extracted with ethyl acetate, and purified through silica gel column chromatography to obtain renieramycin M as an orange solid with an isolation yield of 0.02% w/w relative to the dry sponge [19].

Chemical reactions were carried out at room temperature (25 °C) using oven-dried glassware and magnetically stirred under an argon atmosphere using a balloon. The chemical reagents were purchased from Aldrich (Missouri, USA) and TCI (Tokyo, Japan). Anhydrous solvents were dried over 4Å molecular sieves. All reactions were monitored by thin-layer chromatography (TLC) performed using aluminum silica gel 60F254 (Merck, Darmstadt, Germany). Bands were identified by UV activity. Flash column chromatography was performed using 60 Å silica gel (230–400 mesh) as a stationary phase along with ethyl acetate and hexanes as a mobile phase. Regarding structure elucidations, infrared (IR) spectra were measured on a Perkin Frontier Fourier Transform Infrared Spectrometer. ^{1}H and ^{13}C nuclear magnetic resonance (NMR) spectra were obtained on a Bruker ADVANCE NEO 400 MHz NMR spectrometer, and deuterated chloroform (CDCl3) served as the internal standard for both ^{1}H (7.27 ppm) and ^{13}C (77.0 ppm) spectra. Accurate mass spectra were obtained using an Agilent 6540 UHD Q-TOF LC/MS spectrometer.

Renieramycin M (20 mg, 0.0347 mmol) was weighed into a round-bottom flask and dissolved in dry dichloromethane (30 mL). The orange reaction mixture was irradiated with 18 W fluorescent lamp [39]. The mixture was stirred vigorously at room temperature for 24 h under argon atmosphere. The reaction was monitored by TLC. Once all the starting material was consumed, 1-ethyl-3-(3-dimethylaminopropyl) carbodiimide (EDCI.HCl, 6.65 mg, 0.0347 mmol) and *N*, *N*-4-dimethylaminopyridine (DMAP, 4.24 mg, 0.0347 mmol) were added to the reaction. After stirring for 5 min, *N*-Boc-L-alanine was added (32.83 mg, 0.1735 mmol). The yellow reaction mixture was stirred at room temperature for 3 h under argon atmosphere. Next, the reaction was quenched by addition of water (5 mL). The organic layer was separated by separatory funnel and the aqueous layer was extracted with CH_2Cl_2 (10 mL, 3 times). The organic layers were combined, dried over anhydrous Na_2SO_4, filtered, and concentrated under reduced pressure. Purification by the silica gel flash chromatography eluting with hexanes:EtOAc (1:1) gave 6.1 mg (24%) of 5-*O*-(*N*-Boc-L-alanine)-renieramycin T as a brown amorphous solid. Chemical structure of 5-*O*-(*N*-Boc-L-alanine)-renieramycin T was elucidated by spectroscopic analysis as follows: IR (ATR) λ_{max} in cm^{-1}: 3401.4, 2923.9, 2851.3, 1714.6,1654.0, 1456.7, 1410.0, 1376.8, 1305.7, 1233.5, 1150.6, 1093.7, 1043.8, 955.7, 769.9, 732.8, 557.1. ^{1}H-NMR ($CDCl_3$, 400 MHz) δ_H in ppm: 5.98 (1H, overlapped, 26-H), 5.97 (2H, dd, *J* = 22.4, 1.2, Hz, OCH_2O), 5.01 (1H, br d, *J* = 7.2 Hz, 3′-NH), 4.58 (1H, t, *J* = 6.8 Hz, 2′-H), 4.53 (1H, dd, *J* = 11.6, 3.6 Hz, 22-H_a), 4.02 (1H, dd, *J* = 11.6, 4.4, 22-H_b), 4.16 (1H, overlapped, 1-H), 4.11 (1H, overlapped, 21-H). 3.97 (1H, overlapped, 11-H), 3.96 (3H, s, 17-OCH_3), 3.36 (1H, d, *J* = 7.6, 13-H), 3.23 (1H, dt, *J* = 12.4, 2.8 Hz, 3-H), 2.73 (1H, dd, *J* = 20.8, 7.6 Hz, 14-H_α), 2.55 (1H, m, 4-H_α), 2.32 (1H, dd, *J* = 15.6, 7.6 Hz, 14-H_β), 2.28 (3H, s, NCH_3), 2.04 (3H, s, 6-CH_3), 1.90 (3H, s, 16-CH_3), 1.85 (3H, dq, *J* = 7.6, 1.2 Hz, 27-H_3), 1.70 (3H, d, *J* = 7.2, 7′-H_3), 1.61 (1H, overlapped, 4-H_β), 1.66 (3H, s, 28-H_3), 1.46 (9H, br s, 3 × 6′-CH_3); ^{13}C-NMR ($CDCl_3$, 100 MHz) δ_C in ppm: 186.0 (C-15), 182.7 (C-18), 171.2 (C-1′), 167.0 (C-24), 158.3 (C-4′), 155.2 (C-17), 144.9 (C-7), 141.9 (C-20), 140.9 (C-8), 139.9 (C-5), 140.2 (C-26), 135.3 (C-19), 129.0 (C-16), 126.7 (C-25), 119.9 (C-6), 117.3 (21-CN), 112.3 (C-10), 112.1 (C-9), 101.8 (OCH_2O), 80.1 (C-5′), 63.6 (C-22), 60.9 (17-OCH_3), 59.2 (C-21), 56.3 (C-1), 55.5 (C-3), 54.8 (C-11), 54.7 (C-13), 49.3 (C-2′), 41.4 (NCH_3), 28.3 (3 × 6′-CH_3), 27.6 (C-14), 21.0 (C-4), 20.5 (28-CH_3), 18.6 (7′-CH_3), 15.9 (27-CH_3), 9.5 (6-CH_3), 8.6 (16-CH_3). HR-ESI-MS m/z 747.3231 ($[M+H]^+$, calculated for $C_{39}H_{47}N_4O_{11}$, 747.3236).

4.3. Preparation of the OBA-RT Stock Solution

OBA-RT was prepared by dissolving it in dimethyl sulfoxide (DMSO) solution and then stored at −20 °C. It was freshly diluted with medium to the desired concentrations before use. The final concentration of DMSO in solution was less than 0.5%, which caused no signs of cytotoxicity.

4.4. Cell Lines and Culture

Human non-small cell lung cancer (NSCLC) cell lines, A549 (ATCC® CCL-185™, RRID: CVCL_0023) cells were obtained from the American Type Culture Collection (Manassas, VA, USA). A549 cells were cultured in DMEM. The medium was supplemented with 10% FBS, 2 mM L-glutamine, and 100 units/mL of each penicillin and streptomycin at 37 °C with 5% CO_2 in a humidified incubator.

4.5. Cell Viability

A549 cells were cultured in 96-well plates at a density of 1×10^4 cells/well and incubated overnight at environment 5% CO_2. Cells were treated with OBA-RT at concentrations 0 to 25 μM for 24 h. After treatment, 100 μL of MTT reagent (0.4 mg/mL) was added to each well and incubated for 3 h. The formazan crystals were dissolved in DMSO and measured using a microplate reader (Anthros, Durham, NC, USA) at a wavelength of 570 nm.

4.6. Colony Formation Assay

The survival ability to colonize single cancer cells was investigated by colony formation assay. After treatment, cells were cultured into 6-well plates at density of 300 cells/well and incubated for 7 days. The cells were washed with 1X PBS, fixed with 4% paraformaldehyde (Sigma Chemical, St. Louis, MO, USA) for 30 min, and stained with 0.5% crystal violet solution. Cells were washed with 1 × PBS three times, and the number and sizes of colonies were counted.

4.7. Apoptotic Assay

A549 cells were seeded in 96-well plates at a density of 1×10^4 cells/well and allowed to attach overnight. Cells were incubated with various concentrations of OBA-RT at 0 to 25 μM for 24 h, and then the cells were co-stained with 10 μM of Hoechst 33342 (Sigma, St. Louis, MO, USA) and propidium iodide (PI) (Sigma, St. Louis, MO, USA) for 30 min in darkness. Fluorescence microscopy (Olympus DP70, Melville, NY, USA) was performed to image the apoptotic cells.

In addition, Annexin V-FITC Apoptosis Kit (Thermo Fisher Scientific, Waltham, MA, USA) was assessed to investigate apoptotic and necrotics cells. A549 cells were seeded into 24-well plates at a density of 1.5×10^4 cells/well and incubated overnight. Cells were treated with indicated concentrations of OBA-RT (0–25 μM) for 24 h, then harvested and suspended in the binding buffer followed by incubation with Annexin V and PI for 15 min in darkness. Apoptotic and necrotic cells were assessed by Guava easyCyte™ flow cytometry (EMD Millipore, Hayward, CA, USA).

4.8. Spheroid Formation Assay

A549 cells were pre-treated with concentrations of OBA-RT (0–25 μM) for 24 h. The treated cells were seeded onto ultralow attachment plates at a density 2.5×10^3 cells/well in DMEM containing 1% FBS (*v/v*) (Merck, DA, Germany) for 7 days to form spheroids. On days 3 and 7, the numbers and sizes of spheroids were determined using a phase-contrast microscopy (Nikon ECLIPSE Ts2, Tokyo, Japan).

4.9. CSC-Rich Population

The enrichment of the CSC subpopulation in cancer cells was successfully performed through the three-dimensional (3D) spheroid-formation assay. A549 cells were seeded onto 24-well ultralow attachment plates at approximately 2.5×10^3 cells/well with serum-free medium to form primary spheroids for 7 days. After that, primary spheroids were resuspended into single cells and seeded onto 96-well ultralow attachment plates for 14 days to form CSC-rich spheroids. After 14 days, CSC-rich spheroids were treated with concentrations of OBA-RT (0–25 μM) for 24 h. After treatment, apoptotic cell death was analyzed with Hoechst 33342 and size of single spheroid was captured using phase-contrast microscopy (Nikon ECLIPSE Ts2, Tokyo, Japan).

4.10. Western Blot Analysis

A549 cells were seeded at a density of 4×10^5 cells/well in 6-well plates overnight. Cells were treated with OBA-RT (0–25 μM) for 24 h. Then, cells were washed with cold 1X PBS and incubated in RIPA buffer, 1% Triton X-100, 100 mM PMSF, and a protease inhibitor for 30 min on ice. Protein concentrations were quantified using BCA protein assay kit from Pierce Biotechnology (Rockford, IL, USA). Cell lysates were separated by sodium dodecyl sulfate polyacrylamide gel electrophoresis (SDS-PAGE) and transferred to polyvinylidene difluoride (PVDF) (Bio-Rad Laboratories Inc., Hercules, CA, USA). The membrane was blocked with 5% (*w/v*) non-fat dry milk power (Merck, Darmstadt, Germany) at room temperature for 2 h and each membrane was incubated with the specific primary antibodies for overnight at 4 °C, as well as incubated with horseradish peroxidase (HRP)-conjugated secondary antibodies (Cell Signaling, Danvers, MA, USA) for 2 h at room temperature. The protein expression was observed using chemiluminescence (Supersignal West Pico; Pierce, Rockford, IL, USA) and quantified using ImageJ software (NIH, Bethesda, MD, USA).

4.11. Immunofluorescence Assay

A549 cells were seeded into 96-well plates at a density 1×10^4 cells/well and incubated overnight. After treatment with OBA-RT for 24 h, the cells were fixed with 4% paraformaldehyde for 30 min, permeabilized with 0.5% Triton-X for 5 min, and blocked with 4% BSA for 1 h at room temperature. The cells were incubated with an anti-CD133 antibody overnight at 4 °C and then incubated with secondary antibody for 1 h, stained with Hoechst 33342 (Sigma, St. Louis, MO, USA) for 30 min at room temperature in darkness, and mounted using 50% glycerol (Merck, Darmstadt, Germany). Confocal images were assessed under fluorescence microscope (Nikon ECLIPSE Ts2, Tokyo, Japan) and analyzed by ImageJ software.

4.12. Molecular Docking

The crystal structure of miransertib (ARQ092) in complex with the Akt-1 [40] was retrieved from the Research Collaboratory for Structural Bioinformatics Protein Data Bank (PDB code: 5KCV) [41]. All water molecules and co-crystal ligand were deleted with the UCSF ChimeraX [42]. AutoDockTools version 1.5.7 [43] was used to repair missing atoms and add polar hydrogen atoms. The structure of OBA-RT was constructed utilizing MarvinSketch and optimized with the Gaussian 09 program [44] using density functional theory (DFT) with a B3LYP/6-31G (d,p) basis set. Autodock Vina [45] was performed to investigate an interaction between OBA-RT and the allosteric pocket of Akt-1 using default parameters. A grid box was set with the center of the co-crystal ligand (PDB code: 5KCV). The grid size was set to $20 \times 20 \times 20$ Å with a spacing of 1 Å. Furthermore, visualization of binding interaction patterns was carried out by UCSF ChimeraX.

4.13. Statistical Analysis

All results were compared and expressed as mean ± standard error of the mean (SEM) from at least triplicate independent experiments. Statistical analyses were evaluated using analysis of variance (ANOVA) followed by Tukey's HSD post hoc test. The statistic was calculated by using SPSS version 28 (IBM Corp., Armonk, NY, USA). Statistically significant differences were indicated by * p-values less than 0.05. GraphPad Prism 9 was used for creating graphs in all experiments (GraphPad Software, San Diego, CA, USA).

5. Conclusions

These results provide novel and significant data on the new derivative of RT (OBA-RT) suggesting it can be considered as a potential therapy for lung CSCs. The compound has a potent apoptotic and CSC-suppressing activity in lung cancer cells (Figure 7a,b). In addition, the OBA-RT molecule could exert allosteric inhibition of the Akt protein. As Akt is critical for cancer cell survival and stemness phenotypes, our results might be used in demonstrating OBA-RT as a potential therapy for CSC and Akt-driven cancers.

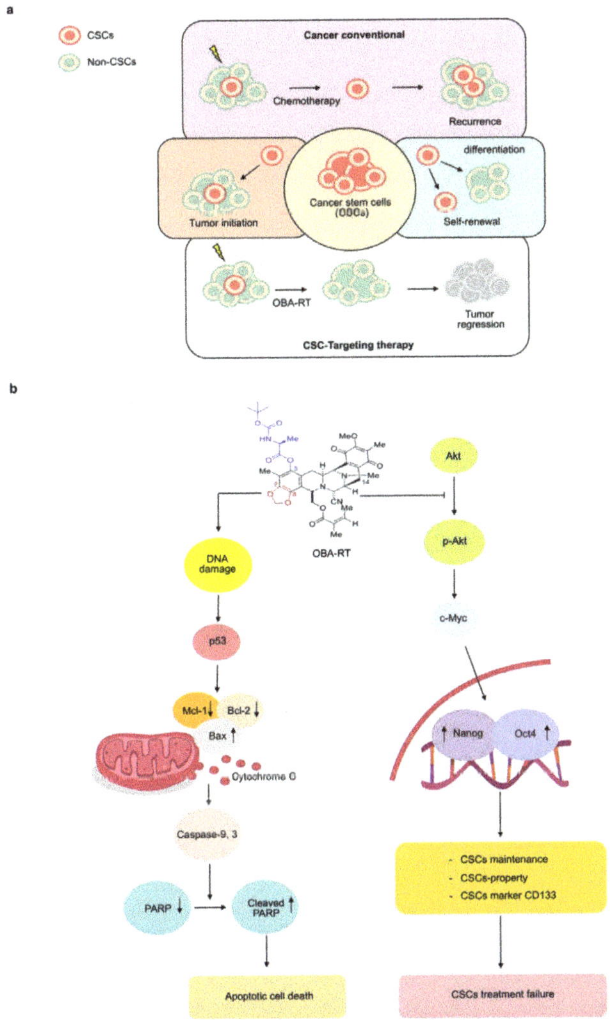

Figure 7. The proposed regulatory pathway of OBA-RT in inhibition of CSC and induction of apoptosis. (**a**) CSCs drive cancer initiation, progression, and therapeutic failure due to their abilities to initiate cancer, induce self-renewal and tumorigenicity, and augment pluripotent signals. CSCs are known to be highly resistant to chemotherapy and cause cancer relapse. Specific treatment to CSCs may induce cancer collapse and prevent the relapse of the disease. (**b**) Akt signaling pathways are critical for CSC properties and apoptotic cell death leading to cancer aggressiveness. OBA-RT could inhibit Akt function, resulting in the induction of apoptosis and cancer stem cell suppression activity in lung cancer cells.

Supplementary Materials: The following are available online at https://www.mdpi.com/article/10.3390/md20040235/s1, Figure S1: ^{1}H-NMR (400 MHz) spectrum of 5-*O*-(*N*-Boc-L-alanine)-renieramycin T in $CDCl_3$; Figure S2: ^{13}C-NMR (400 MHz) spectrum of 5-*O*-(*N*-Boc-L-alanine)-renieramycin T in $CDCl_3$; Figure S3: COSY (400 MHz) spectrum of 5-*O*-(*N*-Boc-L-alanine)-renieramycin T in $CDCl_3$; Figure S4: HSQC (400 MHz) spectrum of 5-O-(*N*-Boc-L-alanine)-renieramycin T in $CDCl_3$; Figure S5: HMBC (400 MHz) spectrum of 5-*O*-(*N*-Boc-L-alanine)-renieramycin T in $CDCl_3$.

Author Contributions: Conceptualization, P.C.; validation, P.C.; formal analysis, P.C., D.S., C.C. (Chatchai Chaotham) and C.C. (Chaisak Chansriniyom); investigation, D.S., S.R., N.S. and P.C.; resources, S.C. and K.S.; synthesized OBA-RT compound, K.A. and A.C.K.L.; writing—original draft preparation, D.S.; writing—review and editing, P.C. All authors have read and agreed to the published version of the manuscript.

Funding: This project is funded by National Research Council of Thailand (NRCT) (N41A640075).

Institutional Review Board Statement: Not applicable.

Data Availability Statement: Data is contained within the article.

Acknowledgments: The authors would like to thank Kittipong Sanookpan for supportive advice and training. We are sincerely grateful for the scholarship from the Graduate School, Chulalongkorn University to commemorate the 72nd anniversary of his Majesty King Bhumibol Adulyadej.

Conflicts of Interest: The authors declare no conflict of interest.

References

1. Tang, Z.; Wang, Q.; Shigdar, S.; Duan, W.; Xiang, D. Cancer Stem Cells—Perspectives and How to Target Them. In *Smart Drug Delivery System*; IntechOpen: London, UK, 2016; pp. 117–137.
2. Pan, Y.; Ma, S.; Cao, K.; Zhou, S.; Zhao, A.; Li, M.; Qian, F.; Zhu, C. Therapeutic approaches targeting cancer stem cells. *J. Cancer Res. Ther.* **2018**, *14*, 1469–1475. [CrossRef] [PubMed]
3. Dragu, D.L.; Necula, L.G.; Bleotu, C.; Diaconu, C.C.; Chivu-Economescu, M. Therapies targeting cancer stem cells: Current trends and future challenges. *World J. Stem Cells* **2015**, *7*, 1185–1201. [CrossRef] [PubMed]
4. Casey, S.C.; Baylot, V.; Felsher, D.W. The MYC oncogene is a global regulator of the immune response. *Blood* **2018**, *131*, 2007–2015. [CrossRef] [PubMed]
5. Chanvorachote, P.; Sriratanasak, N.; Nonpanya, N. C-myc Contributes to Malignancy of Lung Cancer: A Potential Anticancer Drug Target. *Anticancer Res.* **2020**, *40*, 609–618. [CrossRef]
6. Zhang, H.F.; Wu, C.; Alshareef, A.; Gupta, N.; Zhao, Q.; Xu, X.E.; Jiao, J.W.; Li, E.M.; Xu, L.Y.; Lai, R. The PI3K/AKT/c-MYC Axis Promotes the Acquisition of Cancer Stem-Like Features in Esophageal Squamous Cell Carcinoma. *Stem Cells* **2016**, *34*, 2040–2051. [CrossRef]
7. Tan, A.C. Targeting the PI3K/Akt/mTOR pathway in non-small cell lung cancer (NSCLC). *Thorac. Cancer* **2020**, *11*, 511–518. [CrossRef]
8. Demetri, G.D.; Von Mehren, M.; Jones, R.L.; Hensley, M.L.; Schuetze, S.M.; Staddon, A.; Milhem, M.; Elias, A.; Ganjoo, K.; Tawbi, H. Efficacy and safety of trabectedin or dacarbazine for metastatic liposarcoma or leiomyosarcoma after failure of conventional chemotherapy: Results of a phase III randomized multicenter clinical trial. *J. Clin. Oncol.* **2016**, *34*, 786. [CrossRef]
9. Yokoi, E.; Mabuchi, S.; Shimura, K.; Komura, N.; Kozasa, K.; Kuroda, H.; Takahashi, R.; Sasano, T.; Kawano, M.; Matsumoto, Y. Lurbinectedin (PM01183), a selective inhibitor of active transcription, effectively eliminates both cancer cells and cancer stem cells in preclinical models of uterine cervical cancer. *Investig. New Drugs* **2019**, *37*, 818–827. [CrossRef]
10. Hoda, M.A.; Pirker, C.; Dong, Y.; Schelch, K.; Heffeter, P.; Kryeziu, K.; van Schoonhoven, S.; Klikovits, T.; Laszlo, V.; Rozsas, A. Trabectedin is active against malignant pleural mesothelioma cell and xenograft models and synergizes with chemotherapy and Bcl-2 inhibition in vitro. *Mol. Cancer Ther.* **2016**, *15*, 2357–2369. [CrossRef]
11. Martínez-Serra, J.; Maffiotte, E.; Martín, J.; Bex, T.; Navarro-Palou, M.; Ros, T.; Plazas, J.M.; Vögler, O.; Gutiérrez, A.; Amat, J.C. Yondelis®(ET-743, Trabectedin) sensitizes cancer cell lines to CD95-mediated cell death: New molecular insight into the mechanism of action. *Eur. J. Pharmacol.* **2011**, *658*, 57–64. [CrossRef]
12. Powan, P.; Saito, N.; Suwanborirux, K.; Chanvorachote, P. Ecteinascidin 770, a tetrahydroisoquinoline alkaloid, sensitizes human lung cancer cells to anoikis. *Anticancer Res.* **2013**, *33*, 505–512. [PubMed]
13. Scott, J.D.; Williams, R.M. Chemistry and biology of the tetrahydroisoquinoline antitumor antibiotics. *Chem. Rev.* **2002**, *102*, 1669–1730. [CrossRef] [PubMed]
14. Fang, Y.; Li, H.; Ji, B.; Cheng, K.; Wu, B.; Li, Z.; Zheng, C.; Hua, H.; Li, D. Renieramycin-type alkaloids from marine-derived organisms: Synthetic chemistry, biological activity and structural modification. *Eur. J. Med. Chem.* **2021**, *210*, 113092. [CrossRef] [PubMed]

15. Sirimangkalakitti, N.; Chamni, S.; Suwanborirux, K.; Chanvorachote, P. Renieramycin M sensitizes anoikis-resistant H460 lung cancer cells to anoikis. *Anticancer Res.* **2016**, *36*, 1665–1671.
16. Tatsukawa, M.; Punzalan, L.L.C.; Magpantay, H.D.; Villasenor, I.M.; Concepcion, G.P.; Suwanborirux, K.; Yokoya, M.; Saito, N. Chemistry of renieramycins. Part 13: Isolation and structure of stabilized renieramycin type derivatives, renieramycins W–Y, from Philippine blue sponge *Xestospongia* sp., pretreated with potassium cyanide. *Tetrahedron* **2012**, *68*, 7422–7428. [CrossRef]
17. Sirimangkalakitti, N.; Chamni, S.; Suwanborirux, K.; Chanvorachote, P. Renieramycin m attenuates cancer stem cell-like phenotypes in h460 lung cancer cells. *Anticancer Res.* **2017**, *37*, 615–621. [CrossRef]
18. Martinez, E.J.; Owa, T.; Schreiber, S.L.; Corey, E. Phthalascidin, a synthetic antitumor agent with potency and mode of action comparable to ecteinascidin 743. *Proc. Natl. Acad. Sci. USA* **1999**, *96*, 3496–3501. [CrossRef]
19. Chamni, S.; Sirimangkalakitti, N.; Chanvorachote, P.; Suwanborirux, K.; Saito, N. Chemistry of renieramycins. Part 19: Semi-syntheses of 22-O-amino ester and hydroquinone 5-O-amino ester derivatives of renieramycin M and their cytotoxicity against non-small-cell lung cancer cell lines. *Mar. Drugs* **2020**, *18*, 418. [CrossRef]
20. Maiuthed, A.; Pinkhien, T.; Chamni, S.; Suwanborirux, K.; Saito, N.; Petpiroon, N.; Chanvorachote, P. Apoptosis-inducing effect of hydroquinone 5-O-cinnamoyl ester analog of renieramycin M on non-small cell lung cancer cells. *Anticancer. Res.* **2017**, *37*, 6259–6267.
21. Hongwiangchan, N.; Sriratanasak, N.; Wichadakul, D.; Aksorn, N.; Chamni, S.; Chanvorachote, P. Hydroquinone 5-O-Cinnamoyl Ester of Renieramycin M Suppresses Lung Cancer Stem Cells by Targeting Akt and Destabilizes c-Myc. *Pharmaceuticals* **2021**, *14*, 1112. [CrossRef]
22. Daikuhara, N.; Tada, Y.; Yamaki, S.; Charupant, K.; Amnuoypol, S.; Suwanborirux, K.; Saito, N. Chemistry of renieramycins. Part 7: Renieramycins T and U, novel renieramycin–ecteinascidin hybrid marine natural products from Thai sponge *Xestospongia* sp. *Tetrahedron Lett.* **2009**, *50*, 4276–4278. [CrossRef]
23. Petsri, K.; Chamni, S.; Suwanborirux, K.; Saito, N.; Chanvorachote, P. Renieramycin T Induces Lung Cancer Cell Apoptosis by Targeting Mcl-1 Degradation: A New Insight in the Mechanism of Action. *Mar. Drugs* **2019**, *17*, 301. [CrossRef] [PubMed]
24. Chantarawong, W.; Chamni, S.; Suwanborirux, K.; Saito, N.; Chanvorachote, P. 5-O-Acetyl-Renieramycin T from Blue Sponge *Xestospongia* sp. Induces Lung Cancer Stem Cell Apoptosis. *Mar. Drugs* **2019**, *17*, 109. [CrossRef] [PubMed]
25. Yokoya, M.; Toyoshima, R.; Suzuki, T.; Le, V.H.; Williams, R.M.; Saito, N. Stereoselective total synthesis of (−)-renieramycin T. *J. Org. Chem.* **2016**, *81*, 4039–4047. [CrossRef]
26. He, W.; Zhang, Z.; Ma, D. A Scalable Total Synthesis of the Antitumor Agents Et-743 and Lurbinectedin. *Angew. Chem. Int. Ed.* **2019**, *58*, 3972–3975. [CrossRef] [PubMed]
27. Cleves, A.; Jain, A. Knowledge-guided docking: Accurate prospective prediction of bound configurations of novel ligands using Surflex-Dock. *J. Comput.-Aided Mol. Des.* **2015**, *29*, 485–509. [PubMed]
28. Ando, Y.; Suzuki, K. Photoredox reactions of quinones. *Chem.–Eur. J.* **2018**, *24*, 15955–15964. [CrossRef]
29. Andrew, N.; Stephen, P. ATM, ATR, and DNA-PK: The Trinity at the Heart of the DNA Damage Response. *Mol. Cell* **2017**, *66*, 801–817.
30. Nakajima, W.; Tanaka, N. The anti-apoptotic protein MCL1, a novel target of lung cancer therapy. *J. Cancer Treat. Diagn.* **2018**, *2*, 54–58.
31. Yu, J.S.; Cui, W. Proliferation, survival and metabolism: The role of PI3K/AKT/mTOR signalling in pluripotency and cell fate determination. *Development* **2016**, *143*, 3050–3060. [CrossRef]
32. Lin, Y.; Yang, Y.; Li, W.; Chen, Q.; Li, J.; Pan, X.; Zhou, L.; Liu, C.; Chen, C.; He, J.; et al. Reciprocal regulation of Akt and Oct4 promotes the self-renewal and survival of embryonal carcinoma cells. *Mol. Cell* **2012**, *48*, 627–640. [CrossRef] [PubMed]
33. Yoon, C.; Lu, J.; Yi, B.C.; Chang, K.K.; Simon, M.C.; Ryeom, S.; Yoon, S.S. PI3K/Akt pathway and Nanog maintain cancer stem cells in sarcomas. *Oncogenesis* **2021**, *10*, 12. [CrossRef] [PubMed]
34. Rhodes, N.; Heerding, D.A.; Duckett, D.R.; Eberwein, D.J.; Knick, V.B.; Lansing, T.J.; McConnell, R.T.; Gilmer, T.M.; Zhang, S.Y.; Robell, K.; et al. Characterization of an Akt kinase inhibitor with potent pharmacodynamic and antitumor activity. *Cancer Res.* **2008**, *68*, 2366–2374. [CrossRef] [PubMed]
35. Liu, A.; Yu, X.; Liu, S. Pluripotency transcription factors and cancer stem cells: Small genes make a big difference. *Chin. J. Cancer* **2013**, *32*, 483. [CrossRef]
36. Liu, G.; Shi, A.; Wang, N.; Li, M.; He, X.; Yin, C.; Tu, Q.; Shen, X.; Tao, Y.; Wang, Q. Polyphenolic Proanthocyanidin-B2 suppresses proliferation of liver cancer cells and hepatocellular carcinogenesis through directly binding and inhibiting AKT activity. *Redox Biol.* **2020**, *37*, 101701. [CrossRef]
37. Yilmaz, O.G.; Olmez, E.O.; Ulgen, K.O. Targeting the Akt1 allosteric site to identify novel scaffolds through virtual screening. *Comput. Biol. Chem.* **2014**, *48*, 1–13. [CrossRef]
38. Wu, W.I.; Voegtli, W.C.; Sturgis, H.L.; Dizon, F.P.; Vigers, G.P.; Brandhuber, B.J. Crystal structure of human AKT1 with an allosteric inhibitor reveals a new mode of kinase inhibition. *PLoS ONE* **2010**, *5*, e12913. [CrossRef]
39. Yokoya, M.; Takahashi, S.; Saito, N. Preparation of Tricyclic Analog As Cde Ring Model of Renieramycin Marine Natural Product by Novel Photo-Induced Transformation of 6-Methoxy-1,2,3,4-Tetrahydroisoquinoline-5,8-Dione (Dedicated to Professor Tohru Fukuyama on the occasion of his 70th birthday). *Heterocycles Int. J. Rev. Commun. Heterocycl. Chem.* **2019**, *99*, 1276–1303.

40. Lapierre, J.-M.; Eathiraj, S.; Vensel, D.; Liu, Y.; Bull, C.O.; Cornell-Kennon, S.; Iimura, S.; Kelleher, E.W.; Kizer, D.E.; Koerner, S. Discovery of 3-(3-(4-(1-Aminocyclobutyl)phenyl)-5-phenyl-3H-imidazo[4,5-b]pyridin-2-yl) pyridin-2-amine (ARQ 092): An orally bioavailable, selective, and potent allosteric AKT inhibitor. *J. Med. Chem.* **2016**, *59*, 6455–6469. [CrossRef]
41. Burley, S.K.; Bhikadiya, C.; Bi, C.; Bittrich, S.; Chen, L.; Crichlow, G.V.; Christie, C.H.; Dalenberg, K.; Di Costanzo, L.; Duarte, J.M.; et al. RCSB Protein Data Bank: Powerful new tools for exploring 3D structures of biological macromolecules for basic and applied research and education in fundamental biology, biomedicine, biotechnology, bioengineering and energy sciences. *Nucleic Acids Res.* **2021**, *49*, D437–D451. [CrossRef]
42. Pettersen, E.F.; Goddard, T.D.; Huang, C.C.; Meng, E.C.; Couch, G.S.; Croll, T.I.; Morris, J.H.; Ferrin, T.E. UCSF ChimeraX: Structure visualization for researchers, educators, and developers. *Protein Sci.* **2021**, *30*, 70–82. [CrossRef] [PubMed]
43. Morris, G.M.; Huey, R.; Lindstrom, W.; Sanner, M.F.; Belew, R.K.; Goodsell, D.S.; Olson, A.J. AutoDock4 and AutoDockTools4: Automated docking with selective receptor flexibility. *J. Comput. Chem.* **2009**, *30*, 2785–2791. [CrossRef] [PubMed]
44. Frisch, A. *Gaussian 09W Reference;* Gaussian, Inc.: Wallingford, CT, USA, 2009; 25p.
45. Trott, O.; Olson, A.J. AutoDock Vina: Improving the speed and accuracy of docking with a new scoring function, efficient optimization, and multithreading. *J. Comput. Chem.* **2010**, *31*, 455–461. [CrossRef] [PubMed]

marine drugs

MDPI

Article

Bromoditerpenes from the Red Seaweed *Sphaerococcus coronopifolius* as Potential Cytotoxic Agents and Proteasome Inhibitors and Related Mechanisms of Action

Celso Alves [1,*], Joana Silva [1], Susete Pintéus [1], Romina A. Guedes [2], Rita C. Guedes [2], Rebeca Alvariño [3], Rafaela Freitas [1], Márcia I. Goettert [4,5], Helena Gaspar [6], Amparo Alfonso [3], Maria C. Alpoím [7], Luis M. Botana [3] and Rui Pedrosa [8,*]

1 MARE—Marine and Environmental Sciences Centre, ARNET—Aquatic Research Network, Politécnico de Leiria, 2520-630 Peniche, Portugal
2 Research Institute for Medicines (iMed.ULisboa), Faculty of Pharmacy, Universidade de Lisboa, 1649-003 Lisbon, Portugal
3 Department of Pharmacology, Faculty of Veterinary, University of Santiago de Compostela, 27002 Lugo, Spain
4 Cell Culture Laboratory, Postgraduate Programme in Biotechnology, University of Vale do Taquari—Univates, CEP 95914-014 Lajeado, RS, Brazil
5 Department of Pharmaceutical and Medicinal Chemistry, Institute of Pharmacy, Eberhard Karls Universität Tübingen, 72074 Tübingen, Germany
6 BioISI—Biosystems and Integrative Sciences Institute, Faculty of Science, University of Lisbon, 1749-016 Lisbon, Portugal
7 Center for Neuroscience and Cell Biology (CNC), University of Coimbra, 3004-517 Coimbra, Portugal
8 MARE—Marine and Environmental Sciences Centre, ARNET—Aquatic Research Network, ESTM, Politécnico de Leiria, 2520-614 Peniche, Portugal
* Correspondence: celso.alves@ipleiria.pt (C.A.); rui.pedrosa@ipleiria.pt (R.P.); Tel.: +351-262-240-200 (C.A. & R.P.); Fax: +351-262-783-088 (C.A. & R.P.)

Citation: Alves, C.; Silva, J.; Pintéus, S.; Guedes, R.A.; Guedes, R.C.; Alvariño, R.; Freitas, R.; Goettert, M.I.; Gaspar, H.; Alfonso, A.; et al. Bromoditerpenes from the Red Seaweed *Sphaerococcus coronopifolius* as Potential Cytotoxic Agents and Proteasome Inhibitors and Related Mechanisms of Action. *Mar. Drugs* **2022**, *20*, 652. https://doi.org/10.3390/md20100652

Academic Editor: Jose A. Salas

Received: 3 August 2022
Accepted: 17 October 2022
Published: 20 October 2022

Publisher's Note: MDPI stays neutral with regard to jurisdictional claims in published maps and institutional affiliations.

Copyright: © 2022 by the authors. Licensee MDPI, Basel, Switzerland. This article is an open access article distributed under the terms and conditions of the Creative Commons Attribution (CC BY) license (https://creativecommons.org/licenses/by/4.0/).

Abstract: Seaweeds are a great source of compounds with cytotoxic properties with the potential to be used as anticancer agents. This study evaluated the cytotoxic and proteasome inhibitory activities of 12*R*-hydroxy-bromosphaerol, 12*S*-hydroxy-bromosphaerol, and bromosphaerol isolated from *Sphaerococcus coronopifolius*. The cytotoxicity was evaluated on malignant cell lines (A549, CACO-2, HCT-15, MCF-7, NCI-H226, PC-3, SH-SY5Y, and SK-MEL-28) using the MTT and LDH assays. The ability of compounds to stimulate the production of hydrogen peroxide (H_2O_2) and to induce mitochondrial dysfunction, the externalization of phosphatidylserine, Caspase-9 activity, and changes in nuclear morphology was also studied on MCF-7 cells. The ability to induce DNA damage was also studied on L929 fibroblasts. The proteasome inhibitory activity was estimated through molecular docking studies. The compounds exhibited IC_{50} values between 15.35 and 53.34 µM. 12*R*-hydroxy-bromosphaerol and 12*S*-hydroxy-bromosphaerol increased the H_2O_2 levels on MCF-7 cells, and bromosphaerol induced DNA damage on fibroblasts. All compounds promoted a depolarization of mitochondrial membrane potential, Caspase-9 activity, and nuclear condensation and fragmentation. The compounds have been shown to interact with the chymotrypsin-like catalytic site through molecular docking studies; however, only 12*S*-hydroxy-bromosphaerol evidenced interaction with ALA20 and SER169, key residues of the proteasome catalytic mechanism. Further studies should be outlined to deeply characterize and understand the potential of those bromoditerpenes for anticancer therapeutics.

Keywords: terpenes; algae; marine natural products; apoptosis; mitochondrial dysfunction; oxidative stress; anticancer; *Sphaerococcus coronopifolius*

1. Introduction

Marine natural products (MNP) have been revealed to possess uncommon and diverse chemical structures with a great ability to interact with different biological targets, making them excellent candidates to inspire the development of breakthrough pharmacological agents [1,2]. The efforts in discovering new therapeutic entities from marine origin have driven a growing number of marine natural products and derivatives that entered clinical trials, reinforcing their relevance and impact on the pharmaceutical industry [3]. The high success ratio of the approved drugs/MNPs reported (1 in 3500 MNPs) compared with the hit rate (1/5000 to 1/10,000) of non-marine-derived NPs indicates their pharmacological relevance [4,5].

Most of the approved MNP-based drugs and compounds currently in clinical trials, due to distinct factors, have an indication for the treatment of malignant tumors, one of the biggest scourges of human health nowadays, potentiated by the COVID-19 pandemic [5,6]. To date, ten MNP-based drugs (out of fourteen) were clinically approved by different health regulatory agencies to treat cancer—nine of them in the last seventeen years [7]. Despite the advances achieved in the last decades, cancer treatments remain a huge challenge due to the multifactorial complexity of malignant diseases [8]. Cancer diseases possess a diverse and complex cellular machinery supported by a microenvironment that sustains proliferative signalling, deregulates cellular metabolism, activates invasion and metastasis, and resists cell death, among other biological events, ensuring the adaptation of malignant cells to therapeutic regimes, developing chemo-resistance [8]. Consequently, the discovery and development of new anticancer therapeutics is of utmost relevance.

In this field, marine natural products have revealed a capacity to modulate distinct cancer intracellular signalling pathways such as cell proliferation, cell viability, endoplasmic reticulum (ER) stress, the induction of reactive oxygen species (ROS) production, apoptosis, etc [9]. Among MNPs, polyphenols, polysaccharides, alkaloids, peptides, and terpenoids have demonstrated great anticancer activities in in vitro, preclinical, and clinical studies [7,10]. Seaweeds represent the third group from which the highest number of new compounds was obtained in recent decades. These belong to distinct chemical classes such as polysaccharides, sterols, phycocyanins, carotenoids, alkaloids, and terpenoids, among others [11]. Those compounds have exhibited a wide range of biological activities including antimicrobial [12], antioxidant [13], anti-inflammatory [14], antiviral [15], and anticancer activities [16]. Regarding anticancer properties, seaweed metabolites have been shown to prevent tumor growth by inducing apoptosis, blocking cell cycle pathways, and affecting the viability of cancer stem cells, which are major players in angiogenesis, invasion, and metastasis [11]. However, the relevance of seaweeds' bioactive compounds in the treatment of cancer remains underexplored, and their translation to clinical use is not yet a reality.

The chemical profile of the red seaweed *Sphaerococcus coronopifolius* Stackhouse 1797 has revealed the presence of structurally diverse diterpenes, many of them brominated, such as 12*R*-hydroxy-bromosphaerol, 12*S*-hydroxy-bromosphaerol, and bromosphaerol (Figure 1), as a consequence of the abundance of halogen ions in the seawater [11,17]. This chemical feature is rare among secondary metabolites and results predominantly from bromine substitution, which seems to enhance their effects on biological systems [18]. Those compounds have displayed different biological activities, including antimicrobial [19], antifouling [20], and cytotoxicity activities [21–23]. Regarding the antitumor potential, only preliminary screenings were accomplished, and the mechanism of action underlying their cytotoxic effects remains unclear, as well as their ability to interact with the proteasome. Accordingly, the main goal of this work was to evaluate the cytotoxic activities of those bromoditerpenes on several malignant cell lines and related mechanisms of action, also predicting their ability to act as proteasome inhibitors, as evaluated through molecular docking analysis. The proteasome is essential for the maintenance of the intracellular protein homeostasis, and its dysfunction has been associated with the development of several diseases, such as cancer [24].

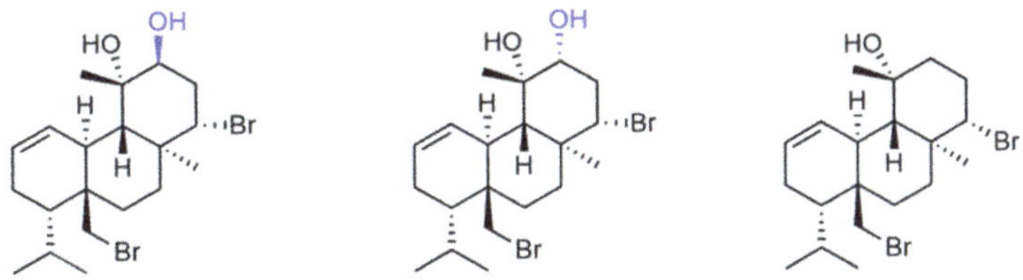

12*S*-hydroxy-bromosphaerol 12*R*-hydroxy-bromosphaerol Bromosphaerol

Figure 1. Chemical structures of *Sphaerococcus coronopifolius* bromoditerpenes.

The bromoditerpenes displayed moderate cytotoxicity on the studied malignant cell lines, which seems to be mediated by an increase in H_2O_2 levels or DNA damage and apoptosis induction.

2. Results

2.1. Interaction with Proteasome—Molecular Docking Studies

The ability of the three bromoditerpenes (bromosphaerol, 12S-hydroxy-bromosphaerol, and 12*R*-hydroxy-bromosphaerol) to inhibit the 20S proteasome was assessed through molecular docking calculations. The crystal structure with the PDB code 4R67 (human constitutive 20S proteasome in complex with carfilzomib) and the chymotrypsin-like (CT-L) catalytic site composed of the β5 catalytic subunit (and the β6 complementary subunit) were prepared for the docking calculations. The interaction profile showed that the three bromoditerpenes are positioned distantly from the Thr1 N-terminal γ hydroxyl group (Thr1Oγ), which acts as a nucleophile in the catalytic mechanism [25–28]: bromosphaerol and 12*R*-hydroxy-bromosphaerol are both at a distance of 10.87 Å from the Thr1Oγ, the 12*S*-hydroxy-bromosphaerol being at 9.26 Å.

The best docking pose for each compound is shown in Figure 2. Bromosphaerol (Figure 2A) interacts with LYS32, TYR130, ARG132, and GLY128 but not with key residues such as THR1, ASP17, ALA20, LYS33, MET45, ALA49, CYS52, SER129, ASP166, and SER169 [29–32]. The bromoditerpene 12*S*-hydroxy-bromosphaerol (Figure 2B) interacts with ALA20 and SER129, but the remaining interactions are established with non-key residues (ALA22, ALA27, TYR107, ILE109, LYS136, and ASP125). At last, the compound 12*R*-hydroxy-bromosphaerol (Figure 2C) interacts with amino acids that are closer to the key residues of the CT-L activity: LYS32, TYR130, GLN131, and ARG132.

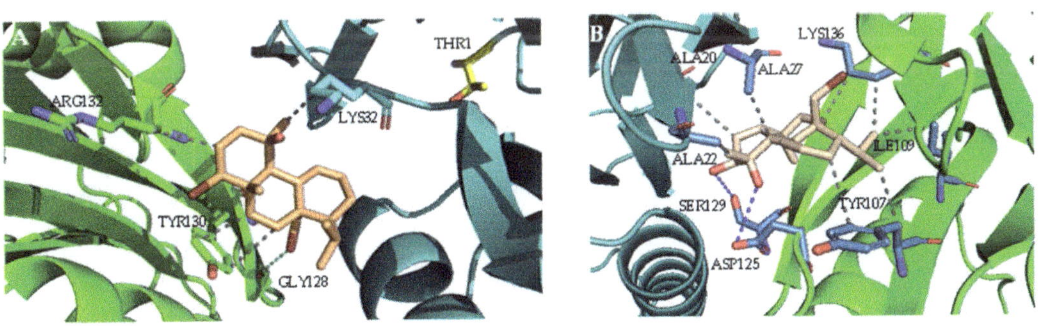

Figure 2. *Cont.*

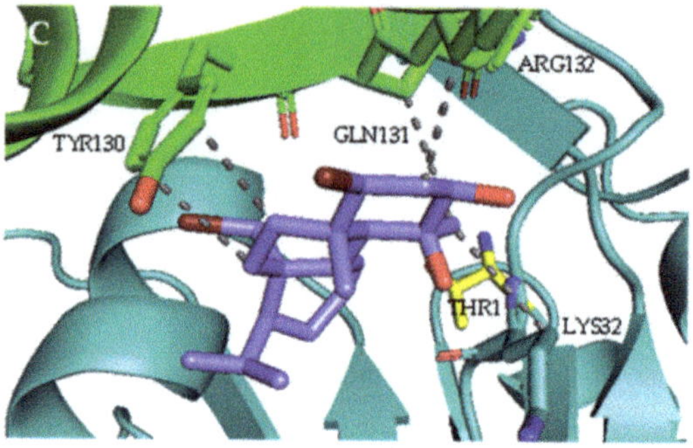

Figure 2. Docking poses of the *Sphaerococcus coronopifolius* bromoditerpenes in the proteasome chymotrypsin-like (CT-L) active site (β5 subunit: cyan; β6 subunit: green; catalytic THR1: yellow). (**A**) Bromosphaerol, (**B**) 12*S*-hydroxy-bromosphaerol, (**C**) 12*R*-hydroxy-bromosphaerol.

2.2. Isolation and Identification of Bromoditerpenes

Sphaerococcus coronopifolius freeze-dried samples were subjected to a sequential extraction and fractionation process by vacuum liquid chromatography, resulting in five fractions (F1–F5). The F3 fraction was purified through successive chromatographic techniques, affording three pure compounds. The analysis of their NMR 1D/2D spectra and the comparison of the chemical shifts and structural assignments (Supplementary Material, Tables S1–S3) with the literature data allowed for the unequivocal identification of the purified compounds known as the bromoterpenes 12*R*-hydroxy-bromosphaerol, 12*S*-hydroxy-bromosphaerol, and bromosphaerol (Figure 1).

2.3. Cytotoxic Activities on Malignant Cells

The cytotoxicity of the compounds was tested on malignant cell lines derived from distinct tissues (A549, CACO-2, HCT-15, MCF-7, NCI-H226, PC-3, SH-SY5Y, and SK-MEL-28), and the results are displayed in Figure 3.

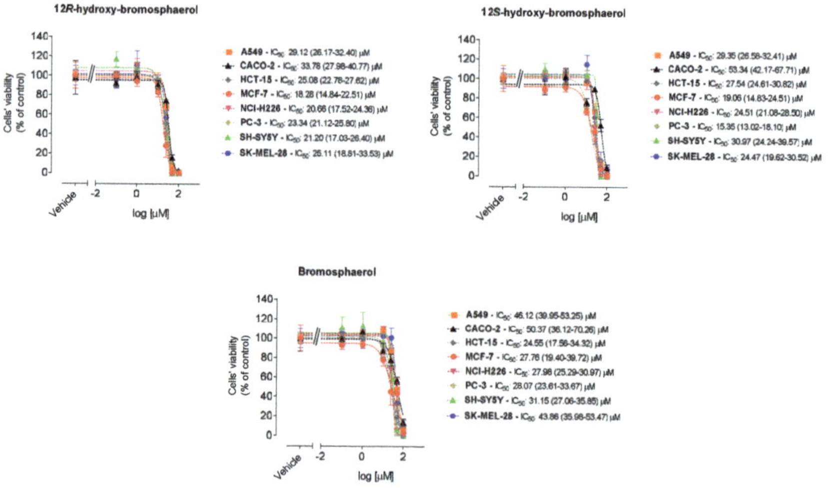

Figure 3. Dose-response analysis (0.1–100 μM) of *Sphaerococcus coronopifolius* bromoditerpenes on malignant cell lines derived from distinct tissues following 24 h of treatment. The effects on cell viability were estimated by the MTT assay. The values in parentheses represent the confidence intervals for 95%.

The 12*R*-hydroxy-bromosphaerol and bromosphaerol displayed a range of IC_{50} values between 18.28/27.76 µM and 33.78/50.37 µM, the lowest value observed on MCF-7 cells and the highest one observed on CACO-2 cells, respectively (Figure 3). 12*S*-hydroxybromosphaerol exhibited IC_{50} values between 15.35 µM and 53.34 µM, the smallest value on cells derived from prostate adenocarcinoma (PC-3), and the highest on CACO-2 cells. Overall, the higher IC_{50} values were observed on malignant cells derived from colorectal adenocarcinoma (CACO-2), these being the most resistant to the bromoditerpenes treatment. In some cases, the compounds exhibited effects more marked than those of the anticancer drugs, especially in colorectal cancer cells, when tested in these experimental conditions (Supplementary Material, Figures S1–S3). Since the compounds presented broad anti-cancer activity in several cell lines, further insights into the mechanisms underlying the observed effects were sought. The MCF-7 cell line was used because breast cancer leads the number of diagnoses in women and is the second most deadly cancer after lung cancer [6].

2.4. Cytotoxicity and Mitochondrial Function

To understand if the effects mediated by the compounds were linked to mitochondrial activity, the lactate dehydrogenase (LDH) release was used as an indicator of cell survival, while the mitochondrial function was assessed by the MTT assay. MCF-7 cells were exposed to compounds (0.1–100 µM) for 24 h, and the results are presented in Figure 4.

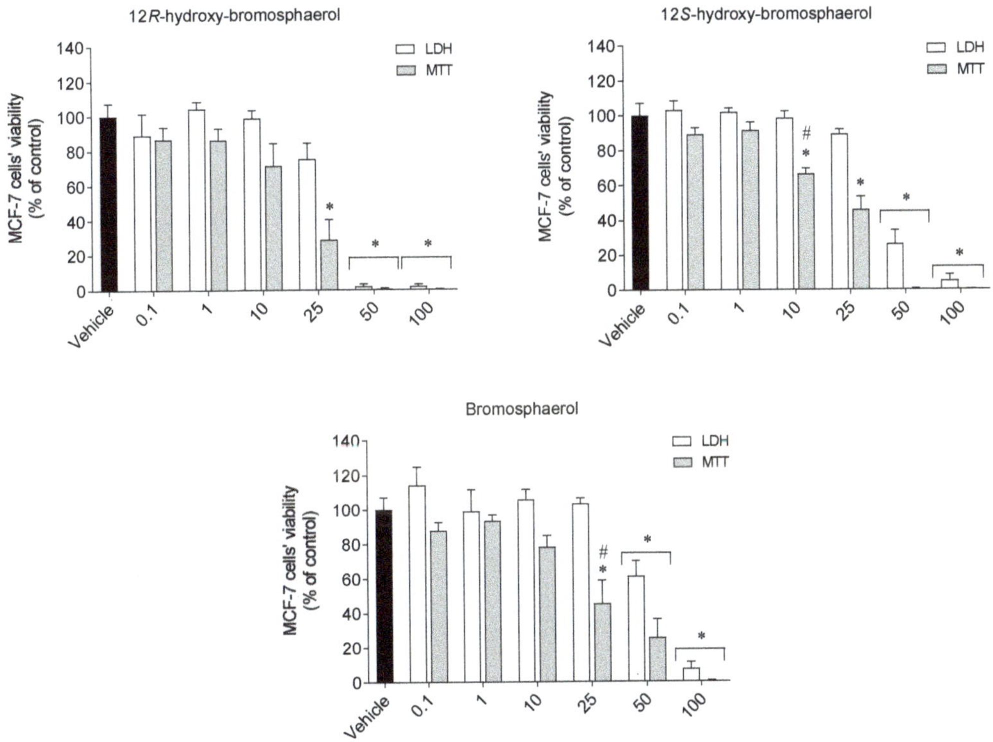

Figure 4. Effects of *Sphaerococcus coronopifolius* bromoditerpenes (0.1–100 µM) on MCF-7 cells' viability, as estimated by the MTT and LDH assays following exposure for 24 h. Symbols represent significant differences ($p < 0.05$) when compared to the * vehicle and # LDH assay.

Overall, the MCF-7 cells treated with the compounds revealed a similar profile on both assays; it was more marked on the MTT assay (Figure 4). Through the MTT assay, all compounds at 25 μM showed significant differences when compared to the vehicle treatment. However, this was not observed on the LDH assay. Furthermore, when tested at 10 and 25 μM of 12*S*-hydroxy-bromosphaerol and bromosphaerol, respectively, the results revealed by the MTT assay displayed significant differences when compared with the effects observed on the LDH assay.

2.5. Hydrogen Peroxide Levels

Hydrogen peroxide (H_2O_2) levels were estimated on MCF-7 cells in real-time following the treatment with the aforementioned compounds (IC_{50}) for 1, 3, and 6 h. The results are presented in Figure 5.

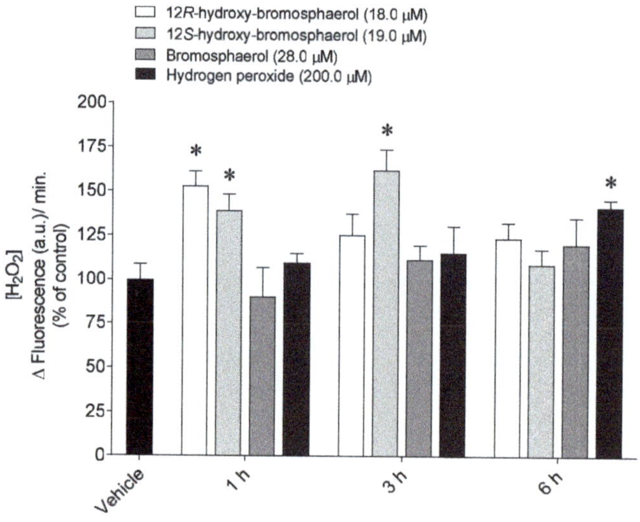

Figure 5. Hydrogen peroxide (H_2O_2) levels generated by MCF-7 cells following treatment with *Sphaerococcus coronopifolius* bromoditerpenes (IC_{50}) for 1, 3, and 6 h. The symbol represents significant differences ($p < 0.05$) compared to the * vehicle.

The treatment with 12*R*-hydroxy-bromosphaerol and 12*S*-hydroxy-bromosphaerol significantly stimulated the production of hydrogen peroxide (H_2O_2) on MCF-7 cells after 1 h of treatment. However, the highest increase was mediated by 12*S*-hydroxy-bromosphaerol on MCF-7 cells after exposure for 3 h. Conversely, bromosphaerol was not able to induce H_2O_2 generation.

2.6. Depolarization of Mitochondrial Membrane Potential

Alterations in the mitochondrial membrane potential were studied following MCF-7 cells' exposure to the aforementioned compounds (IC_{50}) for 15, 30, and 60 min (Figure 6).

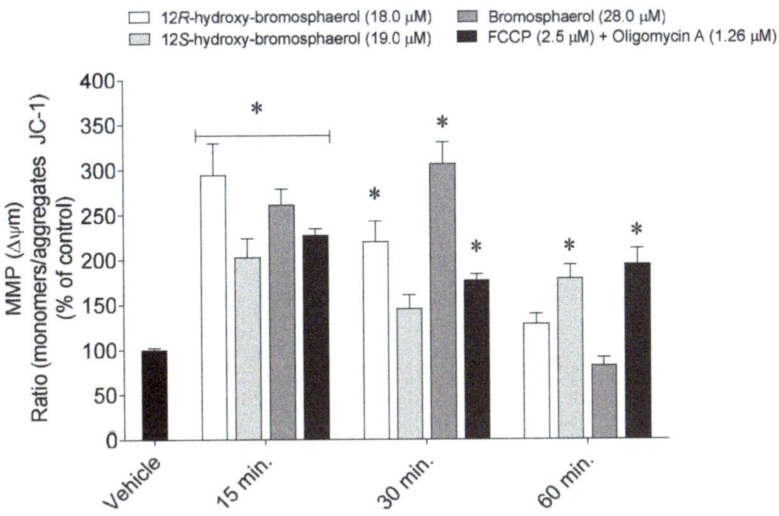

Figure 6. Alterations on the mitochondrial membrane potential of MCF-7 cells following exposure to *Sphaerococcus coronopifolius* bromoditerpenes (IC_{50}) for 15, 30, and 60 min. The symbol (*) represents significant differences ($p < 0.05$) compared to the vehicle.

The treatment of MCF-7 cells with the isolated bromoditerpenes promoted changes in MMP after 15, 30, and 60 min (Figure 6). 12*R*-hydroxy-bromosphaerol and bromosphaerol induced a significant depolarization after 15 and 30 min, while 12*S*-hydroxy-bromosphaerol induced the same effect after 30 and 60 min as compared to the vehicle situation. However, the highest effect was mediated by 12*R*-hydroxy-bromosphaerol and bromosphaerol after 15 min (294.6 ± 34.7%) and 30 min (306.9 ± 23.5%) of treatment, respectively.

2.7. Externalization of Phosphatidylserine, Caspase-9 Activity, and Nuclear Condensation and/or Fragmentation

Apoptosis is characterized by key biological events, including the externalization of phosphatidylserine, caspases activation, and nuclear condensation and fragmentation. Those events were studied on MCF-7 cells following treatment with the compounds (IC_{50}) at different exposition times (Figure 7).

Under controlled conditions, MCF-7 cells were mostly viable, with a small percentage in late apoptosis (Figure 7A). All of the bromoditerpenes promoted a significant decrease in viable cells and cells in the late apoptosis stage compared to the vehicle treatment. As for the apoptosis and necrosis levels, there were no differences between the treated cells and the vehicle. The compounds induced Caspase-9 activity following 6 h exposure, bromosphaerol being the most efficient one (Figure 7B). By analyzing Figure 7C, it is possible to observe changes in MCF-7 cells' nuclear morphology. After 24 h and 48 h of exposition to 12*R*-hydroxy-bromosphaerol, nuclear condensation seemed to be induced; however, the effects were much more expressive with 72 h of exposition. 12*S*-hydroxy-bromosphaerol treatment induced nuclear condensation following 24 h of exposure and extensive nuclear fragmentation for prolonged exposures, i.e., 48 h and 72 h. Similarly, bromosphaerol induced nuclear condensation after 24 h and nuclear fragmentation after 48 and 72 h.

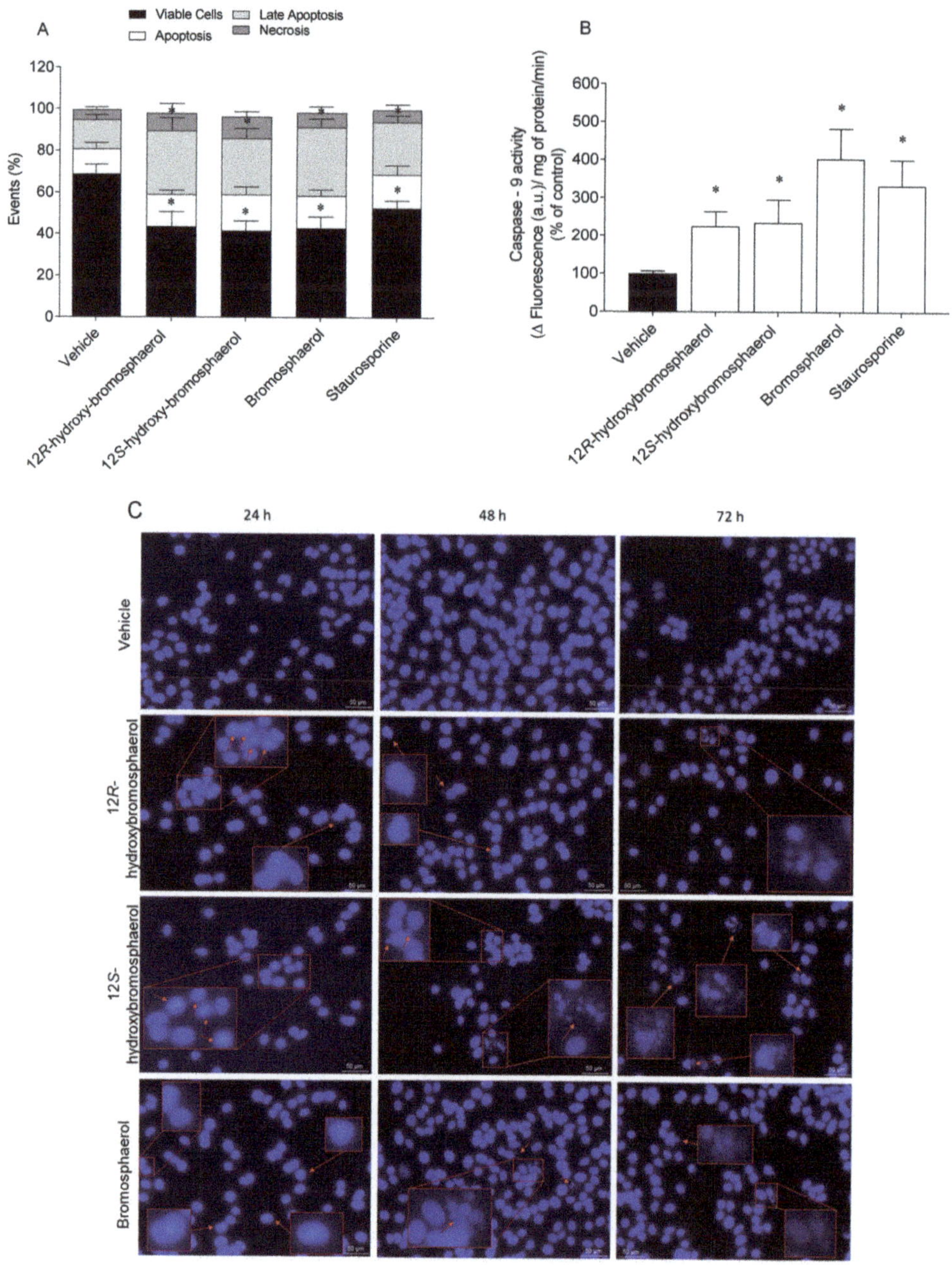

Figure 7. Effects of *Sphaerococcus coronopifolius* bromoditerpenes (IC_{50}) on apoptosis biomarkers: (**A**) externalization of phosphatidylserine (24 h), (**B**) Caspase-9 activity (6 h), and (**C**) nuclear morphology (24, 48, and 72 h). The symbol (*) represents significant differences ($p < 0.05$) compared to the vehicle. Images of DAPI-stained cells were acquired using an inverted fluorescence microscope at ×400. Arrows indicate alterations in DNA compared to the vehicle. The images are representative of one well of each tested condition.

2.8. DNA Damage on L929 Fibroblasts

The ability of bromoditerpenes (25 and/or 50 μM) to affect the DNA integrity was studied on L929 fibroblasts following 3 h of exposure (Figure 8).

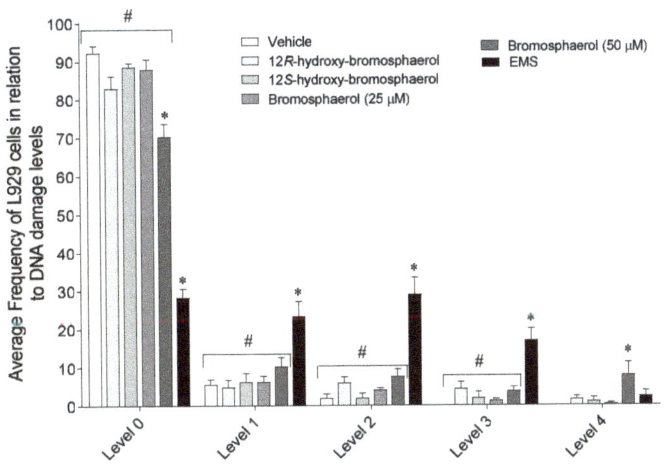

Figure 8. Effects of *Sphaerococcus coronopifolius* bromoditerpenes (25 and/or 50 μM) on the DNA integrity of L929 fibroblasts following 3 h of exposure. Symbols represent significant differences ($p < 0.05$) compared to the * vehicle and # ethyl methanesulfonate (EMS) of the respective DNA damage levels. Damage index: Σ (comet class: 1, 2, 3, 4), 0—nuclei without DNA damage, and 4—nuclei with maximum DNA damage.

Bromosphaerol and ethyl methanesulfonate (EMS)—the positive control for DNA damage—significantly decrease the number of cells at level 0 of the DNA damage index when compared to the vehicle (Figure 8). At levels 1, 2, and 3, only EMS displayed significant differences compared to the vehicle. Particularly, bromosphaerol (50 μM) was the only compound that induced level 4 DNA damage on fibroblasts. However, when tested at 25 μM, this compound exhibited a similar behavior to that of the other tested compounds.

3. Discussion

In the last decades, marine natural products have been shown to be key players in the development of innovative anticancer therapeutic strategies, which is easily proved by the currently approved MNP-derived drugs. The ongoing clinical pipeline presents thirty-three marine-derived molecules, from which twenty-seven are being tested for the treatment of different oncologic diseases [7]. Marine natural products display a great ability to act as biological modulators, exhibiting dissimilar modes of action within typical classes of drugs and establishing new avenues for cancer therapy [33,34]. Despite the efforts, the anticancer potential of several MNPs remains poorly explored, evidencing the relevance of performing studies with molecules that are already described but whose mechanisms affecting malignant cell lines are not fully understood. Thus, the present study aimed to evaluate the potential of three bromoditerpenes isolated from the red seaweed *Sphaerococcus coronopifolius* to interact with the proteasome core and induce cytotoxicity on different cancer cell lines, as well as study their possible mechanisms of action.

Proteasome plays a critical role in the regulation of intracellular protein levels, it being responsible for the degradation of most cellular proteins (80%) in the cytoplasm and nucleus after being tagged with ubiquitin. The malfunction of this system can lead to the degradation of normal proteins while the abnormal ones cannot be degraded, resulting in proteasome-related diseases such as cancer [35]. Furthermore, plasma-increased levels of the 20S proteasome catalytic core have been observed in cancer patients, particularly in the case of solid tumors, which can present values that are 1000-fold higher compared with those of healthy individuals [36,37]. These clinical findings suggest that the 20S proteasome is a hot and challenging target in cancer research. Proteasome inhibitors are able to induce apoptosis in several cancer cells, showing low cytotoxicity in normal cells [38]. Regarding the interaction pattern of the three bromoditerpenes with the proteasome CT-L catalytic site, molecular docking calculations showed that the compounds do not interact with the catalytic THR1. However, 12*S*-hydroxy-bromosphaerol interacts with ALA20 and SER169, which are key residues of proteasome catalytic activity. These interactions may be explained by the distinct conformation adopted by the three compounds, suggesting that the presence of an additional hydroxyl group in derivatives of bromosphaerol, as well as the spatial configuration of 12*S* and 12*R*, can be relevant in the interaction. However, considering these results, the interaction pattern of the three compounds, observed through molecular docking studies, is not very likely to lead to effective proteasome inhibition. Similarly, the marine bromoditerpene sphaerococcenol A also did not establish interactions with key amino acids that are essential for recognition and proteasome inhibition [39]. Nevertheless, several other reports attest to the ability of terpenes obtained from plants and marine organisms (e.g., triptolide, celastrol, pristimerin, withaferin A, petrosapongiolide M, and heteronemin) to interact with key residues of proteasome by molecular modelling, which was confirmed by in vitro and in vivo assays [40–43].

Regarding the cytotoxic effects, the data gathered revealed that those three bromoditerpenes induced a moderate loss of viability in several malignant cell lines with IC_{50} values ranging from 15.35 to 53.34 μM. Regarding A549, PC-3 and SK-MEL-28 tumor cells, the observed IC_{50} range is similar to the IC_{50} values previously reported for those cells (9–35 μM) [23]. By looking to the results attained by the MTT and LDH assays, it is possible to conclude that the effects mediated by 12*S*-hydroxy-bromosphaerol and bromosphaerol were more marked in the MTT assay. Furthermore, despite the treatment with 12*R*-hydroxy-bromosphaerol not promoting significant differences between the assays, the effects on MCF-7 cells' viability were also more noticeable when estimated by the MTT assay compared to the LDH assay at a concentration near their IC_{50} value (25 μM). Those data are particularly interesting since, although the MTT and LDH assays evaluate the effects on cells' viability, the cellular target of each method is distinct. In fact, while the MTT assay evaluates the cells' dehydrogenases activity (both mitochondrial and cytoplasmatic), LDH evaluates the membrane integrity [44]. The results suggest that the compounds may target mitochondrial activity and that their similar effects can be related to the presence of a bromine group in their structures, which is rare in nature and has been associated with their biological activities [18]. Furthermore, 12*R*-hydroxy-bromosphaerol and 12*S*-hydroxy-bromosphaerol are diastereoisomers—specifically, epimers on position 12—which means that the compounds have the same molecular formula and constitutions around the carbon atoms, and the spatial arrangement of the groups around those atoms differ only in terms of the configuration of the stereocenter C12. These spatial differences are enough to mediate distinct pharmacological activities—as observed with thalidomide, a teratogenic drug used in pregnant women in the late 1950s—due to the simultaneous presence of both enantiomers, R and S, in its composition, a fact that was unknown at the time. The (*R*)-enantiomer was responsible for the sedative effects, the therapeutic properties of interest, while the (*S*)-isomer induced teratogenic activities, provoking a range of severe birth defects [45]. However, despite 12*R*-hydroxy-bromosphaerol and 12*S*-hydroxy-bromosphaerol displaying different spatial arrangements around C12, this seemed to not influence the cytotoxic activities, since those compounds exhibited similar activities on all cell lines.

Apoptosis has been a mainstay and a goal of innovative oncology therapeutics to ensure an effective elimination of cancer cells. Apoptotic signaling pathways are triggered by multiple factors, including cellular stress and DNA damage [46]. Several chemotherapeutics, such as cisplatin and doxorubicin, can stimulate the formation of reactive oxygen species (ROS), leading to cancer cells' death by apoptosis [47] and demonstrating that the induction of ROS production could be an appropriate therapeutic strategy. On the other hand, the mechanism of action of other anticancer drugs is associated with the induction of high levels of DNA damage that trigger cell cycle checkpoints, leading to cell cycle arrest and/or cell death [48]. This strategy is based on two fundamental assumptions. The first relies on the fact that cancer cells multiply more often than normal cells; secondly, normal cells have a highly efficient DNA damage response and DNA repair mechanisms, giving normal cells the ability to stop the cell cycle to repair the DNA. Therefore, they have the ability to arrest proliferation for more efficient DNA repair and to avoid the damage mediated by the drug [48,49]. Herein, the ability of compounds to stimulate the production of hydrogen peroxide (H_2O_2) and DNA damage was studied, as well as the capacity to modulate different biomarkers related to apoptosis. The compounds 12*R*-hydroxy-bromosphaerol and 12*S*-hydroxy-bromosphaerol stimulated the production of H_2O_2, and bromosphaerol induced DNA damage, suggesting that the presence of an additional hydroxyl group in the derivatives 12*S* and 12*R* induces a distinct effect between the derivatives and bromosphaerol. These effects were accompanied by changes in mitochondrial membrane potential, more cells in late apoptosis, increased Caspase-9 activity, and nuclear fragmentation/condensation. The ability of marine terpenes to modulate these intracellular signaling pathways has already been reported. The marine sesterterpenoid heteronemin isolated from the sponge *Kyrgios* sp. induced apoptosis and ferroptosis triggered by the production of ROS on several in vitro cancer cellular models [50,51]. Furthermore, previous studies conducted with the bromoditerpenes sphaerococcenol A and sphaerodactylomelol also displayed increased H_2O_2 levels, modulating different apoptotic hallmarks [39,52]. However, further studies need to be accomplished to fully understand the involvement of oxidative stress in MCF-7 cells' death and loss of cell viability. For instance, a pre-treatment with N-acetylcysteine (NAC), known as an ROS scavenging molecule, can be used to understand if the cytotoxic effects mediated by 12*R*-hydroxy-bromosphaerol and 12*S*-hydroxy-bromosphaerol are related to the increase in H_2O_2 levels. Despite the mechanisms of action underlying the activities of these compounds being unexplored, a potential cytostatic effect of 12*S*-hydroxy-bromosphaerol was suggested on U373 GBM cells. Smyrniotopoulos and co-workers [23] observed a marked increase in mitosis length through the computer-assisted phase-contrast microscopy approach. Accordingly, this evidence and our data suggest that 12*S*-hydroxy-bromosphaerol may have the capacity to arrest the cell cycle and trigger apoptosis, two independent physiological processes regulated by a complex network of pathways, including cell cycle regulators, such as P53, that are essential for tissue homeostasis [53].

On the other hand, according to the findings observed following bromosphaerol treatment, it is possible to suppose that its effects may be associated with the induction of DNA damage, leading to the activation of cell death by apoptosis. Among the tested compounds, bromosphaerol was the only one that induced significant DNA damage on L929 cells. However, when tested at a similar concentration (25 μM, the IC_{50} value for MCF-7 cells, 3 h), L929 cells were not affected. However, it is possible that the longer treatment of MCF-7 cells triggered DNA damage repair mechanisms, leading to cells' survival by recovering the effects mediated by bromosphaerol observed on L929 cells after 3 h. Nevertheless, more studies are needed to validate the different hypotheses, including the evaluation of the genotoxic effects over time on L929 cells, carrying out those assays on MCF-7 cells, as well as studying the cell cycle. Although several NPs induce DNA damage, leading to cell cycle arrest and apoptosis [54–56], the present study discloses, for the first time, the potential mechanisms of action underlying the cytotoxic effects of the marine bromoditerpenes 12*R*-hydroxy-bromosphaerol, 12*S*-hydroxy-bromosphaerol, and bromosphaerol, which may be related to increased H_2O_2 levels and DNA damage, leading to cell death by apoptosis. Further experiments are required to understand the involvement of oxidative stress and DNA damage in the cytotoxic activity of these compounds, as well as studies on their effects on normal cells (proliferating or quiescent) in order to define their therapeutic index and understand their antitumor potential.

4. Materials and Methods

4.1. Collection, Extraction, and Purification

Red seaweed specimens of *Sphaerococcus coronopifolius* were collected in the Berlengas Nature Reserve (39°24′44.8″ N 9°30′29.5″ W), Peniche, Portugal by scuba diving and immediately transported to MARE-Polytechnic of the Leiria laboratory, where they were identified by Prof. Teresa Mouga, a biologist with vast experience in the taxonomic identification and ecology of marine seaweeds. The samples were cleaned to remove detritus, sand, and epibionts and freeze-dried. The dry algal material was powdered and then sequentially extracted with methanol and dichloromethane (1:4) for 12 h. The dichloromethane extract was concentrated to dryness in a rotary evaporator and subjected to normal phase vacuum liquid chromatography on silica gel 60 (0.06–0.2 mm), using cyclohexane (VWR, Fontenay-sous-bois, France) with increasing amounts (25%) of ethyl acetate (EtOAc) (VWR, Fontenay-sous-bois, France) as the mobile phase (five fractions). Fraction F3 was purified by the semi-preparative reversed-phase HPLC column (Synergi Fusion-RP 80 Å, Phenomenex, 10 × 250 mm, 4 μm) at a flow rate of 5.19 mL/min (25 °C), using a mixture of H_2O: CH_3CN (VWR, Fontenay-sous-bois, France) as a mobile phase in isocratic conditions from 0 to 5 min (25:75), a linear gradient from 5 to 25 min (from 25:75 to 15:85), and isocratic after 25 min (15: 85). This first purification step afforded 12 sub-fractions (P1–P12), from which only bromosphaerol (P7; tR 23.4 min) was isolated. The sub-fraction P1 was purified on a silica gel 60 column (Sharlau, 0.04–0.06 mm; column height: 19.5 cm; diameter: 2 cm; collection volume: 10 mL) using a mixture of EtOAc/n-Hex (1:9) as a mobile phase, affording 12*S*-hydroxy-bromosphaerol (P1.1, f12 to f15). The sub-fraction P2 was purified by repeating the chromatographic steps: first, by the semi-preparative reversed-phase HPLC column (Synergi Fusion-RP 80 Å, Phenomenex, 10 x 250 mm, 4 μm) using isocratic conditions (60% CH_3CN: 40% H_2O) at a flow rate of 5.0 mL/min (25 °C), affording seven sub-fractions (P2.1–P2.7). Fraction P2.5 was then subjected to preparative column chromatography with silica gel 60 (Sharlau, 0.04–0.06 mm; column height: 19.0 cm; diameter: 2 cm; collection volume: 10 mL) eluted with a mixture of *n*-Hex/EtOAc (8:2) along the first 20 fractions, followed by elution with n-Hex/EtOAc (3:7). This step afforded 12*R*-hydroxy-bromosphaerol (f5 to f9 fraction). The structural elucidation of compounds was attained by NMR spectroscopy analysis, 1D (^1H and ^{13}C Attached Proton Test (APT)) and 2D (COSY, HMBC, HSQC-ed) techniques, and by comparison with previously reported data. For biological evaluation, the compounds were dissolved in DMSO (concentration below 0.2%) and evaluated through a set of in vitro assays. The control situation was always treated with the highest concentration of DMSO as the vehicle.

4.2. In Silico Docking Studies

The receptor structure was retrieved from the Protein Data Bank (www.rcsb.org) through the PDB code 4R67 (Human constitutive 20S proteasome in complex with carfilzomib, 2.89 Å) [32]. To prepare the protein structure for docking calculations, all atoms (i.e., ligand, salts, water, other chains) other than the receptor β5 and β6 subunits (chains L and M, respectively—CT-L active site) were deleted from the X-ray structure using the MOE software package (v.2019.0102) (Molecular Operating Environment; Chemical Computing Group ULC, 1010 Sherbrooke St. West, Suite #910, Montreal, QC, Canada, H3A 2R7, 2021). The AMBER99 forcefield was used to assign atom types and charges to each atom in the receptor. Hydrogen atoms were added, and the appropriate protonation states were assigned using the Protonate-3D tool within the MOE software package (pH 7.4 and T = 310 K). Structures of bromoditerpenes were built and energy-minimized using MOE. Molecular docking simulations were performed using GOLD 5.4 software [43]. The binding site was defined to be centered in the catalytic Thr1Oγ (β5 catalytic subunit) with a 15 Å search radius. Noncovalent docking calculations were performed, with the number of genetic algorithm (GA) runs set to 1000 and the search efficiency set to 100%, and the ten top-ranked solutions were selected. For the other settings, the default parameters were used. First, an initial docking validation step was carried out by performing self-docking calculations using GOLD (scoring functions: GoldScore, Chemscore, ChemPLP, and ASP) and 1000 exhaustive search runs. All protein amino acid residues were kept rigid, whereas all single bonds of the ligands were treated as fully flexible. The docking parameters (scoring function—ChemPLP—and protein 3D structure) selected were able to successfully reproduce the experimental pose (RMSD < 2 Å between the experimental and predicted pose). The docking procedure was subsequently used for the docking calculations. For the analysis of protein–ligand interactions, the top docking poses were submitted to the detection of residue contacts using the docker implementation of PLIP [57]. Images of the compound and the PDB structures were produced using PyMOL v.1.8.4.0.

4.3. Cell Culture Conditions

The cell lines were obtained from the DSMZ and ATCC biobanks. A549 (ATCC: CCL-185) and SH-SY5Y (ATCC: CRL-2266) cells were cultivated in DMEM/F-12 medium (Merck, Germany) supplemented with 10% serum bovine fetal (FBS) (Gibco, USA), GlutaMAX™ (Gibco, USA), 100 IU/mL penicillin, and 100 µg/mL streptomycin (Sigma, USA). CACO-2 (DSMZ: ACC 169), HCT-15 (DSMZ: ACC 357), L929 (DSMZ: ACC 2), MCF-7 (DSMZ: ACC 115), NCI-H226 (Lung squamous cell carcinoma; ATCC: CRL-5826), and PC-3 (Prostate adenocarcinoma; ATCC: CRL-1435) were cultured in RPMI medium supplemented with 10% FBS, 100 IU/mL penicillin, and 100 µg/mL streptomycin. SK-MEL-28 cells (ATCC: HTB-72) were grown in EMEM medium (Sigma, USA) supplemented with 10% FBS, 100 IU/mL penicillin, and 100 µg/mL streptomycin. The cells were dissociated with trypsin (Sigma-Aldrich, USA) and then neutralized with the respective fresh medium and centrifuged at 290 g for 5 min at room temperature. After that, the cells were resuspended in a fresh medium (1:10), seeded in 25 cm^2 T-Flasks, and cultivated in 5% CO_2 and a humidified atmosphere at 37 °C.

4.4. Cytotoxicity Assays

The cells were seeded in 96-well plates (A549: 2.5×10^5 cells/mL; CACO-2: 2.5×10^5 cells/mL; HCT-15: 2.5×10^5 cells/mL; MCF-7: 2.5×10^5 cells/mL; NCI-H226: 7.5×10^4 cells/mL; PC-3: 1.25×10^5 cells/mL; SH-SY5Y: 2.5×10^5 cells/mL; SK-ML-28: 2.5×10^5 cells/mL; AML-12: 5.0×10^4 cell/mL). After 24 h of seeding, the cancer cell lines were exposed to 12*S*-hydroxy-bromosphaerol, 12*R*-hydroxy-bromospherol, and bromosphaerol (0.1–100 µM) for 24 h, and the effects were assessed by the 3-(4,5-dimethylthiazol-2-yl)-2,5-diphenyltetrazolium bromide (MTT) assay [22]. Cisplatin, tamoxifen, and 5-fluorouracil (all from Sigma, Shanghai, China) were used as anticancer standard controls (0.1–500 µM; 24 h). The cell death was measured by the LDH cytotoxicity assay kit (Pierce™ LDH Cytotoxicity Assay Kit; ThermoScientifc, Rockford, USA) according to the manufacturer's instructions. Saponin (Sigma, Darmstadt, Germany) (0.4 mg/mL) was used as the positive control for cell death, reducing the cell viability in 100%.

4.5. Hydrogen Peroxide Levels

The levels of hydrogen peroxide (H_2O_2) were estimated in MCF-7 cells (2.5×10^5 cells/mL) using the Amplex™ Red hydrogen peroxide assay kit (Molecular probes, Eugene, OR, USA), following treatment with the compounds IC_{50} concentration and H_2O_2 (200.0 µM) for 1, 3, and 6 h.

4.6. Mitochondrial Membrane Depolarization

MCF-7 cells (2.5×10^5 cells/mL) were seeded in 96-well plates and treated with the compounds at the IC_{50} concentration and FCCP (2.5 µM) (Sigma, Rehovot, Israel) plus oligomycin A (1.26 µM) (Sigma, St. Louis, MO, USA) conjugate solution for 15, 30, and 60 min. The effects were estimated using the JC-1 (Molecular Probes, Eugene, OR, USA) fluorescent probe [58] through the measurement of JC-1 aggregates (λ excitation: 490 nm; λ emission: 590 nm) and monomers (λ excitation: 490 nm; λ emission: 530 nm) using a plate reader (Bio-Tek Synergy plate reader, Bedfordshire, UK).

4.7. *Translocation of Phosphatidylserine and Membrane Integrity*

MCF-7 cells (1.0×10^6 cells/mL) were seeded in 6-well plates and treated with the compounds at the IC_{50} concentration and staurosporine (1 µg/mL) (Sigma, Rehovot, Israel) for 24 h, and the effects were analyzed by flow cytometry using the Apoptosis Detection Kit (Immunostep, Salamanca, Spain). Ten thousand events were recorded with the AMNIS imaging flow cytometer using the AMNIS INSPIRE™ software. The data were analyzed using the AMNIS IDEAS™ software (Amnis Corporation v6.0, Luminex Corp, Austin, TX, USA).

4.8. *Caspase-9 Activity*

Enzyme activity was estimated in MCF-7 cells (1.0×10^6 cells/mL) previously seeded in 6-well plates following a 6 h treatment with the compounds at the IC_{50} concentration and staurosporine (1 µg/mL). The Caspase 9 Fluorimetric Assay Kit (Biovision, Milpitas, CA, USA) was used.

4.9. *DAPI Staining*

DNA nuclear morphology was evaluated using the DAPI fluorescent probe [58]. MCF-7 cells (1.0×10^6 cells/mL) were seeded in 6-well plates and treated with compounds at the IC_{50} concentration for 24, 48, and 72 h. DNA morphology was analyzed using a fluorescence inverted microscope (ZEISS Axio, VERT. A1, equipped with an AxioCam MRC-ZEISS camera, München, Germany), and a representative image of each treatment was presented.

4.10. *DNA Damage*

L929 mouse fibroblasts (2.0×10^4 cells/mL) were seeded in 12-well plates and cultured overnight. The fibroblasts were then treated with compounds (25 and/or 50 µM) and ethyl methanesulfonate (200 µg/mL) as a positive control for 3 h. The DNA damage was determined according to the protocol established by Singh et al. [59], with slight modifications [52]. One-hundred cells were randomly chosen, analyzed, visually scored, and classified into five levels according to the tail size formed by breaks in the DNA. Non-overlapping was performed.

4.11. *Data and Statistical Analysis*

At least three independent experiments were carried out in triplicate, and the results were presented as the mean ± standard error of the mean (SEM) and the half-maximal inhibitory concentration (IC_{50}). ANOVA with Dunnett's multiple comparison of group means analysis was accomplished, and the Tukey's test was applied for multiple comparisons. When applicable, Student's *t*-test was used. Differences were considered significant at the level of 0.05 ($p < 0.05$). The IBM SPSS Statistics 24 (IBM Corporation, Armonk, NY, USA) and GraphPad v5.1 (GraphPad Software, La Jolla, CA, USA) software were used to accomplish the analysis.

Supplementary Materials: The following supporting information can be downloaded at: https://www.mdpi.com/article/10.3390/md20100652/s1, Figure S1: Dose-response curves of cisplatin (0.1–250 µM; 24 h) on malignant cells' viability (% of control) for IC_{50} determination; Figure S2: Dose-response curve of tamoxifen (0.1–100 µM; 24 h) on MCF-7 cells' viability (% of control) for IC_{50} determination; Figure S3: Dose-response curve of 5-fluorouracil (0.1–500 µM; 24 h) on colorectal cancer cells' viability (% of control) for IC_{50} determination; Table S1: ^1H (400 MHz) and ^{13}C (125 MHz) NMR data ($CDCl_3$) of bromosphaerol; Table S2: ^1H (400 MHz) and ^{13}C (125 MHz) NMR data ($CDCl_3$) of 12*S*-hydroxy-bromosphaerol; Table S3: ^1H (400 MHz) and ^{13}C (125 MHz) NMR data ($CDCl_3$) of 12*R*-hydroxy-bromosphaerol. References [21,60] are cited in the Supplementary Materials.

Author Contributions: Conceptualization, C.A., R.C.G., M.I.G., A.A., M.C.A., L.M.B. and R.P.; Formal analysis, C.A. and J.S.; Funding acquisition, M.I.G., L.M.B. and R.P.; Investigation, C.A., J.S., S.P., R.A.G., R.C.G., R.A., R.F., L.M.B. and R.P.; Methodology, C.A., R.C.G., M.I.G., H.G., A.A., M.C.A., L.M.B. and R.P.; Project administration, R.P.; Resources, R.C.G., M.I.G., H.G., M.C.A., L.M.B. and R.P.; Supervision, M.C.A., L.M.B. and R.P.; Validation, R.C.G., M.I.G., A.A., M.C.A., L.M.B. and R.P.; Visualization, C.A., J.S., S.P., R.C.G., R.F., H.G. and R.P.; Writing—original draft, C.A., J.S., S.P., R.A.G., R.C.G. and R.A.; Writing—review & editing, C.A., J.S., S.P., R.A.G., R.C.G., R.A., R.F., M.I.G., H.G., A.A., M.C.A., L.M.B. and R.P. All authors have read and agreed to the published version of the manuscript.

Funding: This work was funded by the Portuguese Foundation for Science and Technology (FCT) through the strategic projects granted to the MARE—Marine and Environmental Sciences Center (UIDP/04292/2020; UIDB/04292/2020), the BioISI—BioSystems and Integrative Sciences Institute (UIDP/Multi/04046/2020; UIDB/04046/2020), iMed. ULisboa (UIDB/04138/2020; UIDP/04138/2020), and the Associate Laboratory ARNET (LA/P/0069/2020). FCT also support this study through the POINT4PAC project (SAICTPAC/0019/2015-LISBOA-01-0145-FEDER-016405) and through the PDTC/QEQ-MED/7042/2014 and CROSS-ATLANTIC project (PTDC/BIA-OUT/29250/2017), co-financed by COMPETE (PO-CI-01-0145-FEDER-029250). The Spanish part was funded by Conselleria de Cultura, Educacion e Ordenación Universitaria, Xunta de Galicia, GRC (ED431C 2021/01). This work was also supported by the FCT and CAPES cooperation agreement through the project MArTics (FCT/DRI/CAPES 2019.00277.CBM). Rebeca Alvariño is supported by a fellowship from Xunta de Galicia (ED481B-2021-038), Spain.

Institutional Review Board Statement: Not applicable.

Data Availability Statement: The data presented in this study are available on request from the corresponding author.

Acknowledgments: The authors are very grateful for the financial support of the projects and programs described in the funding section. Xunta de Galicia is also acknowledged for the grant attributed to R.A. (ED481B-2021-038).

Conflicts of Interest: The authors declare no conflict of interest.

References

1. Shang, J.; Hu, B.; Wang, J.; Zhu, F.; Kang, Y.; Li, D.; Sun, H.; Kong, D.-X.; Hou, T. Cheminformatic Insight into the Differences between Terrestrial and Marine Originated Natural Products. *J. Chem. Inf. Model.* **2018**, *58*, 1182–1193. [CrossRef] [PubMed]
2. Montaser, R.; Luesch, H. Marine natural products: A new wave of drugs? *Future Med. Chem.* **2011**, *3*, 1475–1489. [CrossRef] [PubMed]
3. Shinde, P.; Banerjee, P.; Mandhare, A. Marine natural products as source of new drugs: A patent review (2015–2018). *Expert Opin. Ther. Pat.* **2019**, *29*, 283–309. [CrossRef] [PubMed]
4. Zhou, Q.; Hotta, K.; Deng, Y.; Yuan, R.; Quan, S.; Chen, X. Advances in Biosynthesis of Natural Products from Marine Microorganisms. *Microorganisms* **2021**, *9*, 2551. [CrossRef]
5. Pereira, F. Have marine natural product drug discovery efforts been productive and how can we improve their efficiency? *Expert Opin. Drug Discov.* **2019**, *14*, 717–722. [CrossRef]
6. Siegel, R.L.; Miller, K.D.; Fuchs, H.E.; Jemal, A. Cancer statistics, 2022. *CA A Cancer J. Clin.* **2022**, *72*, 7–33. [CrossRef]
7. Papon, N.; Copp, B.R.; Courdavault, V. Marine drugs: Biology, pipelines, current and future prospects for production. *Biotechnol. Adv.* **2022**, *54*, 107871. [CrossRef]
8. Hanahan, D. Hallmarks of Cancer: New Dimensions. *Cancer Discov.* **2022**, *12*, 31–46. [CrossRef]
9. Yun, C.W.; Kim, H.J.; Lee, S.H. Therapeutic Application of Diverse Marine-derived Natural Products in Cancer Therapy. *Anticancer. Res.* **2019**, *39*, 5261–5284. [CrossRef]
10. Khalifa, S.A.M.; Elias, N.; Farag, M.A.; Chen, L.; Saeed, A.; Hegazy, M.-E.F.; Moustafa, M.S.; Abd El-Wahed, A.; Al-Mousawi, S.M.; Musharraf, S.G.; et al. Marine Natural Products: A Source of Novel Anticancer Drugs. *Mar. Drugs* **2019**, *17*, 491. [CrossRef]
11. Alves, C.; Silva, J.; Pinteus, S.; Gaspar, H.; Alpoim, M.C.; Botana, L.M.; Pedrosa, R. From Marine Origin to Therapeutics: The Antitumor Potential of Marine Algae-Derived Compounds. *Front. Pharmacol.* **2018**, *9*, 777. [CrossRef] [PubMed]
12. Tang, J.; Wang, W.; Chu, W. Antimicrobial and Anti-Quorum Sensing Activities of Phlorotannins From Seaweed (*Hizikia fusiforme*). *Front. Cell. Infect. Microbiol.* **2020**, *10*, 586750. [CrossRef] [PubMed]
13. Silva, J.; Alves, C.; Freitas, R.; Martins, A.; Pinteus, S.; Ribeiro, J.; Gaspar, H.; Alfonso, A.; Pedrosa, R. Antioxidant and Neuroprotective Potential of the Brown Seaweed *Bifurcaria bifurcata* in an in vitro Parkinson's Disease Model. *Mar. Drugs* **2019**, *17*, 85. [CrossRef] [PubMed]

14. Silva, J.; Alves, C.; Pinteus, S.; Susano, P.; Simões, M.; Guedes, M.; Martins, A.; Rehfeldt, S.; Gaspar, H.; Goettert, M.; et al. Disclosing the potential of eleganolone for Parkinson's disease therapeutics: Neuroprotective and anti-inflammatory activities. *Pharmacol. Res.* **2021**, *168*, 105589. [CrossRef]
15. Liu, J.; Obaidi, I.; Nagar, S.; Scalabrino, G.; Sheridan, H. The antiviral potential of algal-derived macromolecules. *Curr. Res. Biotechnol.* **2021**, *3*, 120–134. [CrossRef]
16. Elhady, S.S.; Habib, E.S.; Abdelhameed, R.F.A.; Goda, M.S.; Hazem, R.M.; Mehanna, E.T.; Helal, M.A.; Hosny, K.M.; Diri, R.M.; Hassanean, H.A.; et al. Anticancer Effects of New Ceramides Isolated from the Red Sea Red Algae *Hypnea musciformis* in a Model of Ehrlich Ascites Carcinoma: LC-HRMS Analysis Profile and Molecular Modeling. *Mar. Drugs* **2022**, *20*, 63. [CrossRef]
17. Smyrniotopoulos, V.; de Andrade Tomaz, A.C.; Vanderlei de Souza, M.d.F.; Leitão da Cunha, E.V.; Kiss, R.; Mathieu, V.; Ioannou, E.; Roussis, V. Halogenated Diterpenes with In Vitro Antitumor Activity from the Red Alga *Sphaerococcus coronopifolius*. *Mar. Drugs* **2020**, *18*, 29. [CrossRef]
18. Cabrita, M.T.; Vale, C.; Rauter, A.P. Halogenated Compounds from Marine Algae. *Mar. Drugs* **2010**, *8*, 2301–2317. [CrossRef]
19. Rodrigues, D.; Alves, C.; Horta, A.; Pinteus, S.; Silva, J.; Culioli, G.; Thomas, O.P.; Pedrosa, R. Antitumor and antimicrobial potential of bromoditerpenes isolated from the red alga, *Sphaerococcus coronopifolius*. *Mar. Drugs* **2015**, *13*, 713–726. [CrossRef]
20. Quémener, M.; Kikionis, S.; Fauchon, M.; Toueix, Y.; Aulanier, F.; Makris, A.M.; Roussis, V.; Ioannou, E.; Hellio, C. Antifouling Activity of Halogenated Compounds Derived from the Red Alga *Sphaerococcus coronopifolius*: Potential for the Development of Environmentally Friendly Solutions. *Mar. Drugs* **2022**, *20*, 32. [CrossRef]
21. Smyrniotopoulos, V.; Quesada, A.; Vagias, C.; Moreau, D.; Roussakis, C.; Roussis, V. Cytotoxic bromoditerpenes from the red alga *Sphaerococcus coronopifolius*. *Tetrahedron* **2008**, *64*, 5184–5190. [CrossRef]
22. Alves, C.; Serrano, E.; Silva, J.; Rodrigues, C.; Pinteus, S.; Gaspar, H.; Botana, L.M.; Alpoim, M.C.; Pedrosa, R. *Sphaerococcus coronopifolius* bromoterpenes as potential cancer stem cell-targeting agents. *Biomed. Pharmacother.* **2020**, *128*, 110275. [CrossRef]
23. Smyrniotopoulos, V.; Vagias, C.; Bruyère, C.; Lamoral-Theys, D.; Kiss, R.; Roussis, V. Structure and in vitro antitumor activity evaluation of brominated diterpenes from the red alga *Sphaerococcus coronopifolius*. *Bioorganic Med. Chem.* **2010**, *18*, 1321–1330. [CrossRef] [PubMed]
24. Cao, Y.; Zhu, H.; He, R.; Kong, L.; Shao, J.; Zhuang, R.; Xi, J.; Zhang, J. Proteasome, a Promising Therapeutic Target for Multiple Diseases Beyond Cancer. *Drug Des. Dev. Ther.* **2020**, *14*, 4327–4342. [CrossRef] [PubMed]
25. Zhu, Y.; Zhao, X.; Zhu, X.; Wu, G.; Li, Y.; Ma, Y.; Yuan, Y.; Yang, J.; Hu, Y.; Ai, L.; et al. Design, Synthesis, Biological Evaluation, and Structure−Activity Relationship (SAR) Discussion of Dipeptidyl Boronate Proteasome Inhibitors, Part I: Comprehensive Understanding of the SAR of α-Amino Acid Boronates. *J. Med. Chem.* **2009**, *52*, 4192–4199. [CrossRef] [PubMed]
26. Diez-Rivero, C.M.; Lafuente, E.M.; Reche, P.A. Computational analysis and modeling of cleavage by the immunoproteasome and the constitutive proteasome. *BMC Bioinform.* **2010**, *11*, 479. [CrossRef]
27. Beck, P.; Dubiella, C.; Groll, M. Covalent and non-covalent reversible proteasome inhibition. *Biol. Chem.* **2012**, *393*, 1101–1120. [CrossRef]
28. Trivella, D.B.; Pereira, A.R.; Stein, M.L.; Kasai, Y.; Byrum, T.; Valeriote, F.A.; Tantillo, D.J.; Groll, M.; Gerwick, W.H.; Moore, B.S. Enzyme inhibition by hydroamination: Design and mechanism of a hybrid carmaphycin-syringolin enone proteasome inhibitor. *Chem. Biol.* **2014**, *21*, 782–791. [CrossRef]
29. Unno, M.; Mizushima, T.; Morimoto, Y.; Tomisugi, Y.; Tanaka, K.; Yasuoka, N.; Tsukihara, T. The Structure of the Mammalian 20S Proteasome at 2.75 Å Resolution. *Structure* **2002**, *10*, 609–618. [CrossRef]
30. Borissenko, L.; Groll, M. 20S Proteasome and Its Inhibitors: Crystallographic Knowledge for Drug Development. *Chem. Rev.* **2007**, *107*, 687–717. [CrossRef]
31. Huber, E.M.; Basler, M.; Schwab, R.; Heinemeyer, W.; Kirk, C.J.; Groettrup, M.; Groll, M. Immuno- and constitutive proteasome crystal structures reveal differences in substrate and inhibitor specificity. *Cell* **2012**, *148*, 727–738. [CrossRef] [PubMed]
32. Harshbarger, W.; Miller, C.; Diedrich, C.; Sacchettini, J. Crystal structure of the human 20S proteasome in complex with carfilzomib. *Structure* **2015**, *23*, 418–424. [CrossRef] [PubMed]
33. Yoshida, T.; Ozawa, Y.; Kimura, T.; Sato, Y.; Kuznetsov, G.; Xu, S.; Uesugi, M.; Agoulnik, S.; Taylor, N.; Funahashi, Y.; et al. Eribulin mesilate suppresses experimental metastasis of breast cancer cells by reversing phenotype from epithelial–mesenchymal transition (EMT) to mesenchymal–epithelial transition (MET) states. *Br. J. Cancer* **2014**, *110*, 1497–1505. [CrossRef]
34. Erba, E.; Bergamaschi, D.; Bassano, L.; Damia, G.; Ronzoni, S.; Faircloth, G.T.; D'Incalci, M. Ecteinascidin-743 (ET-743), a natural marine compound, with a unique mechanism of action. *Eur. J. Cancer* **2001**, *37*, 97–105. [CrossRef]
35. Jang, H.H. Regulation of Protein Degradation by Proteasomes in Cancer. *J. Cancer Prev.* **2018**, *23*, 153–161. [CrossRef]
36. Dutaud, D.; Aubry, L.; Henry, L.; Levieux, D.; Hendil, K.B.; Kuehn, L.; Bureau, J.P.; Ouali, A. Development and evaluation of a sandwich ELISA for quantification of the 20S proteasome in human plasma. *J. Immunol. Methods* **2002**, *260*, 183–193. [CrossRef]
37. Hoffmann, O.; Heubner, M.; Anlasik, T.; Winterhalter, M.; Dahlmann, B.; Kasimir-Bauer, S.; Kimmig, R.; Wohlschlaeger, J.; Sixt, S.U. Circulating 20S proteasome in patients with non-metastasized breast cancer. *Anticancer. Res.* **2011**, *31*, 2197–2201.
38. Almond, J.B.; Cohen, G.M. The proteasome: A novel target for cancer chemotherapy. *Leukemia* **2002**, *16*, 433–443. [CrossRef]
39. Alves, C.; Silva, J.; Afonso, M.B.; Guedes, R.A.; Guedes, R.C.; Alvariño, R.; Pinteus, S.; Gaspar, H.; Goettert, M.I.; Alfonso, A.; et al. Disclosing the antitumour potential of the marine bromoditerpene sphaerococcenol A on distinct cancer cellular models. *Biomed. Pharmacother.* **2022**, *149*, 112886. [CrossRef]

40. Margarucci, L.; Tosco, A.; De Simone, R.; Riccio, R.; Monti, M.C.; Casapullo, A. Modulation of Proteasome Machinery by Natural and Synthetic Analogues of the Marine Bioactive Compound Petrosaspongiolide M. *Chembiochem* **2012**, *13*, 982–986. [CrossRef]
41. Schumacher, M.; Cerella, C.; Eifes, S.; Chateauvieux, S.; Morceau, F.; Jaspars, M.; Dicato, M.; Diederich, M. Heteronemin, a spongean sesterterpene, inhibits TNF alpha-induced NF-kappa B activation through proteasome inhibition and induces apoptotic cell death. *Biochem. Pharmacol.* **2010**, *79*, 610–622. [CrossRef] [PubMed]
42. Yang, H.; Chen, D.; Cui, Q.C.; Yuan, X.; Dou, Q.P. Celastrol, a triterpene extracted from the Chinese "Thunder of God Vine," is a potent proteasome inhibitor and suppresses human prostate cancer growth in nude mice. *Cancer Res.* **2006**, *66*, 4758–4765. [CrossRef] [PubMed]
43. Yang, H.; Ping Dou, Q. Targeting Apoptosis Pathway with Natural Terpenoids: Implications for Treatment of Breast and Prostate Cancer. *Curr. Drug Targets* **2010**, *11*, 733–744. [CrossRef] [PubMed]
44. Menyhárt, O.; Harami-Papp, H.; Sukumar, S.; Schäfer, R.; Magnani, L.; de Barrios, O.; Győrffy, B. Guidelines for the selection of functional assays to evaluate the hallmarks of cancer. *Biochim. Biophys. Acta (BBA)-Rev. Cancer* **2016**, *1866*, 300–319. [CrossRef]
45. Vargesson, N. Thalidomide-induced teratogenesis: History and mechanisms. *Birth Defects Res. Part C Embryo Today: Rev.* **2015**, *105*, 140–156. [CrossRef]
46. Carneiro, B.A.; El-Deiry, W.S. Targeting apoptosis in cancer therapy. *Nat. Rev. Clin. Oncol.* **2020**, *17*, 395–417. [CrossRef]
47. Nakamura, H.; Takada, K. Reactive oxygen species in cancer: Current findings and future directions. *Cancer Sci.* **2021**, *112*, 3945–3952. [CrossRef]
48. Swift, L.; Golsteyn, R. Genotoxic Anti-Cancer Agents and Their Relationship to DNA Damage, Mitosis, and Checkpoint Adaptation in Proliferating Cancer Cells. *Int. J. Mol. Sci.* **2014**, *15*, 3403–3431. [CrossRef]
49. Liu, B.; Ezeogu, L.; Zellmer, L.; Yu, B.; Xu, N.; Joshua Liao, D. Protecting the normal in order to better kill the cancer. *Cancer Med.* **2015**, *4*, 1394–1403. [CrossRef]
50. Chang, W.T.; Bow, Y.D.; Fu, P.J.; Li, C.Y.; Wu, C.Y.; Chang, Y.H.; Teng, Y.N.; Li, R.N.; Lu, M.C.; Liu, Y.C.; et al. A Marine Terpenoid, Heteronemin, Induces Both the Apoptosis and Ferroptosis of Hepatocellular Carcinoma Cells and Involves the ROS and MAPK Pathways. *Oxidative Med. Cell. Longev.* **2021**, *2021*, 7689045. [CrossRef]
51. Lee, M.G.; Liu, Y.C.; Lee, Y.L.; El-Shazly, M.; Lai, K.H.; Shih, S.P.; Ke, S.C.; Hong, M.C.; Du, Y.C.; Yang, J.C.; et al. Heteronemin, a Marine Sesterterpenoid-Type Metabolite, Induces Apoptosis in Prostate LNcap Cells via Oxidative and ER Stress Combined with the Inhibition of Topoisomerase II and Hsp90. *Mar. Drugs* **2018**, *16*, 204. [CrossRef]
52. Alves, C.; Silva, J.; Pinteus, S.; Alonso, E.; Alvariño, R.; Duarte, A.; Marmitt, D.; Goettert, M.I.; Gaspar, H.; Alfonso, A.; et al. Cytotoxic Mechanism of Sphaerodactylomelol, an Uncommon Bromoditerpene Isolated from *Sphaerococcus coronopifolius*. *Mar. Drugs* **2021**, *26*, 1374. [CrossRef] [PubMed]
53. Wiman, K.G.; Zhivotovsky, B. Understanding cell cycle and cell death regulation provides novel weapons against human diseases. *J. Intern. Med.* **2017**, *281*, 483–495. [CrossRef] [PubMed]
54. Srivastava, S.; Somasagara, R.R.; Hegde, M.; Nishana, M.; Tadi, S.K.; Srivastava, M.; Choudhary, B.; Raghavan, S.C. Quercetin, a Natural Flavonoid Interacts with DNA, Arrests Cell Cycle and Causes Tumor Regression by Activating Mitochondrial Pathway of Apoptosis. *Sci. Rep.* **2016**, *6*, 24049. [CrossRef]
55. Choi, Y.; Kim, J.; Lee, K.; Choi, Y.-J.; Ye, B.-R.; Kim, M.-S.; Ko, S.-G.; Lee, S.-H.; Kang, D.-H.; Heo, S.-J. Tuberatolide B Suppresses Cancer Progression by Promoting ROS-Mediated Inhibition of STAT3 Signaling. *Mar. Drugs* **2017**, *15*, 55. [CrossRef] [PubMed]
56. Chung, T.-W.; Lin, S.-C.; Su, J.-H.; Chen, Y.-K.; Lin, C.-C.; Chan, H.-L. Sinularin induces DNA damage, G2/M phase arrest, and apoptosis in human hepatocellular carcinoma cells. *BMC Complement. Altern. Med.* **2017**, *17*, 62. [CrossRef]
57. Salentin, S.; Schreiber, S.; Haupt, V.J.; Adasme, M.F.; Schroeder, M. PLIP: Fully automated protein-ligand interaction profiler. *Nucleic Acids Res.* **2015**, *43*, W443–W447. [CrossRef]
58. Silva, J.; Alves, C.; Pinteus, S.; Mendes, S.; Pedrosa, R. Neuroprotective effects of seaweeds against 6-hydroxidopamine-induced cell death on an in vitro human neuroblastoma model. *BMC Complement. Altern. Med.* **2018**, *18*, 58. [CrossRef]
59. Singh, N.P.; McCoy, M.T.; Tice, R.R.; Schneider, E.L. A simple technique for quantitation of low levels of DNA damage in individual cells. *Exp. Cell Res.* **1988**, *175*, 184–191. [CrossRef]
60. De Rosa, S.; de Stefano, S.; Scarpelli, P.; Zavodnik, N. Terpenes from the red alga Sphaerococcus coronopifolius of the North Adriatic Sea. *Phytochemistry* **1988**, *27*, 1875–1878. [CrossRef]

marine drugs

Article

Laminaria japonica Peptides Suppress Liver Cancer by Inducing Apoptosis: Possible Signaling Pathways and Mechanism

Yingzi Wu [1,2,†], Yuanhui Li [3,†], Wenhai Guo [1,†], Jie Liu [4], Weiguo Lao [5], Penghui Hu [6], Yiguang Lin [1,7,*] and Hongjie Chen [1,*]

1 Department of Traditional Chinese Medicine, The Third Affiliated Hospital of Sun Yat-sen University, Guangzhou 510630, China
2 School of Chinese Medicine, Hong Kong Baptist University, Hong Kong 999077, China
3 National Marketing Center, Sinopharm Group Pharmaceutical Co., Ltd., Guangzhou 510010, China
4 State Key Laboratory of Respiratory Disease for Allergy and Shenzhen Key Laboratory of Allergy & Immunology, Shenzhen University School of Medicine, Shenzhen 518060, China
5 Department of Biochemistry, Douglass Hanly Moir Pathology, Macquarie Park, NSW 2113, Australia
6 Department of Oncology, Jiangmen Central Hospital, Jiangmen 529030, China
7 School of Life Sciences, University of Technology Sydney, Broadway, NSW 2007, Australia
* Correspondence: yiguang.lin@hotmail.com (Y.L.); chenhj63@mail.sysu.edu.cn (H.C.)
† These authors contributed equally to this work.

Abstract: The anticancer properties of *Laminaria japonica* peptides (LJPs) have never been studied. Here, we extracted LJPs from fresh seaweed and explored their anti-liver cancer activity (in vivo and in vitro). LJPs were isolated/purified by HPLC-ESI-MS. HepG2 cell apoptosis and cell cycle were evaluated. MTT assays were used to examine the cytotoxicity of LJPs. Caspase activation of caspases 3 and 9, cleaved caspases 3 and 9, and cleaved PARP was examined by Western blotting. The PI3K/AKT pathway and the phosphorylation states of MAPKs (p38 and JNK) were examined. We found that the LJP-1 peptide had the most antiproliferative activity in H22 cells in vitro. LJP-1 blocked H22 cells in the G0/G1 phase, accompanied by inhibition of cyclin expression. LJP-1 induced apoptosis through caspase activation and regulation of the ASK1/MAPK pathway. Concurrent in vivo studies demonstrated that LJP-1 significantly inhibited tumor growth and induced tumor cell apoptosis/necrosis. In conclusion, LJPs, particularly LJP-1, exert strong inhibitory effects on liver cancer growth in vivo and in vitro. LJP-1 induces HCC cell apoptosis through the caspase-dependent pathway and G0/G1 arrest. LJP-1 induces caspase-dependent apoptosis, in part by inhibiting PI3K, MAPK signaling pathways, and cell cycle proteins. LJP-1 has the potential to be a novel candidate for human liver cancer therapeutics.

Keywords: seaweed; *Laminaria japonica*; *Laminaria japonica* peptides; cancer; liver; cell cycle; apoptosis

Citation: Wu, Y.; Li, Y.; Guo, W.; Liu, J.; Lao, W.; Hu, P.; Lin, Y.; Chen, H. *Laminaria japonica* Peptides Suppress Liver Cancer by Inducing Apoptosis: Possible Signaling Pathways and Mechanism. *Mar. Drugs* **2022**, *20*, 704. https://doi.org/10.3390/md20110704

Academic Editors: Marc Diederich and Celso Alves

Received: 10 October 2022
Accepted: 5 November 2022
Published: 10 November 2022

Publisher's Note: MDPI stays neutral with regard to jurisdictional claims in published maps and institutional affiliations.

Copyright: © 2022 by the authors. Licensee MDPI, Basel, Switzerland. This article is an open access article distributed under the terms and conditions of the Creative Commons Attribution (CC BY) license (https://creativecommons.org/licenses/by/4.0/).

1. Introduction

Hepatocellular carcinoma (HCC) is one of the most common forms of primary hepatic carcinoma and represents between 85% and 90% of primary liver cancers worldwide [1–3]. The incidence of HCC has almost tripled in recent decades. HCC poses a particularly serious sociomedical problem in Asia and sub-Saharan Africa, where the number of deaths is almost equal to the number of cases diagnosed annually (approximately 600,000), and the 5-year survival rate is below 9% [2,4]. Basic treatments for HCC include surgical resection, liver transplantation, percutaneous ablation, chemotherapy, and targeted therapy. However, the cure rate for patients who undergo resection is relatively low, and among patients who are not eligible for surgical or percutaneous procedures, only chemoembolization improves survival. Locally applied external radiation therapy, alone or in combination with chemotherapy, frequently leads to a significant improvement in primary and metastatic

HCC [5,6], with a palliative effect in metastatic disease and possibly playing an equally palliative role in unresectable primary liver tumors [5]. Therefore, the development of new effective and more therapeutic agents remains urgently needed for the treatment of HCC.

Natural products have been and are currently a valuable source of anticancer drugs in drug discovery [6,7]. It is widely accepted that intricate architectures generally composed of natural products offer numerous opportunities and clues for the exploration of novel drugs. Recent studies have demonstrated that seaweed contains various bioactive components that have strong anticancer properties [8–15]. Various edible seaweed extracts have been shown to have protective effects against some types of cancer, demonstrating suppressive effects against chemically induced tumorigenesis through suppression in the initiation and promotion phases [16]. *Laminaria japonica* (*L. japonica*), a brown seaweed, is one of the most important seaweeds and has been widely used as a health food and a traditional oriental herbal medicine for more than a thousand years [17–19]. Many studies have shown that fucoidan, a complex polysaccharide extracted from brown seaweed, has promising anticancer effects against multiple types of cancer through various anticancer mechanisms, such as cell cycle arrest, apoptosis evocation, and stimulation of cytotoxic natural killer cells and macrophages [12,13,15]. In addition to its anticancer properties, fucoidan possess other pharmacological properties, including antioxidant, anticoagulant, anti-inflammatory, and immunomodulatory activities [20–22]. Fucoxanthin, another major active component extracted from *L. japonica*, has recently been reported to have an anti-lung cancer effect [19] and anti-liver cancer activities [9]. Importantly, a novel glycoprotein isolated from *L. japonica* has been shown to stimulate normal gastrointestinal cell growth by activating the epidermal growth factor receptor (EGFR) signaling pathway [23]. On the contrary, the isolated glycoprotein inhibits colon cancer cell proliferation, demonstrated in HT-29 cells, by inducing cell cycle arrest and apoptosis [4].

Research is currently being conducted on polysaccharides (such as fucoidan) and the main carotenoids (fucoxanthin) derived from *L. japonica*, as stated above. However, studies on the protein and peptide moieties present in *L. japonica* are limited, despite the fact that *L. japonica* is composed of more than 10% proteins and peptides [24]. No studies investigating the anticancer properties of *L. japonica* peptides have been reported to date. Therefore, in the present study, we first isolated the peptides from *L. japonica* and then screened and investigated the anticancer effects and possible underlying anticancer mechanisms of the *L. japonica* peptides through in vivo and in vitro experiments using various human liver cancer cell lines and a liver cancer animal model.

2. Results

2.1. Isolation and Analysis of LJPs

In the current study, 158 g of total protein was isolated from *L. japonica*. Then, ultrafiltration, hydrophobic chromatography, anion exchange chromatography, gel filtration chromatography, and RP-HPLC were performed in conjunction with anticancer activity tracking detection. Finally, four pentapeptides, seven hexapeptides, and a heptapeptide were isolated, and the amino acid sequence was identified (Table 1). After the LJPs were obtained, HPLC-ESI-MS and Edman degradation experiments were carried out to analyze the amino acid sequence of the LJPs.

LJP-1 was analyzed using HPLC-ESI-MS for molecular mass determination and peptide characterization. As shown in Figure 1, the fragment of ion m/z 602.2921 was considered a fragment $[M+H]^+$. The fragment of ion m/z 471.1991 was considered the y4 ion, whereas m/z 425.1929 was considered the $[b4\text{-}COOH+H]^+$ fragment, m/z 416.2296 was considered the b3 ion, m/z 285.1349 was considered the b3-b1 ion, and m/z 269.1602 was considered b2. The ion (m/z 251.1500) was considered the $[b2\text{-}H_2O+H]^+$ fragment, the ion (m/z 223.1553) was the $[b2\text{-}COOH+H]^+$ fragment, m/z 156.0767 was the $[His\text{-}H_2O+H]^+$ fragment, and m/z 110.0705 was the $[His\text{-}COOH+H]^+$ fragment. Based on HPLC-ESI-MS data and corresponding by Edman degradation results, we concluded that the LJP-1 sequence was EGFHL. The rest of the LJPs were identified using the same method as LJP-1; their amino acid sequences are listed in Table 1.

Table 1. In vitro antiproliferative activity of 12 LJPs.

Comp.	Amino Acid Sequence	IC_{50} (mM)		
		HuH7	HepG2	H22
LJP-1	EGFHL	0.48 ± 0.05	0.45 ± 0.05	0.36 ± 0.03
LJP-2	LWEHSH	2.25 ± 0.22	1.71 ± 0.13	0.62 ± 0.05
LJP-3	FSHRGH	1.42 ± 0.12	>4.0	1.70 ± 0.15
LJP-4	EGHGF	0.62 ± 0.07	0.65 ± 0.07	0.68 ± 0.07
LJP-5	FSTHGG	2.44 ± 0.22	2.78 ± 0.26	1.49 ± 0.13
LJP-6	FKEHGY	>4.0	3.06 ± 0.31	>4.0
LJP-7	HAGYSWA	2.53 ± 0.24	1.66 ± 0.11	1.44 ± 0.12
LJP-8	FSHTYV	0.44 ± 0.04	0.63 ± 0.05	0.76 ± 0.08
LJP-9	FEHSG	0.53 ± 0.05	0.69 ± 0.08	0.51 ± 0.07
LJP-10	HASWEH	3.52 ± 0.35	2.69 ± 0.22	3.53 ± 0.34
LJP-11	YEHSHG	0.49 ± 0.05	0.61 ± 0.07	0.70 ± 0.07
LJP-12	TFKHG	0.41 ± 0.04	0.60 ± 0.08	0.72 ± 0.05

IC_{50} values are shown as mean ± standard error of the mean (SD) from at least three independent experiments.

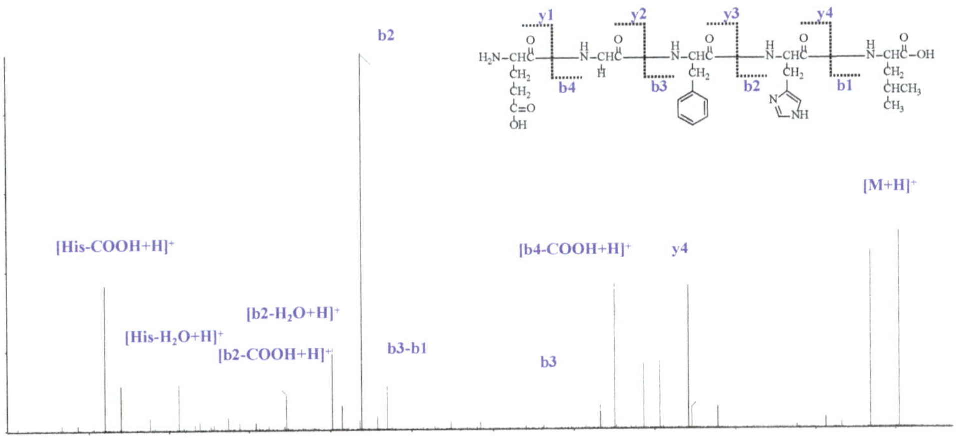

Figure 1. ESI-MS spectrum and structure of LJP-1. Electrospray ionization mass spectrometry (ESI-MS) was performed using a SCIEX X500R Q-TOF mass spectrometer equipped with an ESI source. The amino acid sequences of the LJPs were identified on the basis of ESI-MS data and accompanied by Edman degradation results.

2.2. LJPs Inhibited HCC Cell Growth In Vitro

Three representative liver cancer cell lines, HuH7, HepG2, and H22, were specifically chosen to explore the effects of LJPs in in vitro liver cancer studies. As shown in Table 1, six LJPs (LJP-1, LJP-4, LJP-8, LJP-9, LJP-11, and LJP-12) exhibited significant antiproliferative activity against the three liver cancer cell lines. LJP-1 showed significant antiproliferative activity in HuH7, HepG2, and H22 cell lines, with IC_{50} values of 0.48 ± 0.05 mM, 0.45 ± 0.05 mM, and 0.36 ± 0.03 mM, respectively. Among the cell lines tested, the H22 cell line had the lowest IC_{50} value and was therefore chosen for further experiments. The results indicated that LJP-1 showed a wide range of growth-inhibitory activity against liver cancer cells.

With promising results showing antiproliferative activity of LJP-1 in the three liver cancer cell lines tested, we then investigated cytotoxicity in normal cells using the same technique. We found that the cytotoxicity of LJP-1 in normal cells was significantly less than in cancer cells. Cytotoxicity, or killing effect, in the human liver cell line HL-7702 required much higher doses of LJP-1 (IC_{50} value of 7.76 ± 0.71 mM for HL-7702) compared to tumor cells, suggesting that LJP-1 was a suitable candidate as an anticancer drug for further study.

2.3. *LJP-1 Induced Cell Cycle Arrest by Regulating Cyclin Expression*

To investigate the anticancer activity of LJP-1 in cell cycle arrest, we measured the cell cycle phases of H22 cells by flow cytometry using propidium iodide (PI) staining after LJP-1 treatments. As shown in Figure 2A, H22 cells in phase G0/G1 were significantly blocked by 38.8% (control), 44.3% (0.36 mM, vs. control, * $p < 0.05$), and 56.1% (1.80 mM, vs. control, * $p < 0.05$).

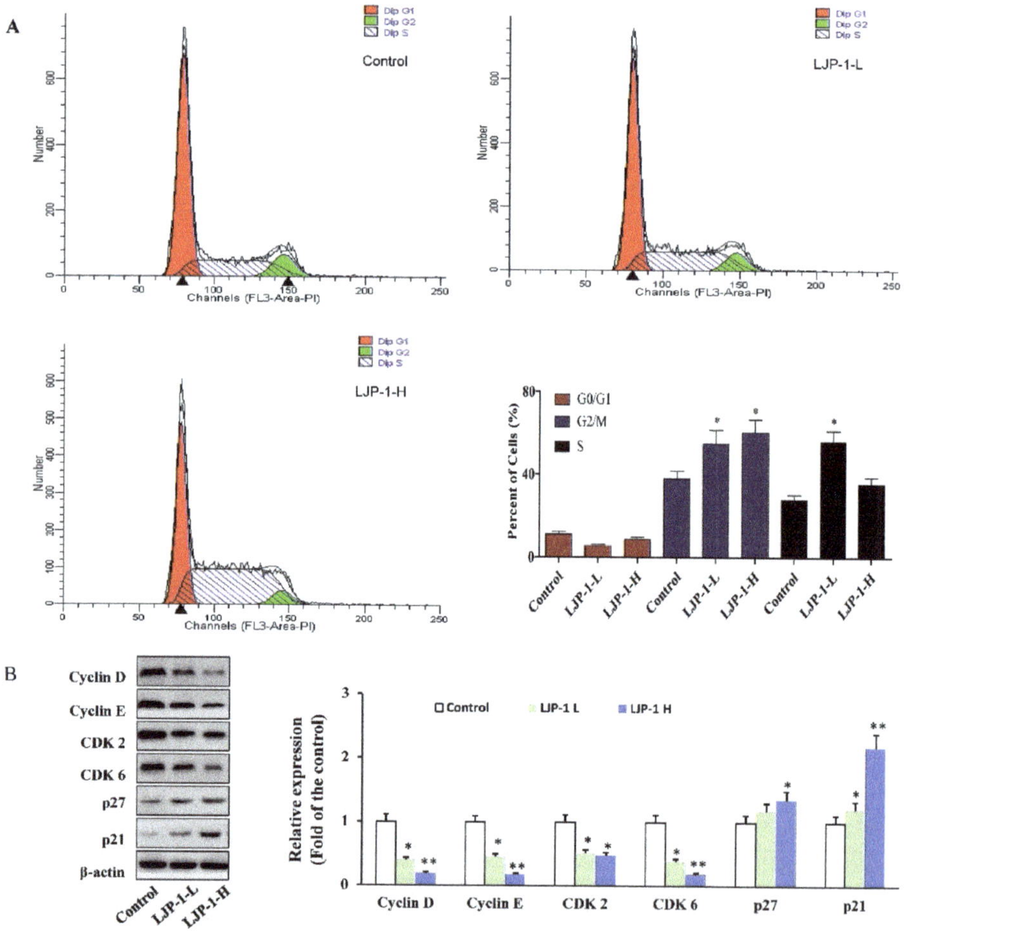

Figure 2. LJP-1 induces G0/G1 cell cycle arrest in H22 cells. Following LJP-1 treatments, H22 cells were harvested. (**A**) Cell cycle profiles were measured by flow cytometry. (**B**) Western blotting was performed to detect p27, p21, cyclin D, cyclin E, CDK2, and CDK6. β-actin was used as a loading control. The blots were quantified using ImageJ software. Data are expressed as the mean ± SD of three independent experiments. * $p < 0.05$, ** $p < 0.01$ compared to the control group.

We analyzed the expression of proteins involved in cell cycle regulation to examine the molecular events of LJP-1 inhibition of the G0/G1 transition; the results are shown in

Figure 2B. LJP-1 suppressed the expression of cyclin D and cyclin E and attenuated the expression of both CDK2 and CDK6. Furthermore, the expression of both p21 and p27 was upregulated by LJP-1 treatments, indicating that LJP-1 is related to cell cycle arrest and dependent on p21 and p27. In particular, these results indicate that LJP-1 modulates the G0/G1 phase proteins, resulting in cycle arrest.

2.4. LJP-1 Induced Caspase-Dependent Apoptosis in H22 Cells

To investigate whether LJP-1 induced arrest in the G0/G1 phase in H22 cells through the apoptotic pathway, we first performed an annexin V-FITC/PI double-staining assay. As shown in Figure 3A, LJP-1 induced significant apoptosis in H22 cells. After LJP-1 treatments, the percentage of apoptotic cells increased from 3.42% (Control) to 21.0% (0.36 mM, * $p < 0.05$) and 34.0% (1.80 mM, * $p < 0.05$).

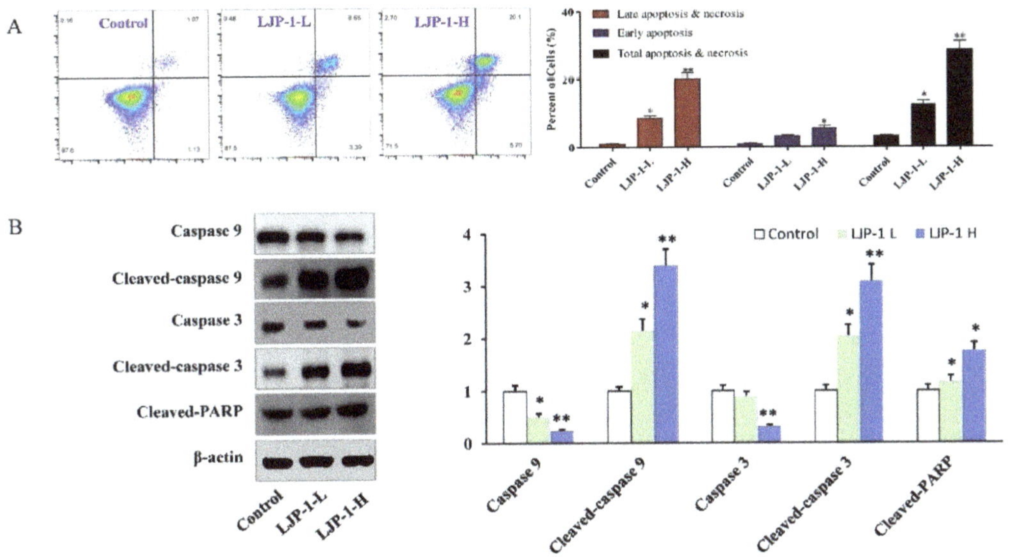

Figure 3. LJP-1 induced caspase-dependent apoptosis in H22 cells. (**A**) Representative scatter diagrams. After the LJP-1 treatments, H22 cells were harvested and stained with annexin V and PI and evaluated by flow cytometry. In each scatter diagram, the abscissa represents the fluorescence intensity of the cells dyed by annexin V, and the ordinate represents the fluorescence intensity of the cells dyed by PI. The lower left quadrant shows the viable cells, the upper left shows the necrotic cells, the lower right shows the early apoptotic cells, and the upper right shows the late apoptotic cells. (**B**) LJP-1 activates caspase cleavage. After the LJP-1 treatments, H22 cells were collected and prepared for Western blot analysis. Equal amounts of whole-cell extracts were separated by 10% SDS-PAGE, electro-transferred onto PVDF membranes, and analyzed by Western blotting using the indicated antibodies against proteins related to caspase-dependent apoptosis. β-actin was used as a loading control. Data are expressed as the mean ± SD of three independent experiments. * $p < 0.05$, ** $p < 0.01$ compared to the control group.

In the experiment examining whether caspase activation is involved in LJP-1-induced cell apoptosis, we found that, as shown in Figure 3B, LJP-1 increased the expression of cleaved caspase-9 and cleaved caspase-3. The cleaved poly-ADP ribose polymerase (PARP) was also strongly activated. The above results suggest that LJP-1 induces programmed apoptosis by activating the caspase cell death pathway.

2.5. LJP-1 Induced Apoptosis of H22 Cells by Regulating p38-MAPK and PI3K/AKT Pathways

The PI3K/AKT pathway acts as a key regulator of cellular survival and apoptosis in most cancers. We therefore evaluated whether PI3K/AKT played a central role in LJP-1-mediated apoptotic cell death. LJP-1 treatments (both LJP-1-L and LJP-1-H) significantly downregulated PI3K expression and increased p-AKT expression (Figure 4A), indicating that the PI3K/AKT pathway also played a key role in LJP-1-mediated apoptosis. LJP-1 also decreased apoptosis signal-regulating kinase 1 (ASK1). Furthermore, we investigated whether LJP-1 treatments regulated MAPK phosphorylation states (p38 and JNK). As shown in Figure 4B, both p38 and JNK phosphorylation were activated in H22 cells after LJP-1 treatments.

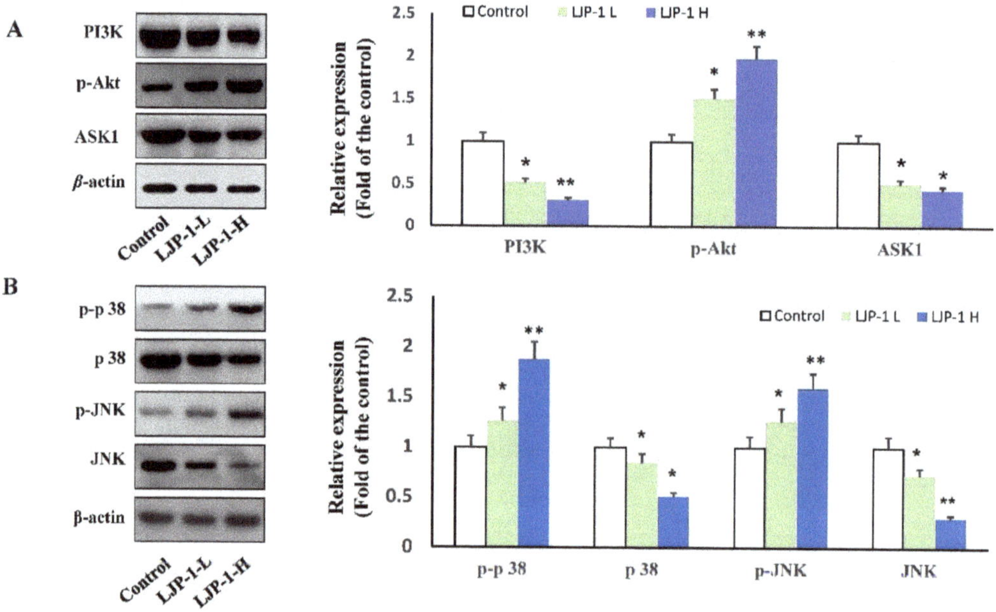

Figure 4. Effects of LJP-1 on the expression of proteins involved in the MAPK and PI3K/AKT signaling pathways in tumor cells (H22 cells). After LJP-1 treatments, H22 cells were lysed and quantitated, and equal protein concentrations were subjected to SDS-PAGE, followed by Western blot analysis. β-actin was used as a protein loading control. (**A**) Western blot of H22 cells treated with LJP-1 expressing proteins in the PI3K/AKT pathway: p-Akt, PI3K, and ASK1 and β-actin. (**B**) Western blot of the expression of p-p38, p38, p-JNK, JNK, and β-actin. The blots were quantified using ImageJ software. Data are expressed as the mean ± SD of three independent experiments. * $p < 0.05$, ** $p < 0.01$ compared to the control group.

2.6. LJP-1 Inhibited Tumor Growth In Vivo

Because LJP-1 exhibited significant in vitro anticancer activity in H22 cells, further experiments were carried out to investigate the in vivo antitumor effect of LJP-1. Tumors were induced in mice by injecting H22 cells. When tumor volume reached 300 mm^3, mice were randomly divided into three groups as described in Section 2.5. The animals were treated with saline or LJP-1 for 3 weeks. To evaluate tumor growth in mice, tumor volume was calculated, and tumor weight was recorded (Figure 5).

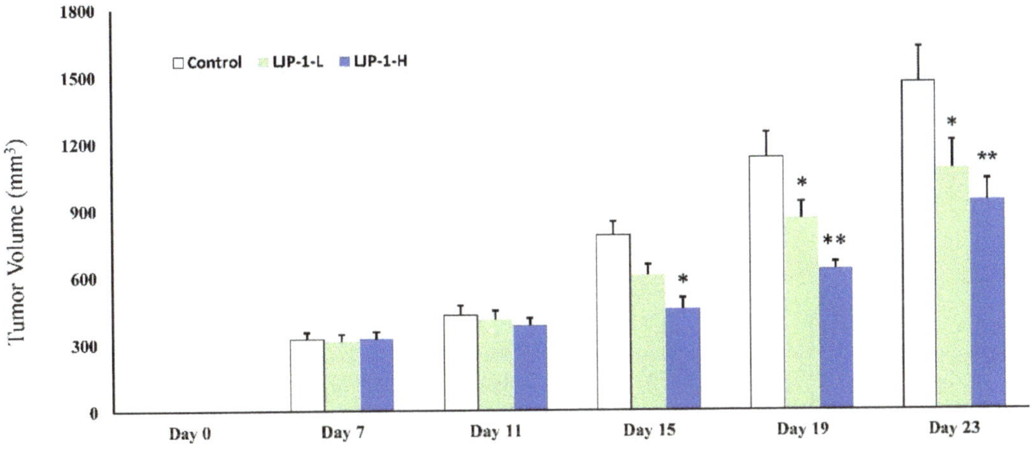

Figure 5. Effect of LJP-1 injection on tumor growth. Liver-cancer-bearing mice were injected with either 200 μL saline (control), 2 mg/kg LJP-1 (LJP-1-L), or 10 mg/kg LJP-1 (LJP-1-H) every 4 days around tumor tissue. Tumor volume was measured on days 7, 11, 15, 19, and 23. Data are expressed as mean ± SD. * $p < 0.05$, ** $p < 0.01$ compared to the control group.

As shown in Figure 5, tumor growth inhibition was observed in the LJP-1 treatment groups (both treated with 2 mg/kg and 10 mg/kg) compared to the control group. Tumor volume was significantly decreased in LJP-1-H treatment groups from day 15 after LJP-1 treatment. The magnitude of inhibition, measured as tumor volume, was very significant and up to 50% on day 19 and day 23 at a dose of 10 mg/kg.

2.7. LJP-1 Induced Cell Apoptosis and Tumore Necrosis

In the current experiment, cancer tissue was stained with ordinary TUNEL staining to detect whether LJP-1 treatment inhibited tumor growth through cell apoptosis. The results are shown in Figure 6A; the apoptotic cells are stained brown. Apoptotic cells in the LJP-1-H group were significantly higher than in the control group. The results showed that approximately 34% more apoptotic cells were observed in the LJP-1-H-treated group than in the control group. Tumor tissue was fixed with formalin, and paraffin sections were stained with H&E. As shown in Figure 6B, there were large necrotic cells in the tumor tissue, as well as pyknosis fragmentation and nuclei dissolution. The necrotic area of tumor tissue in the LJP-1-H-treated group was significantly greater than in the control group. Furthermore, the intercellular space between tissues was significantly widened. In the current experiment, the number of apoptotic cells was counted in six visual fields for each group. After TUNEL fluorescent staining, apoptotic cells were stained green and observed under a fluorescence microscope (Figure 6C). Compared to the control group, the results showed that LJP-1-H treatments induced significant cell apoptosis ($p < 0.05$).

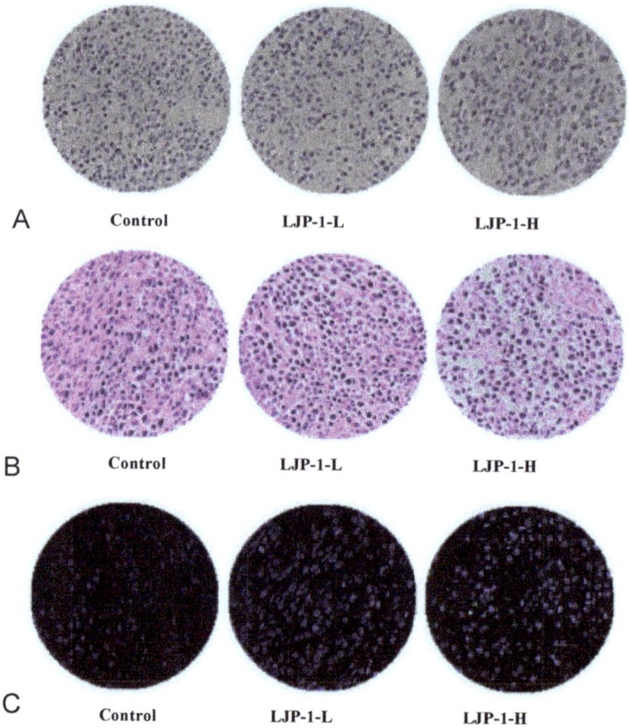

Figure 6. LJP-1 induced cell apoptosis and necrosis in experimental mice. Tumor tissues were fixed in formalin. Paraffin sections were prepared and stained with the appropriate procedures as described in the Materials and Methods. (**A**) TUNEL ordinary staining; TUNEL-positive cells are stained in brown, indicating apoptosis of the central cells. (**B**) H&E staining; the paraffin sections were prepared and stained with H&E, indicating the edema around the necrotic focus of tumor tissue. (**C**) TUNEL fluorescence staining; TUNEL-positive cells are stained green.

3. Discussion

Previous studies have shown that isolated *L. japonica glycoprotein* inhibits cancer cell proliferation by inducing cell cycle arrest and apoptosis [25,26]. However, studies on the anticancer effect of *L. japonica* peptides have not been carried out. In the present study, we isolated *L. japonica* peptides (LJP-1 to LJP-12) using an activity-tracking method; subsequently, we screened the anticancer (HCC) properties of these peptides. We found that six LJPs (LJP-1, LJP-4, LJP-8, LJP-9, LJP-11, and LJP-12) exhibited significant antiproliferative activity against the three cancer cells tested. We then further investigated the anticancer properties of LJP-1 and the underlying mechanism using the H22 liver cancer cell line and an in vivo animal model. For the first time, we demonstrated that LJP-1 has strong inhibitory effects on liver cancer growth, significantly suppressing tumor growth and decreasing tumor volume by more than 50% at a dose of 10 mg/kg on day 23 compared to the control (Figure 5). Furthermore, we found that the underlying mechanism is associated with apoptosis of HCC cells through the caspase-dependent pathway and through phase arrest G0/G1 by regulating cell cycle checkpoint proteins. Furthermore, LJP-1 inhibited the PI3K/AKT and MAPK signaling pathways.

Deregulation of cell cycle progression is a common feature of liver cancer cells. Therefore, targeting regulatory cyclins has been proposed as an important strategy for the treatment of human liver cancer [27,28]. In our in vitro experiments, H22 cells were shown to accumulate significantly in the G0/G1 phase. The cell cycle is regulated by multifaceted proteins, including two classes of molecules: cyclin-dependent kinases (CDK) and cyclin-binding partners. Cyclin D and cyclin E (along with CDK2 and CDK6) play a central role in the G0/G1 phase of the cell cycle [29]. Our studies demonstrated suppression of cyclin D and E expression and attenuation of CDK 2 and 6 expression in cells treated with LJP-1, suggesting that these proteins are involved in the LJP-1-induced cell inhibitory pathway in cancer. P21 and p27 are potent cyclin-dependent kinase inhibitors that bind to and inhibit the activities of CDKs; thus, increased expressions of these proteins indicate the induction of G0/G1 cell cycle arrest [30]. In the current study, we also demonstrated up-regulation of p21 and p27 expression after LJP-1 treatments, supporting that hypothesis that LJP-1 is related to p21- and p27-dependent cell cycle arrest. It should be noted that LJP-1 modulated the expression of the G0/G1 phase protein, resulting in cycle arrest.

The results of the cell cycle analysis revealed that LJP-1 arrested H22 cells in the G0/G1 phase, indicating the occurrence of apoptosis. The results of cell apoptosis were further confirmed by flow cytometry detection. Caspase activation is usually accompanied by PARP activation, which indicates activation of the DNA repair mechanism. Caspase activation is considered a hallmark of apoptosis [31,32]. In the current study, LJP-1 significantly increased the expressions of cleaved caspase-9, -3, and PARP was strongly activated (Figure 3B), suggesting that LJP-1 induced cell apoptosis through caspase activation, a mitochondrial apoptosis pathway.

The ASK1/MAPK pathway is involved in cell cycle regulation and apoptosis. A variety of stresses, such as ROS accumulation, can activate ASK1. ASK1 phosphorylation can lead to downstream activation of the p38 MAPK pathway [33]. Furthermore, the phosphatidylinositol-3-kinase (PI3K)/AKT pathways are common in human cancer, and there is increasing evidence that PI3K/AKT is involved in the development of many types of cancers. Previous studies suggested that PI3K/AKT and its downstream pathways are promising targets for therapeutic intervention [3,27,34].

An interesting finding of the current study is that we found that LJP-1 negatively regulated PI3K expression and simultaneously increased (not decreased) the expression of p-AKT (Figure 4A). How is AKT activation related to apoptosis activation and inhibition of tumor growth? One possible explanation is that activated AKT promotes autophagy, leading to autophagic cell death, resulting in tumor suppression and inhibition of tumor cell proliferation due to the dual effects (suppression and promotion) of autophagy in liver cancer [35]. The AKT/mTOR pathway is known to be a key regulator of autophagy, and AKT activation can stimulate downstream targets through the AKT/mTOR pathway; subsequent dephosphorylation of human homologues Unc-51-like autophagy-activating kinase-1 (ULK1) and Unc-51-like autophagy-activating kinase-2 (ULK2) leads to the promotion of autophagy [36]. Suppression of the mTOR pathway can also initiate autophagy [36]. Many studies have shown that autophagy functions as a tumor suppressor in liver cancer, and compromised autophagy could promote liver tumorigenesis [37]. Therefore, it is possible that the activation of AKT as a result of LJP-1 treatment can promote autophagy, leading to apoptosis/tumor suppression. We cannot confirm the molecular events that link AKT activation with the proposed autophagic cell death, as they are beyond the scope of this study. It would be interesting to conduct further studies investigating the molecular role of autophagy in controlling apoptosis in HCC.

Furthermore, LJP-1 activated p38 and JNK (MAPK phosphorylation states) of H22 cells, as shown in Figure 4B. These results indicate that LJP-1-induced H22 cell apoptosis may occur through the regulation of the MAPK pathway and possibly the PI3K/AKT pathway. Multiple apoptotic pathways work together through cross talk, leading to tumor suppression, since cross-talk of pathways is common in cancer signaling [35,37–41].

An important finding of our study was that LJP-1 exhibited very strong in vivo antitumor activity against HCC in tumor-bearing mice. Tumor volume was decreased significantly in animals treated with either a low dose of 2 mg/kg or a high dose of 10 mg/kg of LJP-1, as shown in Figure 5. The inhibitory effect was more prominent in the group treated with high doses, and a significant decrease was observed from day 15 after LJP-1 treatments, with a further decrease on days 19 and 23, indicating its potential therapeutic application for the treatment of human liver cancer. Mechanistically, we found that in our experiments, LJP-1 treatment significantly induced cancer cell apoptosis in liver cancer tissue (Figure 6), reaffirming that the underlying mechanism of the anticancer property of LJP is apoptosis-related.

Because no previous studies have been conducted on the anticancer effect of *L. japonica* peptides, the most relevant supporting data could be those from studies using the *L. japonica* glycoprotein (LJGP) and the *L japonica*-derived polysaccharide, fucoidan. Go et al. found that an LJGP from brown seaweed inhibited the proliferation of several cancer cell lines, including AGS, HepG2, and HT-29, in a dose-dependent manner by inducing apoptosis [26]. Furthermore, it increased cell growth in normal intestinal cells through the EGFR signaling pathway [23]. Mechanistically, they found that LJGP induced Akt/ERK activation and downregulated JNK/p38, which is similar to the findings of the current study using LJP-1. Increasing evidence supports the notion that fucoidan has strong antitumor actions, inhibiting the growth of various cancer cells by inducing cell cycle arrest and apoptosis and regulating growth-signaling molecules [12,13,15]. Duan et al. recently reported that fucoidan effectively suppressed HCC by inducing apoptosis through the p38 MAPK/ERK and PI3K/AKT signal pathways [10]. We demonstrated here that the PI3K/AKT and MARK pathways play a key role in LJP-1-mediated apoptosis. Our findings, together with previous work on LJGP and fucoidan, suggest that these bioactive components derived from *L japonica*, i.e., fucoidan, LJGP, and LJPs, share a similar mechanism of action in their anticancer activities, although they are structurally very different.

Our work provides original evidence to support the potential of LJP as a natural derivative of seaweed with significant anti-liver cancer activities, highlighting it potential for novel treatment of liver cancer. Our findings add another component derived from *L. japonica* to the list of anticancer bioactive substances derived seaweed. LJP shares a mechanism of action similar to that of fucoidan and LJGP in their anticancer actions. However, the link between LJPs, LJGP, and fucoidan is unknown. Current understanding the anticancer effect of LJPs is very limited. Furthermore, it would be interesting to explore the basic pharmacokinetics of LJP as an anticancer agent. Therefore, further work is needed to elucidate the potential of LJP as a new and effective natural therapy for liver cancer.

4. Materials and Methods

4.1. Materials and Cell Culture

Liver cancer cells (HuH7, HepG2, and H22) and human liver cells (HL-7702) were obtained from the Cell Bank of the Chinese Academy of Sciences (Shanghai, China). Fresh *L. japonica* was acquired from the South China Agricultural University (Guangzhou, China) and identified by Professor C. Wang (South China Agricultural University, Guangzhou, China). The annexin V-FITC/PI staining assay kit and propidium iodide (PI) reagents were supplied by Beyotime (Shanghai, China). Dulbecco's modified Eagle medium (DMEM), fetal bovine serum (FBS), and penicillin-streptomycin (PS) were purchased from Gibco BRL (Life Technologies, Grand Island, NY, USA). The antibodies used in the current study were acquired from Cell Signaling Technology, Inc. (Manchester, NH, USA). Cell lines were grown in specific medium supplemented with 10% FBS. Cells were grown in a humidified atmosphere with 5% CO_2 in incubators maintained at 37 °C. Balb/c mice (6–8 weeks old, 20 ± 2 g) were acquired from the Guangdong Experimental Animal Center.

4.2. Isolation and Amino Acid Sequence Analysis of LJPs

All isolation procedures were conducted at 4 °C. Fresh *L. japonica* (8 kg) was minced in a homogenate mixed with isopropanol in a ratio of 1:6 (w/v) and stirred uninterrupted for 4 h. Subsequently, the sediment was collected and lyophilized. The defatted precipitate (732 g) was dissolved (5%, w/v) in 0.50 M phosphate buffer solution (PBS, pH 7.5). After centrifugation (8000× g, 10 min), the supernatant was collected and freeze-dried as the total protein.

Total protein was fractionated using ultrafiltration with a membrane cutoff of 1 kDa molecular weight (MW) (Millipore, Wanchai, China). Two peptide fractions, LJP-A (MW < 1 kDa) and LJP-B (MW > 1 kDa), were collected and freeze-dried.

4.2.1. Hydrophobic Chromatography

LJP-A was dissolved in 1.20 M $(NH_4)_2SO_4$ prepared with 30 mM phosphate buffer (pH 7.5) and loaded onto a hydrophobic column of phenyl sepharose CL-4B (3.0 cm × 120 cm). A stepwise elution with decreasing concentrations of $(NH_4)_2SO_4$ (1.20, 0.60, and 0 M) was dissolved in 30 mM phosphate buffer (pH 7.5) at a flow rate of 3.0 mL / min. Each 100 mL fraction was collected and monitored at 280 nm. Five fractions (LJP-A-1~LJP-A-5) were collected, and antiproliferative activity was detected against the three cancer cells. The fraction with significant anticancer activity was collected and prepared for anion-exchange chromatography.

4.2.2. Anion-Exchange Chromatography

The LJP-A-3 fraction was collected (LJP-A-3, 6 mL, 4.42 g/mL) and injected into a DEAE-52 cellulose (Sigma-Aldrich, Shanghai, China) anion-exchange column (2.0 × 100 cm) equilibrated with deionized water and stepwise eluted with distilled water solutions of 0.30, 0.60, and 1.20 M (NH_4) $2SO_4$ at a flow rate of 2.0 mL/min. Each eluted fraction (50 mL) was collected and monitored at 280 nm. Seven fractions (LJP-A-3-1~LJP-A-3-7) were collected, and antiproliferative activity was detected against the three cancer cells. The fraction with the highest antiproliferative activity was collected and prepared for gel filtration chromatography.

4.2.3. Gel Filtration Chromatography

The LJP-A-3-5 fraction was collected and fractionated in a Sephadex G-25 column (Sigma-Aldrich, Shanghai, China) (2.0 × 100 cm) with a flow rate of 2.0 mL/min. Each eluate (50 mL) was collected and monitored at 280 nm. Five fractions (LJP-A-3-5-1~LJP-A-3-5-5) were collected, and antiproliferative activity against the three cancer cells was detected. The fraction with significant antiproliferative activity was collected and prepared for reversed-phase high-performance liquid chromatography (RP-HPLC).

4.2.4. RP-HPLC and HPLC-ESI-MS Analysis

The LJP-A-3-5-3 fraction was collected. Subsequently, LJP-A-3-5-3 was separated by RP-HPLC (Agilent 1200) on a Zorbax SB C-18 column (4.6 × 250 mm, 5 μm). The elution solvent system was composed of water-trifluoroacetic acid (solvent A; 100:0.1, v/v) and acetonitrile-trifluoroacetic acid (solvent B; 100:0.1, v/v). The peptides were separated using a 30% to 70% gradient elution of solvent B for 45 min at a flow rate of 1.0 mL/min, with the detection wavelength set at 280 nm.

HPLC-ESI-MS was performed on a SCIEX X500R Q-TOF mass spectrometer (Framingham, MA, USA). The MS conditions were as follows: ESI-MS analysis was performed using a SCIEX X500R Q-TOF mass spectrometer equipped with an ESI source. The mass range was set to m/z 100–1200. The Q-TOF MS data were acquired in positive mode, and the MS analysis conditions were as follows: CAD gas flow rate, 7 L/min; drying gas temperature, 550 °C; ion spray voltage, 5500 V; declustering potential, 80 V; software-generated data file: SCIEX OS 1.0. The peptide is usually protonated under ESI-MS/MS conditions, and fragmentations occur mostly at the amide bonds because it is difficult to break the chemical bonds of the side chains at such low energy. Hence, on the basis of the HPLC-ESI-MS data and accompanied by the Edman degradation results, the amino acid sequences of the LJPs were identified.

4.2.5. Summary of Key Steps

The key steps involved in the isolation of LJPs and the identification of amino acid sequences of LJPs are summarized in Scheme 1.

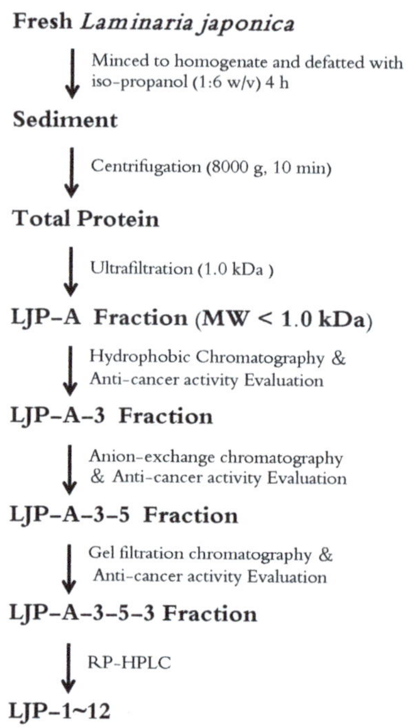

Scheme 1. Key Steps in the isolation of LJPs (LJP-1~12).

4.3. *Cell Apoptosis and Cell Cycle Assays*

Ab MTT assay was used to detect the cytotoxicity activity of LJPs in vitro [42]. Briefly, 5×10^3 cells/well were seeded in 96-well plates, and varying concentrations of LJP were added. After 48 h, the MTT solution (5 mg/mL) was added for an additional 4 h. The absorbance was measured at 570 nm using a microplate reader (Bio-Rad; Hercules, CA, USA) after 100 μL of DMSO was added. The IC^{50} values were determined by the non-linear multipurpose curve-fitting program.

After treatment with LJP-1 (0, 0.36, and 1.80 mM representing control, low dose of LJP-1 and LJP-1-L, and high dose of LJP-1 and LJP-1-H, respectively) for 48 h, the apoptosis of H22 cells was evaluated by flow cytometry. Briefly, after LJP-1 treatment, H22 cells were collected, washed with cold PBS, suspended in binding buffer (100 μL) (BD Biosciences, San Jose, CA, USA), treated with annexin V and propidium iodide (PI) (BD Biosciences), and incubated in the dark for 15 min. Then, another 300 μL binding buffer was added, and flow cytometry analysis was performed for 1 h to measure the rate of apoptosis. The percentages of cells in the G0/G1, S, and G2/M phases were determined using a cell cycle detection kit (BD Biosciences, Haryana, India) using a Beckman Coulter EPICS ALTRA II cytometer (Beckman Coulter, Brea, CA, USA).

4.4. *Western Blot Analysis*

After treatment with LJP-1 (0, 0.36, and 1.80 mM representing control, low dose of LJP-1 and LJP-1-L, and high dose of LJP-1 and LJP-1-H, respectively) for 48 h, H22 cells were collected, and protein was collected and measured with a Bradford protein assay to calculate the amount of protein. Equal amounts of protein were separated by sodium dodecyl sulfate polyacrylamide gel electrophoresis (SDS-PAGE) and electroblotted onto a polyvinylidene difluoride (PVDF) membrane. Immunoblots were blocked with 5% non-fat milk and incubated with primary antibody (1:1000) at 4 °C overnight, followed by incubation with the second conjugated peroxidase antibody (1:5000) at room temperature for 2 h [43].

Protein bands were measured, and β-actin was used as an internal standard of process control. The blot band densitometry was analyzed with ImageJ software, version 1.53t.

4.5. Immunization of Liver-Cancer-bearing Mice

The procedures for the animal study were approved by the Animal Ethics Committee of Shenzhen University. Mice were kept in a specific pathogen-free facility with free access to food and water. H22 cells were cultured and suspended in PBS, and 18 Balb/c mice were subcutaneously injected with H22 cells (1×10^6) in the right back near the skin of the underarm. Tumor growth was measured every 2 days. When tumor volume reached 300 mm^3, mice were randomly divided into three groups and treated with the following procedures: Group 1 (Control): mice were injected with 200 μL saline every 4 days around tumor tissue; Group 2 (LJP-1-L): mice were injected with LJP-1 (in 200 μL saline) 2 mg/kg every 4 days (4 days in a cycle, four times) around tumor tissue; Group 3 (LJP-1-H): mice were injected with LJP-1 (in 200 μL saline) 10 mg/kg every 4 days (4 days in a cycle, four times) around tumor tissue. All mice were sacrificed on day 23. The subcutaneous tumors were excised, and the tumor index was calculated. Furthermore, tumor tissues were cut into small woven pieces and fixed with polyformaldehyde, and paraffin sections were made later.

4.6. Evaluation of Tumor Apoptosis and Hematoxylin and Eosin (H&E) Staining

Apoptotic cells in cancer tissue sections were stained with a TUNEL reagent kit following the manufacturer's instructions. Hematoxylin and eosin (H&E) staining was performed according to the routine procedure. The paraffin section was dewaxed and dehydrated with xylene and gradient alcohol, then stained with hematoxylin solution for 5 min, soaked in 1% acid ethanol (1% HCL in 70% ethanol) for 2 min, and rinsed in distilled water. Slices were stained with eosin solution for 3 min, dehydrated with graded alcohol, and cleaned with xylene.

4.7. Statistical Analysis

Data are presented as mean ± standard deviation (SD). GraphPad Prism 5.0 (Graph Pad Software, La Jolla, CA, USA) was used for statistical analysis. Statistical analysis was performed with one-way analysis of variance (ANOVA). $p < 0.05$ was considered statistically significant.

5. Conclusions

In conclusion, our study demonstrates that LJP-1 isolated from *L. japonica* possesses strong antitumor effects against HCC-based on evidence from both in vitro and in vivo studies. In vivo experiments show that LJP-1 strongly suppressed tumor growth on day 14 after treatment at doses of 2 and10 mg/kg. Our data supports that LJP-1 controls liver cancer proliferation by inducing HCC cell apoptosis through the caspase-dependent pathway and by arresting cells in the G0/G1 phase by regulating cell cycle checkpoint proteins. Furthermore, LJP-1 induces caspase-dependent apoptosis, in part, by inhibiting MAPK signaling pathways. The PI3K/AKT pathway and possibly other pathways may be involved. In addition, our screening study shows that other LJPs, namely LJP-4, LJP-8, LJP-9, LJP-11, and LJP-12, also exhibit antitumor activities. Therefore, *L. japonica peptides* (not just LJP-1) could be potential drug candidates for the novel treatment of human liver cancer and warrant further investigation.

Author Contributions: Conceptualization, Y.L. (Yiguang Lin) and H.C.; methodology, software, and validation, Y.W., Y.L. (Yuanhui Li), W.G., J.L., W.L. and P.H.; formal analysis, investigation, and data curation, Y.W., Y.L. (Yuanhui Li), W.G. and J.L.; writing—original draft preparation, Y.L. (Yiguang Lin), J.L. and Y.W.; writing—review and editing, Y.W., Y.L. (Yuanhui Li), W.G., J.L., W.L., P.H., Y.L. (Yiguang Lin) and H.C.; visualization, Y.W., J.L., Y.L. (Yiguang Lin) and H.C.; supervision, H.C. and Y.L. (Yiguang Lin); project administration, Y.L. (Yiguang Lin) and H.C.; funding acquisition, H.C. All authors have read and agreed to the published version of the manuscript.

Funding: This research received no external funding.

Institutional Review Board Statement: The procedures for the animal study were approved by the Animal Ethics Committee of Shenzhen University (No: 2017-0113).

Informed Consent Statement: Not applicable.

Data Availability Statement: The data (figures and tables) used to support the findings of this study are included within the article.

Conflicts of Interest: The authors declare no conflict of interest.

References

1. Wild, C.; Weiderpass, E.; Stewart, B.W. *World Cancer Report: Cancer Research for Cancer Prevention*; IARC Press: Lyon, France, 2020.
2. Siegel, R.L.; Miller, K.D.; Jemal, A. Cancer statistics, 2018. *CA Cancer J. Clin.* **2018**, *68*, 7–30. [CrossRef] [PubMed]
3. Wang, F.; Bank, T.; Malnassy, G.; Arteaga, M.; Shang, N.; Dalheim, A.; Ding, X.; Cotler, S.J.; Denning, M.F.; Nishimura, M.I.; et al. Inhibition of insulin-like growth factor 1 receptor enhances the efficacy of sorafenib in inhibiting hepatocellular carcinoma cell growth and survival. *Hepatol. Commun.* **2018**, *2*, 732–746. [CrossRef] [PubMed]
4. Kaseb, A.O. Beyond the basics: The differential effects of demographics and hepatitis status on treatment outcome in hepatocellular carcinoma. *Oncology* **2013**, *85*, 41–43. [CrossRef] [PubMed]
5. Maduro, J.H.; Pras, E.; Willemse, P.H.B.; Vries, E.G.E.D. Acute and long-term toxicity following radiotherapy alone or in combination with chemotherapy for locally advanced cervical cancer. *Cancer Treat. Rev.* **2004**, *29*, 471–488. [CrossRef]
6. Chen, Z.; Xie, H.; Hu, M.; Huang, T.; Hu, Y.; Sang, N.; Zhao, Y. Recent progress in treatment of hepatocellular carcinoma. *Am. J. Cancer Res.* **2020**, *10*, 2993–3036.
7. Rodrigues, T.; Sieglitz, F.; Bernardes, G.J.L. Natural product modulators of transient receptor potential (TRP) channels as potential anti-cancer agents. *Chem. Soc. Rev.* **2016**, *45*, 6130–6137. [CrossRef]
8. Mabate, B.; Daub, C.D.; Malgas, S.; Edkins, A.L.; Pletschke, B.I. Fucoidan Structure and Its Impact on Glucose Metabolism: Implications for Diabetes and Cancer Therapy. *Mar. Drugs* **2021**, *19*, 30. [CrossRef]
9. Jin, X.; Zhao, T.; Shi, D.; Ye, M.B.; Yi, Q. Protective role of fucoxanthin in diethylnitrosamine-induced hepatocarcinogenesis in experimental adult rats. *Drug Dev. Res.* **2019**, *80*, 209–217. [CrossRef]
10. Duan, Y.; Li, J.; Jing, X.; Ding, X.; Yu, Y.; Zhao, Q. Fucoidan Induces Apoptosis and Inhibits Proliferation of Hepatocellular Carcinoma via the p38 MAPK/ERK and PI3K/Akt Signal Pathways. *Cancer Manag. Res.* **2020**, *12*, 1713–1723. [CrossRef]
11. Du, X.; Xiao, S.; Luo, Q.; Liu, X.; Liu, J. Laminaria japonica cyclic peptides exert anti-colorectal carcinoma effects through apoptosis induction in vitro and in vivo. *J. Pept. Sci.* **2022**, *28*, e3385. [CrossRef]
12. Senthilkumar, K.; Manivasagan, P.; Venkatesan, J.; Kim, S.K. Brown seaweed fucoidan: Biological activity and apoptosis, growth signaling mechanism in cancer. *Int. J. Biol. Macromol.* **2013**, *60*, 366–374. [CrossRef] [PubMed]
13. Jin, J.O.; Chauhan, P.S.; Arukha, A.P.; Chavda, V.; Dubey, A.; Yadav, D. The Therapeutic Potential of the Anticancer Activity of Fucoidan: Current Advances and Hurdles. *Mar. Drugs* **2021**, *19*, 265. [CrossRef]
14. Hsu, W.J.; Lin, M.H.; Kuo, T.C.; Chou, C.M.; Mi, F.L.; Cheng, C.H.; Lin, C.W. Fucoidan from Laminaria japonica exerts antitumor effects on angiogenesis and micrometastasis in triple-negative breast cancer cells. *Int. J. Biol. Macromol.* **2020**, *149*, 600–608. [CrossRef]
15. Lin, Y.; Qi, X.; Liu, H.; Xue, K.; Xu, S.; Tian, Z. The anti-cancer effects of fucoidan: A review of both in vivo and in vitro investigations. *Cancer Cell Int.* **2020**, *20*, 154. [CrossRef] [PubMed]
16. Jimenez-Escrig, A.; Goni Cambrodon, I. Nutritional evaluation and physiological effects of edible seaweeds. *Arch. Latinoam. Nutr.* **1999**, *49*, 114–120. [PubMed]
17. Oshima, E. Medicinal Uses of Seaweed in Traditional Chinese Medicine. In *Traditional Chinese Medicine: Scientific Basis for Its Use*; Royal Society of Chemistry, Thomas Graham House: Cambridge, UK, 2013; p. 238.
18. Huang, H.; Fang, J.; Fan, X.; Miyata, T.; Hu, X.; Zhang, L.; Zhang, L.; Cui, Y.; Liu, Z.; Wu, X. Advances in Molecular Mechanisms for Traditional Chinese Medicine Actions in Regulating Tumor Immune Responses. *Front. Pharmacol.* **2020**, *11*, 1009. [CrossRef] [PubMed]
19. Ming, J.X.; Wang, Z.C.; Huang, Y.; Ohishi, H.; Wu, R.J.; Shao, Y.; Wang, H.; Qin, M.Y.; Wu, Z.L.; Li, Y.Y.; et al. Fucoxanthin extracted from Laminaria Japonica inhibits metastasis and enhances the sensitivity of lung cancer to Gefitinib. *J. Ethnopharmacol.* **2021**, *265*, 113302. [CrossRef]
20. Thomas, N.V.; Kim, S.K. Fucoidans from Marine Algae as Potential Matrix Metalloproteinase Inhibitors. *Adv. Food Nutr. Res.* **2014**, *72*, 177–193.
21. Duarte, M.E.R.; Cardoso, M.A.; Noseda, M.D.; Cerezo, A.S. Structural studies on fucoidans from the brown seaweedSargassum stenophyllum. *Carbohydr. Res.* **2001**, *333*, 281–293. [CrossRef]
22. Apostolova, E.; Lukova, P.; Baldzhieva, A.; Katsarov, P.; Nikolova, M.; Iliev, I.; Peychev, L.; Trica, B.; Oancea, F.; Delattre, C.; et al. Immunomodulatory and Anti-Inflammatory Effects of Fucoidan: A Review. *Polymers* **2020**, *12*, 2338. [CrossRef]
23. Go, H.; Hwang, H.J.; Nam, T.J. Glycoprotein extraction from Laminaria japonica promotes IEC-6 cell proliferation. *Int. J. Mol. Med.* **2009**, *24*, 819–824. [CrossRef] [PubMed]

24. Cho, D.-M.; Kim, D.-S.; Lee, D.-S.; Kim, H.-R.; Pyeun, J.-H. Trace components and functional saccharides in seaweed-1-changes in proximate composition and trace elements according to the harvest season and places. *Korean J. Fish. Aquat. Sci.* **1995**, *28*, 49–59.
25. Han, M.H.; Kim, G.Y.; Moon, S.K.; Kim, W.J.; Nam, T.J.; Choi, Y.H. Apoptosis induction by glycoprotein isolated from Laminaria japonica is associated with down-regulation of telomerase activity and prostaglandin E2 synthesis in AGS human gastric cancer cells. *Int. J. Oncol.* **2011**, *38*, 577–584. [CrossRef] [PubMed]
26. Go, H.; Hwang, H.J.; Nam, T.J. A glycoprotein from Laminaria japonica induces apoptosis in HT-29 colon cancer cells. *Toxicol. Vitr.* **2010**, *24*, 1546–1553. [CrossRef] [PubMed]
27. Frezza, C. The role of mitochondria in the oncogenic signal transduction. *Int. J. Biochem. Cell Biol.* **2014**, *48*, 11–17. [CrossRef]
28. Malumbres, M.; Carnero, A. Cell cycle deregulation: A common motif in cancer. *Prog. Cell Cycle Res.* **2003**, *5*, 5–18.
29. Scaglione-Sewell, B.A.; Bissonnette, M.; Skarosi, S.; Abraham, C.; Brasitus, T. A vitamin D3 analog induces a G1-phase arrest in CaCo2 Cells by inhibiting Cdk2 and Cdk6: Roles of cyclin E, p21(Waf1), and p27(Kip1). *Endocrinology* **2000**, *141*, 3931–3939. [CrossRef]
30. Hall, M.; Bates, S.; Peters, G. Evidence for different modes of action of cyclin-dependent kinase inhibitors: p15 and p16 bind to kinases, p21 and p27 bind to cyclins. *Oncogene* **1995**, *11*, 1581–1588.
31. Estaquier, J.; Vallette, F.; Vayssiere, J.L.; Mignotte, B. The mitochondrial pathways of apoptosis. *Adv. Exp. Med. Biol.* **2012**, *942*, 157–183. [CrossRef]
32. Choudhary, G.S.; Al-Harbi, S.; Almasan, A. Caspase-3 activation is a critical determinant of genotoxic stress-induced apoptosis. In *Apoptosis and Cancer*; Springer: Berlin/Heidelberg, Germany, 2015; pp. 1–9. [CrossRef]
33. Kong, A.N.; Yu, R.; Chen, C.; Mandlekar, S.; Primiano, T. Signal transduction events elicited by natural products: Role of MAPK and caspase pathways in homeostatic response and induction of apoptosis. *Arch. Pharm. Res.* **2000**, *23*, 1–16. [CrossRef]
34. Noorolyai, S.; Shajari, N.; Baghbani, E.; Sadreddini, S.; Baradaran, B. The relation between PI3K/AKT signalling pathway and cancer. *Gene* **2019**, *698*, 120–128. [CrossRef] [PubMed]
35. Yazdani, H.O.; Huang, H.; Tsung, A. Autophagy: Dual Response in the Development of Hepatocellular Carcinoma. *Cells* **2019**, *8*, 91. [CrossRef] [PubMed]
36. Ryu, H.Y.; Kim, L.E.; Jeong, H.; Yeo, B.K.; Lee, J.-W.; Nam, H.; Ha, S.; An, H.-K.; Park, H.; Jung, S. GSK3B induces autophagy by phosphorylating ULK1. *Exp. Mol. Med.* **2021**, *53*, 369–383. [CrossRef] [PubMed]
37. Qian, H.; Chao, X.; Williams, J.; Fulte, S.; Li, T.; Yang, L.; Ding, W.X. Autophagy in liver diseases: A review. *Mol. Asp. Med.* **2021**, *82*, 100973. [CrossRef] [PubMed]
38. Garcia-Pras, E.; Fernandez-Iglesias, A.; Gracia-Sancho, J.; Perez-Del-Pulgar, S. Cell Death in Hepatocellular Carcinoma: Pathogenesis and Therapeutic Opportunities. *Cancers* **2021**, *14*, 48. [CrossRef]
39. Sun, E.J.; Wankell, M.; Palamuthusingam, P.; McFarlane, C.; Hebbard, L. Targeting the PI3K/Akt/mTOR Pathway in Hepatocellular Carcinoma. *Biomedicines* **2021**, *9*, 1639. [CrossRef]
40. Peng, Y.; Wang, Y.; Zhou, C.; Mei, W.; Zeng, C. PI3K/Akt/mTOR Pathway and Its Role in Cancer Therapeutics: Are We Making Headway? *Front. Oncol.* **2022**, *12*, 819128. [CrossRef]
41. Hoxhaj, G.; Manning, B.D. The PI3K-AKT network at the interface of oncogenic signalling and cancer metabolism. *Nat. Rev. Cancer* **2020**, *20*, 74–88. [CrossRef]
42. Stec, J.; Szczotka, M.; Kuźmak, J. Cytotoxicity of feed-borne mycotoxins to animal cell lines in vitro using the MTT assay. *Bull. Vet. Inst. Pulawy* **2007**, *51*, 679–684.
43. Liu, J.; Zhou, F.; Zhang, L.; Wang, H.; Chen, H. DMXAA-pyranoxanthone hybrids enhance inhibition activities against human cancer cells with multi-target functions. *Eur. J. Med. Chem.* **2017**, *143*, 1768. [CrossRef]

marine drugs

Article

7S,15R-Dihydroxy-16S,17S-epoxy-docosapentaenoic Acid Overcomes Chemoresistance of 5-Fluorouracil by Suppressing the Infiltration of Tumor-Associated Macrophages and Inhibiting the Activation of Cancer Stem Cells in a Colorectal Cancer Xenograft Model

Yan Su [1,2], Hack Sun Choi [3], Jong Hyun Choi [1], Hee-Sik Kim [4], Yong-Suk Jang [2,*] and Jeong-Woo Seo [1,*]

[1] Microbial Biotechnology Research Center, Korea Research Institute of Bioscience and Biotechnology (KRIBB), Jeongeup-si 56212, Republic of Korea
[2] Department of Bioactive Material Sciences, The Institute for Molecular Biology and Genetics, Jeonbuk National University, Jeonju-si 54896, Republic of Korea
[3] Faculty of Biotechnology, College of Applied Life Sciences, Jeju National University, Jeju-si 63243, Republic of Korea
[4] Cell Factory Research Center, Korea Research Institute of Bioscience and Biotechnology (KRIBB), Daejeon-si 34141, Republic of Korea
* Correspondence: yongsuk@jbnu.ac.kr (Y.-S.J.); jwseo@kribb.re.kr (J.-W.S.); Tel.: +82-63-570-5160 (J.-W.S.)

Abstract: Although the tumor bulk is initially reduced by 5-fluorouracil (5-FU), chemoresistance developed due to prolonged chemotherapy in colorectal cancer (CRC). The enrichment of cancer stem cells (CSCs) and the infiltration of tumor-associated macrophages (TAMs) contribute to chemoresistance and poor outcomes. A docosahexaenoic acid derivative developed by our group, 7S,15R-dihydroxy-16S,17S-epoxy-docosapentaenoic acid (diHEP-DPA), exerts antitumor effects against TAMs infiltration and CSCs enrichment in our previous study. The current study aimed to investigate whether diHEP-DPA was able to overcome chemoresistance to 5-FU in CRCs, together with the potential synergistic mechanisms in a CT26-BALB/c mouse model. Our results suggested that although 5-FU inhibited tumor growth, 5-FU enriched CSCs via the WNT/β-catenin signaling pathway, resulting in chemoresistance in CRCs. However, we revealed that 5-FU promoted the infiltration of TAMs via the NF-kB signaling pathway and improved epithelial–mesenchymal transition (EMT) via the signal transducer and activator of the transcription 3 (STAT3) signaling pathway; these traits were believed to contribute to CSC activation. Furthermore, supplementation with diHEP-DPA could overcome drug resistance by decreasing the CSCs, suppressing the infiltration of TAMs, and inhibiting EMT progression. Additionally, the combinatorial treatment of diHEP-DPA and 5-FU effectively enhanced phagocytosis by blocking the CD47/signal regulatory protein alpha (SIRPα) axis. These findings present that diHEP-DPA is a potential therapeutic supplement to improve drug outcomes and suppress chemoresistance associated with the current 5-FU-based therapies for colorectal cancer.

Keywords: colorectal cancer; 5-fluorouracil; 7S,15R-dihydroxy-16S,17S-epoxy-docosapentaenoic acid; tumor-associated macrophages; chemoresistance

Citation: Su, Y.; Choi, H.S.; Choi, J.H.; Kim, H.-S.; Jang, Y.-S.; Seo, J.-W. 7S,15R-dihydroxy-16S,17S-epoxy-Docosapentaenoic Acid Overcomes Chemoresistance of 5-Fluorouracil by Suppressing the Infiltration of Tumor-Associated Macrophages and Inhibiting the Activation of Cancer Stem Cells in a Colorectal Cancer Xenograft Model. *Mar. Drugs* **2023**, *21*, 80. https://doi.org/10.3390/md21020080

Academic Editors: Celso Alves and Marc Diederich

Received: 19 December 2022
Revised: 20 January 2023
Accepted: 20 January 2023
Published: 24 January 2023

Copyright: © 2023 by the authors. Licensee MDPI, Basel, Switzerland. This article is an open access article distributed under the terms and conditions of the Creative Commons Attribution (CC BY) license (https://creativecommons.org/licenses/by/4.0/).

1. Introduction

Colorectal cancer (CRC) is a highly malignant cancer that, with the aging of the population and changes in lifestyle, accounts for a third of the cancer-related deaths worldwide [1]. One of the most important first-line medicines in clinical CRC therapy is 5- fluorouracil (5-FU). However, chemoresistance and the associated adverse effects have limited the clinical benefits; thus, it is imperative to find alternative therapies to overcome chemoresistance and improve outcomes with less toxicity for patients with CRC [2].

Several studies have reported that long-term treatment with 5-FU may cause a cytokine storm in the tumor microenvironment (TME), induce macrophages to produce proinflammatory mediators, and enrich cancer stem cells (CSCs), resulting in poor outcomes and chemoresistance [3–5]. Therefore, the biological factors involved in mediating resistance to 5-FU-based therapy must be extensively examined.

The TME, which comprises tumor cells and stromal cells, including fibroblasts, endothelial cells, and immune cells, plays a crucial role in tumor progression, including metastasis, invasion, stemness, and acquired chemoresistance [6,7]. Tumor-associated macrophages (TAMs) are major components of the TME. Macrophages are classified as M1 and M2 subtypes, depending on their immune responses [8]. M2-like macrophages are the main subsets of TAMs, and they produce various growth factors and cytokines, such as vascular endothelial growth factor (VEGF), interleukin-6 (IL-6), and tumor necrosis factor-α (TNF-α). These not only promote tumor growth but also confer chemoresistance [9,10].

During the epithelial–mesenchymal transition (EMT) procession, epithelial cancer cells acquire the features of mesenchymal cells by downregulating epithelial markers (E-cadherin) and upregulating mesenchymal markers (vimentin and N-cadherin) [11]. Cancer cells undergoing EMT reportedly possess enhanced metastatic and invasive abilities, express high levels of stem surface markers, and strongly resist radio- or chemotherapy [12]. Several cytokines, chemokines, and growth factors secreted by TAMs likely contribute to EMT and chemoresistance by activating the signal transducer and activator of the transcription 3 (STAT3) pathway in many tumors [13,14].

CD47 is a common mechanism through which cells protect themselves from phagocytosis. CD47 functions as a ligand for signal regulatory protein-α (SIRPα), a protein expressed on macrophages and dendritic cells. SIRPα binds with CD47 to initiate a signaling cascade which results in the inhibition of phagocytosis, a critical "do not eat me" signal for the innate immune system which is overexpressed on many kinds of tumor cells [15,16].

CSCs, a subpopulation of cells, are characterized by some key markers, such as CD133, CD166, CD44, CD24, SOX2, OCT4, and ALDH, which are associated with tumor initiation, growth, and therapy resistance [17]. Some studies also showed that massive populations of CSCs correlate with poor overall survival rates after chemotherapy in advanced patients with CRC [18]. One of the mechanisms of activation of CSCs involves the WNT/β-catenin pathway [17]. Treatment using 5-FU activated CSCs via p53-induced WNT3 transcription, followed by the activation of the WNT/β-catenin pathway in CRC cell lines and xenograft tumors as well as patient avatar models [19].

The novel resolvin, 7S,15R-dihydroxy-16S,17S-epoxy-docosapentaenoic acid (diHEP-DPA) (Figure 1), is synthesized by cyanobacterial lipoxygenase from DHA (purity > 98%). In our previous study, we showed the generation and structure of diHEP-DPA and demonstrated that diHEP-DPA regulated the polarization of TAMs, EMT, and CSCs activation in HCT116 and HT26 cells [20]. In the current study, we further investigated the effects of diHEP-DPA on 5-FU-induced chemoresistance in colorectal xenograft tumors via TAMs, CSCs, and EMT. Our results collectively indicated that diHEP-DPA reversed the challenges caused by prolonged chemotherapy, such as the infiltration of M2-like TAMs, the enrichment of CSCs, and the progression of EMT in colorectal tumors, suggesting that diHEP-DPA is a promising therapy to overcome 5-FU resistance and improve 5-FU treatment outcomes in colon cancer.

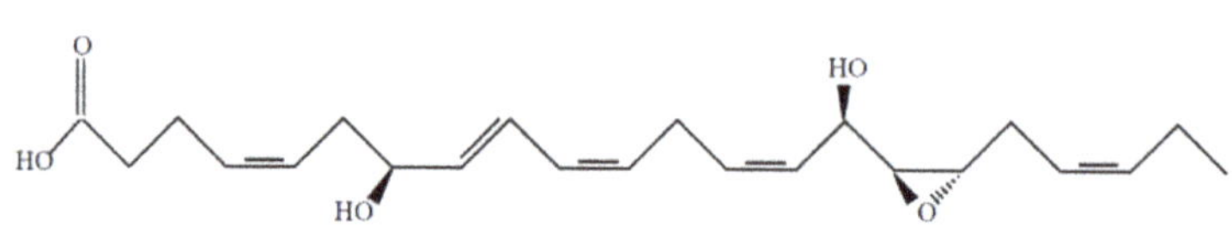

Figure 1. The structure of 7*S*,15*R*-dihydroxy-16*S*,17*S*-epoxy-docosapentaenoic acid (diHEP-DPA).

2. Results

2.1. diHEP-DPA and 5-FU Inhibited Tumor Growth in the CRC Xenograft Model

The combined treatment of diHEP-DPA and 5-FU synergistically inhibited tumor growth and size (Figure 2). Briefly, the tumor volume in control mice was ~1791 mm^3 (2.80 ± 0.30 g), as measured on day 30 post-cell injection. The corresponding volumes in the diHEP-DPA, 5-FU, and combined treatment groups were ~1221 mm^3 (2.07 ± 0.34 g), ~887 mm^3 (1.48 ± 0.23 g), and ~636 mm^3 (0.96 ± 0.13 g). These findings indicated that, compared with diHEP-DPA or 5-FU alone, the combination of the two inhibited colorectal tumor growth and size more effectively.

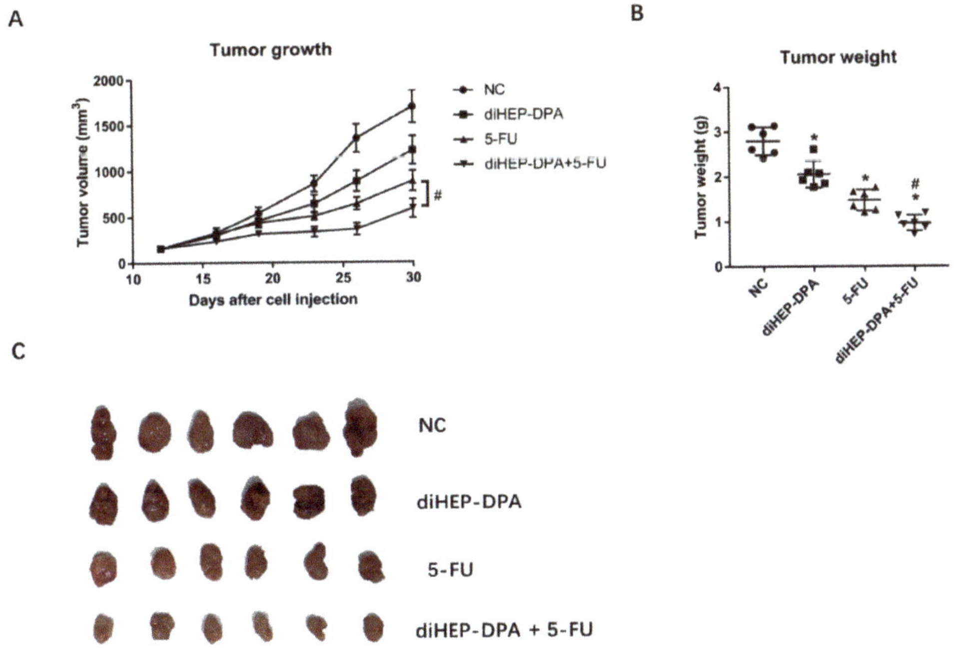

Figure 2. Effects of diHEP-DPA and 5-FU on tumor growth and tumor weight. (**A**) Tumor mass volumes in BALB/c mice intraperitoneally injected with saline (control), diHEP-DPA (10 μg/kg/day), 5-FU (20 mg/kg/five times a week), or both diHEP-DPA (10 μg/kg/day) and 5-FU (20 mg/kg/five times a week). (**B**) Tumor weight after sacrifice on day 30. (**C**) Tumors excised after sacrifice on day 30. Data are expressed as mean ± SD; $n = 6$ per group. * $p < 0.05$ compared with the control group; # $p < 0.05$ compared with the 5-FU group.

2.2. diHEP-DPA Suppressed 5-FU-Induced CSCs Activation via the WNT/β-Catenin Pathway

As shown in Figure 3A–C, diHEP-DPA significantly decreased the expression of CSC markers, including CD133, CD44, and SOX2. However, the expression of CD133 was significantly inhibited, whereas the expressions of CD44 and SOX2 were markedly increased in the 5-FU group. Combination treatment with diHEP-DPA and 5-FU reversed the 5-FU-induced activation of CSC markers. To confirm the above results, these protein levels were evaluated via western blotting. Similarly, diHEP-DPA significantly decreased the protein levels of all CSC markers. Although the 5-FU treatment decreased the expression of CD133, it significantly increased the protein expressions of CD44 and SOX2. Moreover, the combined treatment decreased the levels of these CSC markers more effectively than the 5-FU treatment (Figure 3D). We assumed that 5-FU enriched CSCs by the activation of the WNT/β-catenin pathway. diHEP-DPA caused a significant decrease in the β-catenin level. However, the 5-FU treatment significantly increased the β-catenin level, which was reversed via the additional diHEP-DPA treatment (Figure 3D). It predominantly suggested that diHEP-DPA overcame 5-FU-induced CRC activation via the WNT/β-catenin signaling pathway.

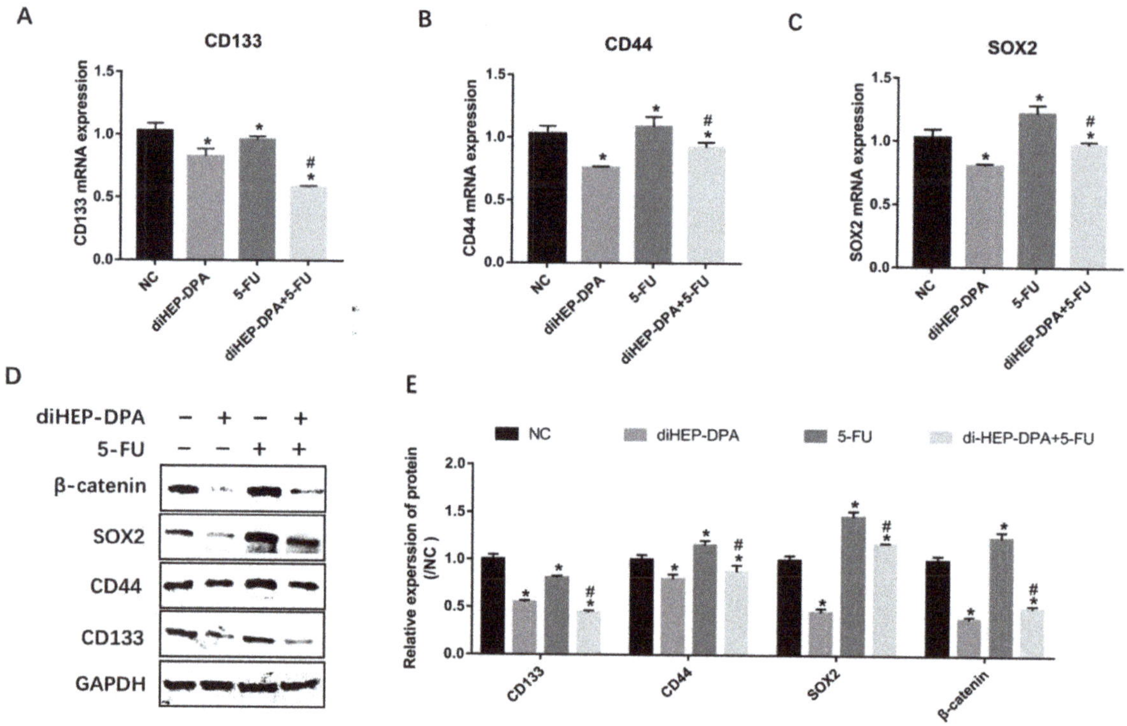

Figure 3. Effects of diHEP-DPA and 5-FU on cancer stem cells via the WNT/β-catenin signaling pathway. Relative mRNA levels of (**A**) CD133, (**B**) CD44, and (**C**) SOX2 were determined by qRT-PCR in isolated tumors. (**D**) The protein levels of CD133, CD44, SOX2, and β-catenin were detected by western blotting in isolated tumors. (**E**) The relative levels of CD133, CD44, SOX2, and β-catenin were calculated by ImageJ. Data are expressed as mean ± SD; $n = 3$ per group. * $p < 0.05$ compared with the control group; # $p < 0.05$ compared with the 5-FU group.

2.3. *diHEP-DPA Inhibited 5-FU-Induced Infiltration of M2-likeTAMs*

The crucial proteolytic enzymes, growth factors, and inflammatory cytokines secreted by TAMs, including MMP2, MMP9, VEGF, IL-6, and TNF-α, were significantly downregulated by diHEPA-DPA but upregulated by the 5-FU treatment. The combination treatment, again, significantly lowered the expression of these factors compared to the 5-FU treatment (Figure 4A–E). Furthermore, the treatment with diHEP-DPA significantly downregulated the expression of CD206, a specific marker of M2-likeTAMs, indicating that it could suppress the infiltration of M2-like TAMs into tumor tissue. In contrast, the 5-FU treatment significantly increased CD206 levels, which were decreased by the combination treatment (Figure 4F,G,H). The NF-κB signaling pathway, which includes NF-kB1 (p50), NF-kB2 (p52), RelA (p65), RelB, and c-Rel, plays a crucial role in immune responses, cellular growth, apoptosis, and inflammation [20]. The phosphorylation of NF-kB (pp65) was significantly reduced in diHEP-DPA, but elevated in 5-FU-treated tumors, and subsequently reduced after the additional diHEP-DPA treatment (Figure 4G,I). All these findings suggested that diHEP-DPA inhibited the 5-FU-induced infiltration of M2-like TAMs and the NF-κB signaling pathway.

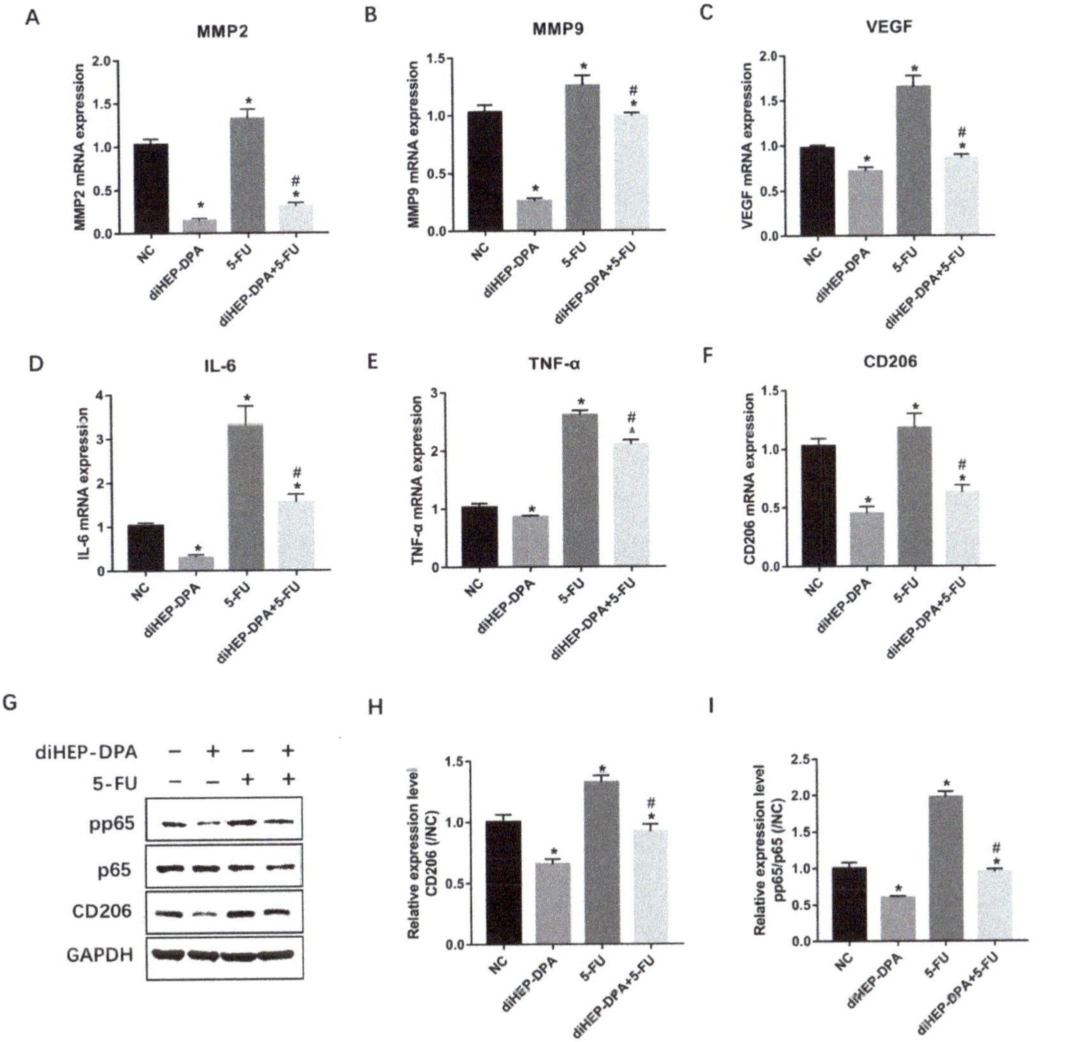

Figure 4. Effects of diHEP-DPA and 5-FU on the infiltration of M2-like TAMs and the NF-κB signaling pathway. Relative mRNA levels of TAMs secretions including (**A**) MMP2, (**B**) MMP9, (**C**) VEGF, (**D**) IL-6, and (**E**) TNF-α in isolated tumors. Relative mRNA levels of (**F**) CD206 were determined via qRT-PCR. (**G**) The protein levels of CD206, p65, and pp65 were detected by western blotting in isolated tumors. The relative levels of (**H**) CD206 and (**I**) pp65/p65 were calculated using ImageJ. Data are expressed as mean ± SD; n = 3 per group. * $p < 0.05$ compared with the control group; # $p < 0.05$ compared with the 5-FU group.

2.4. diHEP-DPA Impeded EMT via the STAT3 Signaling Pathway

EMT is closely related to increased chemoresistance and tumor metastasis [21]. As shown in Figure 5A–D, diHEP-DPA upregulated the expression of the epithelial marker E-cadherin, and downregulated mesenchymal markers N-cadherin and vimentin, while 5-FU treatment enhanced the expression of N-cadherin and vimentin and declined the expressions of E-cadherin. Furthermore, we observed a significantly decreased expression of N-cadherin and vimentin and an increased expression of E-cadherin in the combination treatment group compared with the 5-FU group.

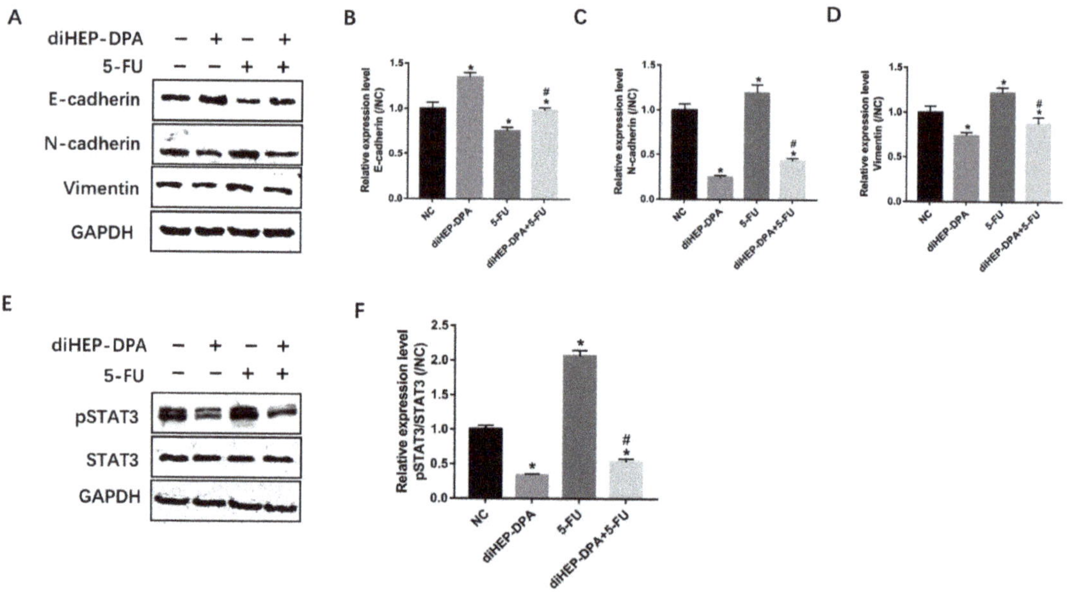

Figure 5. Effects of diHEP-DPA and 5-FU on EMT via the STAT3 signaling pathway. (**A**) The level of E-cadherin, N-cadherin, and vimentin were detected by western blotting. The relative expression of (**B**) E-cadherin (**C**) N-cadherin, and (**D**) vimentin were calculated by ImageJ. (**E**) The level of STAT3 and pSTAT3 were detected by western blotting in isolated tumors and (**F**) were calculated by ImageJ. Data are expressed as mean ± SD; $n = 3$ per group. * $p < 0.05$ compared with the control group; # $p < 0.05$ compared with the 5-FU group.

The STAT3 signaling pathway has been shown to stimulate EMT progression [22,23]. To assess the mechanism by which this stimulation occurs, we examined the expression of pSTAT3 via western blotting. We observed that diHEP-DPA alone could significantly downregulate the expression of pSTAT3, while the 5-FU treatment significantly enhanced it. The combination treatment decreased pSTAT3 levels compared with the 5-FU treatment (Figure 5E,F), showing that diHEP-DPA suppressed 5-FU-induced EMT progression by inhibiting the STAT3 signaling pathway.

2.5. diHEP-DPA and 5-FU Enhanced Macrophage Phagocytic Activity via CD47/SIRPα

The disruption of the CD47/SIRPα axis reduces the ability of the tumor to escape phagocytosis [24]. Hence, we evaluated the effects of diHEP-DPA and 5-FU on SIRPα and CD47 expression in tumor tissues. diHEP-DPA alone significantly reduced the gene levels of CD47 and SIRPα compared with the control; 5-FU downregulated the expression of CD47 but upregulated the expression of SIRPα; the combination of diHEP-DPA and 5-FU was proven to downregulate the expression of CD47 and SIRPα compared with the 5-FU group (Figure 6A,B). Accordingly, the western blotting results showed similar trends (Figure 6C). These findings demonstrated the powerful effect of diHEP-DPA combined with the 5-FU on phagocytic activity via the CD47/SIRPα axis.

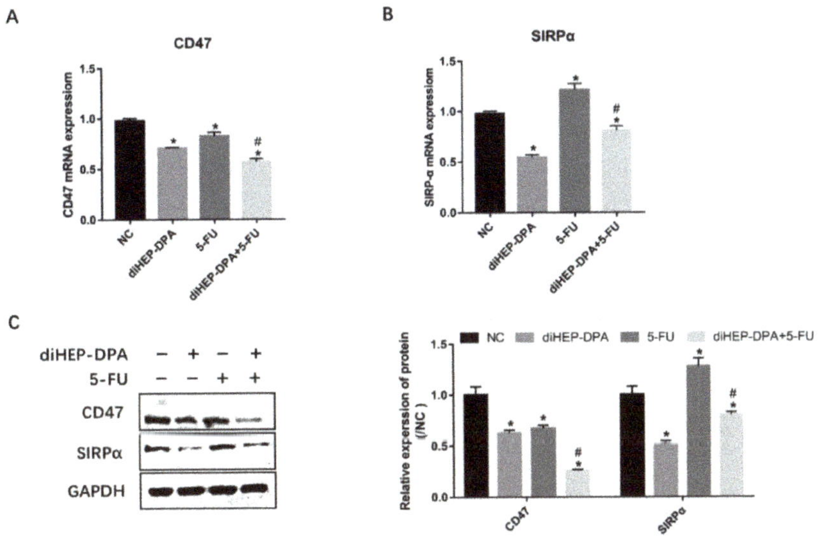

Figure 6. Effects of diHEP-DPA and 5-FU on phagocytic activity via the CD47/SIRPα axis. Relative mRNA levels of (**A**) CD47 and (**B**) SIRPα were determined by qRT-PCR in isolated tumors. (**C**) The protein levels of CD47 and SIRPα were detected by western blotting and calculated by ImageJ in isolated tumors. Data are expressed as mean ± SD; n = 3 per group. * $p < 0.05$ compared with the control group; # $p < 0.05$ compared with the 5-FU group.

3. Discussion

Since the 1950s, 5-FU has been an antitumor drug widely used to treat different types of cancer, including colorectal cancer and breast cancer [2]. However, because post-chemotherapy recurrence reduces clinical outcomes even for those who initially react to chemotherapy, there is an urgent need to develop new medications [19].

Cancer progression depends on many different molecular pathways, which hints at the complexity of the complex mechanisms of treatment resistance [25]. Additionally, most drug resistance studies have focused on the genetics and epigenetics of cancer cells, while ignoring the cellular components of the TME, among which macrophages are the most prominent innate immune cells [26]. Our present study uncovered important mechanisms of resistance to 5-FU therapy related to CSCs and TAMs. Firstly, we found that the resistance of 5-FU therapy involves the enrichment of CSCs related to the activation of WNT/β-catenin signaling in the CT-26-BALB/c model. Moreover, we identified that 5-FU induced the infiltration of M2-like macrophages and promoted the EMT progression, which contribute to the resistance of 5-FU in CRC. Importantly, diHEP-DPA could overcome the chemoresistance caused by 5-FU via depleting CSCs, inhibiting the infiltration of M2-like TAMs, and suppressing the EMT progression. Moreover, combinatorial treatment with diHEP-DPA and 5-FU enhanced macrophage phagocytosis and effectively repressed tumor regrowth.

Although the 5-FU treatment could effectively inhibit colorectal tumor growth, we observed an enrichment of CSCs in 5-FU-treated tumors supported by the upregulation of CSC markers (CD44, SOX2), which could be responsible for the observed chemoresistance. Interestingly, although the 5-FU treatment downregulated the expression of CD133, it is reported that CD133 expression is not restricted to cancer-initiating cells; further, during the metastatic transition, $CD133^{+}$ tumor cells may give rise to the more aggressive $CD133^{-}$ subset (such as CD44+/CD24−/CD133−), taking away the necessity for CD133 in tumor initiation [27]. The level of SOX2 expression in CRC is believed to confer to tumor metastasis and lymph node infiltration [28]. The WNT/β-catenin signaling pathway activates CSCs, contributing to tumor initiation and tumor recurrence [19,28]. Indeed, we found that the 5-FU treatment upregulated the expression of β-catenin, the center of the WNT/β-catenin signaling pathway, further activating CSCs. Similarly, another previous study demonstrated that 5-FU activated CSCs via the p53-mediated WNT/β-catenin pathway in CRC cell lines, xenograft tumors, and patient avatar models [19]. Interestingly, diHEP-DPA could reverse the upregulation of β-catenin expression caused by 5-FU and then reduce the enrichment of CSCs, minimizing recurrence as an expansion of CSCs. The tankyrase inhibitor XAV939 reversed 5-fluorouracil chemoresistance by targeting the WNT/β-catenin signaling pathway in colorectal cancer cells [29]. Our results have provided an experimental basis for the clinical application of diHEP-DPA in combination with 5-Fu-based chemotherapeutics for CRC patients, especially for those with a poor chemotherapy tolerance.

TAMs are another key factor for chemoresistance, which has been previously recognized by many researchers; TAMs release several enzymes, cytokines, chemokines, and growth factors which contribute to tumor growth and chemoresistance, making them potential targets to inhibit tumor recurrence [8,30,31]. Recently, it has been proposed that CSCs can directly or indirectly interact with several immune cell populations within the tumor microenvironment, which are thought to markedly influence tumor progression [32,33]. Therefore, strategies aimed at depleting TAMs carry the promise of increasing chemotherapy efficiency and decreasing anti-cancer drug resistance [3,9,34]. In this study, we found that diHEP-DPA significantly inhibited the infiltration of TAMs and decreased the secretion of MMP2, MMP9, VEGF, IL-6, and TNF-α in tumor tissue. Nevertheless, the 5-FU treatment increased the infiltration of TAMs and secreted higher levels of these factors, which contributed to the upregulation of CSCs. Similarly, the 5-FU treatment significantly increased the infiltration of TAMs, and produced ornithine decarboxylase-dependent putrescine to confer resistance to further chemotherapy with 5-FU in CRC [7]. The 5-FU treatment induced the activation of NF-κB and upregulated CSCs in HCT116 high-density tumor microenvironment co-cultures, which were abolished by curcumin [34]. NF-κB is overactivated in tumors and controls tumor survival, metastasis, and chemoresistance. It has been proven that blocking the NF-κB signaling pathway could restore the sensitivity towards 5-FU in CRC [35,36]. We observed that 5-FU promoted the phosphorylation of p65, which may be activated by proinflammatory cytokines secreted by TAMs, such as IL-6 and TNFα, which were then abolished by diHEP-DPA. Based on these results, we hypothesized that the aberrant activation of NF-κB induced by 5-FU was one of the major causes leading to CRC chemoresistance and that diHEPA-DPA possibly abolished the 5-FU-induced abnormal activation of NF-κB. Similarly, aspirin enhanced the sensitivity to 5-FU in CRC by suppressing the NF-κB pathway both in vivo and in vitro [37]. The combination of curcumin and 5-FU has synergistic anti-tumor or modulatory effects on HCT116 and their 5-FU-chemoresistant counterparts via blocking the activity of NF-κB [38]. These results indicate that the interaction between the tumor and TAMs is crucial in promoting CSCs and that there is a strong chemotherapy sensitivity of diHEP-DPA by blocking NF-κB and suppressing TAMs infiltration.

Cytokines secreted by TAMs also stimulate EMT progression, which contributes to tumor invasion, metastasis, and chemoresistance [3,21,39]. We evaluated the effect of diHEP-DPA, 5-FU, and the combined use of both on the EMT process. Interestingly, we found that diHEP-DPA suppressed EMT by upregulating the epithelial cell marker E-cadherin and downregulating the mesenchymal cell markers (vimentin and N-cadherin), which is consistent with the findings of our previous in vitro study [20]. Moreover, it is reported that M2-like macrophages regulated 5-FU resistance in CRC cells through the epithelial–mesenchymal transition (EMT) program [40]. In current study, we observed that 5-FU increased the infiltration of M2-like TAMs in tumor tissue; thus, we assumed that 5-FU treatment might promote the EMT process. We revealed that 5-FU strongly decreased the expression of E-cadherin and increased the expression of vimentin and N-cadherin in the colorectal tumor tissue, indicating a promotion of the EMT status. Importantly, diHEP-DPA could significantly inhibit 5-FU-induced EMT progression. Curcumin enhanced the inhibitory effects of 5-FU against the cell growth on 5-FU resistant HCT-116 cells by regulating the TET1-NKD-Wnt signal pathway to inhibit the EMT progress [41]. Enalapril has been shown to enhance the antitumor efficacy of 5-FU and counter chemoresistance in CRC by suppressing cell proliferation, EMT, and chemoresistance via the NF-κB/STAT3 pathway in cells and nude mice [22]. As expected, we observed the overexpression of pp65 and pSTAT3 in 5-FU-treated tumors. Combined treatment with diHEP-DPA effectively inhibited the activation of NF-κB and STAT3, subsequently enhancing the effects of chemotherapy and preventing chemoresistance in CRC. These results strongly support that diHEP-DPA blocks the STAT3 signaling pathway, thus inhibiting the EMT progression indued by 5-FU.

The CD47/SIRPα interaction is another therapeutic target for human solid tumors: CD47 is a unique cell-surface marker expressed by human cancers; SIRPα is a protein expressed on macrophages and dendritic cells [15,16,24]. In this study, we demonstrated that diHEP-DPA inhibited the expression of CD47 and SIRPα. The expression of CD47 was only decreased by 5-FU; however, it increased the expression of SIRPα. The upregulation of SIRPα might be correlated with the infiltration of TAMs; in turn, high levels of SIRPα promote TAMs polarization [42]. However, the combined treatment of diHEP-DPA and 5-FU resulted in a synergistic suppression of the CD47/SIRPα axis. Our data clearly suggests the synergistic increase of phagocytosis between diHEP-DPA and 5-FU by blocking the CD47/ SIRPα axis.

4. Materials and Methods

4.1. Materials

The mouse colon cancer cell line CT26 was purchased from the Korean Cell Line Bank (Seoul, Korea). The bicinchoninic acid assay kit was purchased from Sango Company (San Diego, CA, USA). Antibodies were purchased from Abcam (Cambridge, MA, USA). The enhanced chemiluminescence (ECL) substrate kit was purchased from Bio-Rad Laboratories Inc. (Tewksbury, MA, USA).

4.2. Animals and Cell Culture

Five-week-old female mice obtained from Orient bio (Gyeonggi, Korea) were housed at a constant temperature (21–23 °C) and a relative humidity (60–70%) under a 12 h light/dark cycle. The study was reviewed by the Institutional Animal Care and the Use Committee of the Korea Research Institute of Bioscience and Biotechnology (Daejeon, Korea), and was approved by the Institutional Animal Ethics Committee (KRIBB-AEC-22140).

CT26 cells were maintained in Roswell Park Memorial Institute 1640 medium, supplemented with 10% fetal bovine serum (HyClone, Thermofisher Scientific, Waltham, MA, USA), 100 U/mL penicillin, and 100 μg/mL streptomycin (Gibco, Thermofisher Scientific), at 37 °C in 5% CO_2.

4.3. CRC Xenograft Model in BALB/c Mice

Female mice were injected subcutaneously in the right flank with CT26 cells (3×10^4 cells/mouse), suspended in 100 μL of phosphate-buffered saline. When the mean tumor size reached between 100–150 mm^3, the mice were randomly divided into four groups: (1) control, intraperitoneally administered with sterile saline; (2) diHEP-DPA, intraperitoneally administered 10 μg/kg of diHEP-DPA dissolved in saline daily; (3) 5-FU, intraperitoneally administered 20 mg/kg of 5-FU dissolved in saline, five times a week; (4) diHEP-DPA + 5-FU, intraperitoneally administered 10 μg/kg of diHEP-DPA daily and 20 mg/kg of 5-FU five times a week. The tumor size was calculated twice a week and the mice were sacrificed when the tumor volume without treatment grew to approximately 2000 mm^3.

4.4. Quantitative Reverse Transcription PCR (qRT-PCR)

Total RNA was isolated using a TaKaRa MiniBEST kit (TaKaRa, Tokyo, Japan), according to the manufacturer's protocol. The levels of transcripts were measured with a One-Step AccuPower GreenStar RT-qPCR PreMix kit (Bioneer Corporation, Daejeon, Korea) using SYBR Green, according to the manufacturer's instructions. RT-PCR was performed in a reaction volume of 50 μL. qRT-PCR was performed in the CFX Connect system (Bio-Rad, CA, USA). The glyceraldehyde-3-phosphate dehydrogenase (GAPDH) gene was used as a housekeeping control. The relative mRNA expression of target genes was calculated by the $2^{-\Delta\Delta CT}$ method. All specific primers are listed in Table 1.

Table 1. Primer sequences.

Gene (Mouse)	Sequence (5′ → 3′)
CD133	Forward: CTGCGATAGCATCAGACCAAGC Reverse: CTTTTGACGAGGCTCTCCAGATC
CD44	Forward: CGGAACCACAGCCTCCTTTCAA Reverse: TGCCATCCGTTCTGAAACCACG
SOX2	Forward: AACGGCAGCTACAGCATGATGC Reverse: CGAGCTGGTCATGGAGTTGTAC
CD206	Forward: GTTCACCTGGAGTGATGGTTCTC Reverse: AGGACATGCCAGGGTCACCTTT
VEGF	Forward: CTGCTGTAACGATGAAGCCCTG Reverse: GCTGTAGGAAGCTCATCTCTCC
MMP2	Forward: CAAGGATGGACTCCTGGCACAT Reverse: TACTCGCCATCAGCGTTCCCAT
MMP9	Forward: GCTGACTACGATAAGGACGGCA Reverse: TAGTGGTGCAGGCAGAGTAGGA
IL-6	Forward: TACCACTTCACAAGTCGGAGGC Reverse: CTGCAAGTGCATCATCGTTGTTC
TNF-α	Forward: GGTGCCTATGTCTCAGCCTCTT Reverse: GCCATAGAACTGATGAGAGGGAG
CD47	Forward: GGTGGGAAACTACACTTGCGAAG Reverse: CTCCTCGTAAGAACAGGCTGATC
SIRPα	Forward: TCATCTGCGAGGTAGCCCACAT Reverse: ACTGTTGGGTGACCTTCACGGT
GAPDH	Forward: CATCACTGCCACCCAGAAGACTG Reverse: ATGCCAGTGAGCTTCCCGTTCAG

CD, cluster of differentiation; SOX2, SRY-Box transcription factor 2; VEGF, vascular endothelial growth factor; MMP, matrix metalloproteinase; IL-6, interleukin-6; TNF-α, tumor necrosis factor-α; SIRPα, signal regulatory protein alpha; GAPDH, glyceraldehyde-3-phosphate hydrogenase.

4.5. PROTEIN Preparation and Western Blotting

The protein was obtained from tumor tissue homogenates using a RIPA lysis buffer (Biosolution, Seoul, Korea) supplemented with 1:100 each of protease inhibitor cocktail, phenylmethyl sulfonyl fluoride, and phosphatase inhibitor. The tissue homogenates were incubated on ice for 30 min and the concentration of the protein was estimated using a bicinchoninic acid assay kit (Abcam, Cambridge, MA, USA). The samples were heated with a loading buffer (Solarbio, Beijing, China) for 10 min at 100 °C. Equal amounts of proteins (~80 μg) were separated on 7.5% or 10% sodium dodecyl sulfate–polyacrylamide gels and transferred onto 0.45 μm polyvinylidene fluoride membranes (Millipore, Bedford, MA, USA) at 20 V for 120 min. The membranes were blocked for 45 min with Tris-buffered saline/Tween 20 (TBST) containing 5% skim milk and incubated overnight at 4 °C with primary antibodies against the following proteins: β-catenin (ab223075, 1:10,000), CD133 (ab284389, 1:5000), CD44 (ab189524, 1:1000), SOX2 (ab92494, 1:1000), CD206 (ab64693, 1:5000), p65 (ab16502, 1:10,000), pp65 (ab76302, 1:1000), STAT3 (ab68153, 1:1000), pSTAT3 (ab76315, 1:2000), E-cadherin (ab231303, 1:1000), N-cadherin (ab76011, 1:5000), vimentin (ab92547, 1:1000), CD47 (ab214453, 1:1000), SIRPα (ab191419, 1:1000), and GAPDH (ab181602, 1:20,000). The membranes were washed thrice with TBST before being incubated at room temperature for 2 h with the appropriate secondary antibodies (ab205718, 1:50,000). After being rinsed with TBST, the membranes were incubated with the Clarity Western ECL Substrate (Bio-Rad, Hercules, CA, USA). The CL-XPosure film was then exposed to the polyvinylidene fluoride membranes (Thermo Scientific, Rockford, IL, USA).

4.6. Statistical Analysis

The data were expressed as means $\pm$ standard deviation. Statistical analysis was performed by one-way ANOVA analysis of variance using GraphPad Prism 7.0 (GraphPad, San Diego, CA, USA). The results were considered statistically significant for p-values < 0.05.

5. Conclusions

This study aimed to evaluate the effects of diHEP-DPA on 5-FU-induced chemoresistance in CRC. Per our findings, diHEP-DPA could be an ideal CRC therapy to strongly restore chemosensitivity and significantly boost the antitumor effect of 5-FU. Our results have provided an experimental basis for the clinical application of diHEP-DPA in combination with 5-FU-based chemotherapeutics for patients with CRC, especially for those with poor chemotherapeutic tolerance. Considering the low toxicity and the better economic effectiveness of the combination therapy, this study is of high clinical value. Further clinical studies are necessary to confirm our findings in patients with CRC to precede a translation of our treatment strategy to clinical oncology.

Author Contributions: Conceptualization, J.-W.S. and Y.S.; methodology, Y.S. and J.-W.S.; validation, Y.S.; formal analysis, Y.S., Y.-S.J.; investigation, Y.S., J.-W.S., and H.S.C.; resources, Y.S. and J.-W.S.; data curation, Y.S.; writing—original draft preparation, Y.S.; writing—review and editing, J.-W.S., Y.-S.J., H.-S.K., J.H.C., and H.S.C.; visualization, Y.S. and J.-W.S.; supervision, J.-W.S. and Y.-S.J.; project administration, J.-W.S.; funding acquisition, J.-W.S. All authors have read and agreed to the published version of the manuscript.

Funding: This research was funded by the Microbial Biotechnology Research Center, Korea Research Institute of Bioscience and Biotechnology (KRIBB) from Ministry of Science and ICT (KGM5482221).

Institutional Review Board Statement: The animal study protocol was reviewed by the Institutional Animal Care and Use Committee of the Korea Research Institute of Bioscience and Biotechnology (Daejeon, Korea), and was approved by the Institutional Animal Ethics Committee (KRIBB-AEC-22140).

Data Availability Statement: The data presented in this study are available on request from the corresponding author.

Conflicts of Interest: The authors declare no conflict of interest.

References

1. Siegel, R.L.; Miller, K.D.; Jemal, A. Cancer Statistics, 2019. *CA Cancer J. Clin.* **2019**, *69*, 7–34. [CrossRef]
2. Blondy, S.; David, V.; Verdier, M.; Mathonnet, M.; Perraud, A.; Christou, N. 5-Fluorouracil Resistance Mechanisms in Colorectal Cancer: From Classical Pathways to Promising Processes. *Cancer Sci.* **2020**, *111*, 3142–3154. [CrossRef]
3. Dean, M.; Fojo, T.; Bates, S. Tumour Stem Cells and Drug Resistance. *Nat. Rev. Cancer* **2005**, *5*, 275–284. [CrossRef]
4. Erin, N.; Grahovac, J.; Brozovic, A.; Efferth, T. Tumor Microenvironment and Epithelial Mesenchymal Transition as Targets to Overcome Tumor Multidrug Resistance. *Drug Resist. Updates* **2020**, *53*, 100715. [CrossRef]
5. Sethy, C.; Kundu, C.N. 5-Fluorouracil (5-FU) Resistance and the New Strategy to Enhance the Sensitivity against Cancer: Implication of DNA Repair Inhibition. *Biomed. Pharmacother.* **2021**, *137*, 111285. [CrossRef]
6. Acharyya, S.; Oskarsson, T.; Vanharanta, S.; Malladi, S.; Kim, J.; Morris, P.G.; Manova-Todorova, K.; Leversha, M.; Hogg, N.; Seshan, V.E.; et al. A CXCL1 Paracrine Network Links Cancer Chemoresistance and Metastasis. *Cell* **2012**, *150*, 165–178. [CrossRef]
7. Zhang, X.; Chen, Y.; Hao, L.; Hou, A.; Chen, X.; Li, Y.; Wang, R.; Luo, P.; Ruan, Z.; Ou, J.; et al. Macrophages Induce Resistance to 5-Fluorouracil Chemotherapy in Colorectal Cancer through the Release of Putrescine. *Cancer Lett.* **2016**, *381*, 305–313. [CrossRef]
8. Azwar, S.; Seow, H.F.; Abdullah, M.; Jabar, M.F.; Mohtarrudin, N. Recent Updates on Mechanisms of Resistance to 5-Fluorouracil and Reversal Strategies in Colon Cancer Treatment. *Biology* **2021**, *10*, 854. [CrossRef]
9. Shih, J.-Y.; Yuan, A.; Chen, J.J.-W.; Yang, P.-C. Tumor-Associated Macrophage: Its Role in Cancer Invasion and Metastasis. *J. Cancer Mol.* **2006**, *2*, 101–106.

10. Ding, L.; Liang, G.; Yao, Z.; Zhang, J.; Liu, R.; Chen, H.; Zhou, Y.; Wu, H.; Yang, B.; He, Q. Metformin Prevents Cancer Metastasis by Inhibiting M2-like Polarization of Tumor Associated Macrophages. *Oncotarget* **2015**, *6*, 36441–36455. [CrossRef]
11. Wei, H.; Liang, F.; Cheng, W.; Zhou, R.; Wu, X.; Feng, Y.; Wang, Y. The Mechanisms for Lung Cancer Risk of PM2.5: Induction of Epithelial-Mesenchymal Transition and Cancer Stem Cell Properties in Human Non-Small Cell Lung Cancer Cells. *Environ. Toxicol.* **2017**, *32*, 2341–2351. [CrossRef]
12. Wang, W.; Zhao, Y.; Yao, S.; Cui, X.; Pan, W.; Huang, W.; Gao, J.; Dong, T.; Zhang, S. Nigericin Inhibits Epithelial Ovarian Cancer Metastasis by Suppressing the Cell Cycle and Epithelial−mesenchymal Transition. *Biochem. Mosc.* **2017**, *82*, 933–941. [CrossRef]
13. Kong, L.; Zhou, Y.; Bu, H.; Lv, T.; Shi, Y.; Yang, J. Deletion of Interleukin-6 in Monocytes/Macrophages Suppresses the Initiation of Hepatocellular Carcinoma in Mice. *J. Exp. Clin. Cancer Res.* **2016**, *35*, 131. [CrossRef]
14. Storr, S.J.; Safuan, S.; Ahmad, N.; El-Refaee, M.; Jackson, A.M.; Martin, S.G. Macrophage-Derived Interleukin-1beta Promotes Human Breast Cancer Cell Migration and Lymphatic Adhesion in Vitro. *Cancer Immunol. Immunother.* **2017**, *66*, 1287–1294. [CrossRef]
15. Willingham, S.B.; Volkmer, J.-P.; Gentles, A.J.; Sahoo, D.; Dalerba, P.; Mitra, S.S.; Wang, J.; Contreras-Trujillo, H.; Martin, R.; Cohen, J.D.; et al. The CD47-Signal Regulatory Protein Alpha (SIRPa) Interaction Is a Therapeutic Target for Human Solid Tumors. *Proc. Natl. Acad. Sci. USA* **2012**, *109*, 6662–6667. [CrossRef]
16. Arrieta, O.; Aviles-Salas, A.; Orozco-Morales, M.; Hernández-Pedro, N.; Cardona, A.F.; Cabrera-Miranda, L.; Barrios-Bernal, P.; Soca-Chafre, G.; Cruz-Rico, G.; de Lourdes Peña-Torres, M.; et al. Association between CD47 Expression, Clinical Characteristics and Prognosis in Patients with Advanced Non-small Cell Lung Cancer. *Cancer Med.* **2020**, *9*, 2390–2402. [CrossRef]
17. Cherciu, I.; Bărbălan, A.; Pirici, D.; Mărgăritescu, C.; Săftoiu, A. Stem Cells, Colorectal Cancer and Cancer Stem Cell Markers Correlations. *Curr. Health Sci. J.* **2014**, *40*, 153–161. [CrossRef]
18. Eppert, K.; Takenaka, K.; Lechman, E.R.; Waldron, L.; Nilsson, B.; van Galen, P.; Metzeler, K.H.; Poeppl, A.; Ling, V.; Beyene, J.; et al. Stem Cell Gene Expression Programs Influence Clinical Outcome in Human Leukemia. *Nat. Med.* **2011**, *17*, 1086–1093. [CrossRef]
19. Cho, Y.-H.; Ro, E.J.; Yoon, J.-S.; Mizutani, T.; Kang, D.-W.; Park, J.-C.; Il Kim, T.; Clevers, H.; Choi, K.-Y. 5-FU Promotes Stemness of Colorectal Cancer via P53-Mediated WNT/β-Catenin Pathway Activation. *Nat. Commun.* **2020**, *11*, 5321. [CrossRef]
20. Wang, L.F.; Choi, H.S.; Su, Y.; Lee, B.; Song, J.J.; Jang, Y.-S.; Seo, J.-W. 7S,15R-Dihydroxy-16S,17S-Epoxy-Docosapentaenoic Acid, a Novel DHA Epoxy Derivative, Inhibits Colorectal Cancer Stemness through Repolarization of Tumor-Associated Macrophage Functions and the ROS/STAT3 Signaling Pathway. *Antioxidants* **2021**, *10*, 1459. [CrossRef]
21. Wang, K.; Song, K.; Ma, Z.; Yao, Y.; Liu, C.; Yang, J.; Xiao, H.; Zhang, J.; Zhang, Y.; Zhao, W. Identification of EMT-Related High-Risk Stage II Colorectal Cancer and Characterisation of Metastasis-Related Genes. *Br. J. Cancer* **2020**, *123*, 410–417. [CrossRef]
22. Yang, Y.; Ma, L.; Xu, Y.; Liu, Y.; Li, W.; Cai, J.; Zhang, Y. Enalapril Overcomes Chemoresistance and Potentiates Antitumor Efficacy of 5-FU in Colorectal Cancer by Suppressing Proliferation, Angiogenesis, and NF-KB/STAT3-Regulated Proteins. *Cell Death Dis.* **2020**, *11*, 477. [CrossRef]
23. Liu, H.; Ren, G.; Wang, T.; Chen, Y.; Gong, C.; Bai, Y.; Wang, B.; Qi, H.; Shen, J.; Zhu, L.; et al. Aberrantly Expressed Fra-1 by IL-6/STAT3 Transactivation Promotes Colorectal Cancer Aggressiveness through Epithelial–Mesenchymal Transition. *Carcinogenesis* **2015**, *36*, 459–468. [CrossRef]
24. Oldenborg, P.-A.; Zheleznyak, A.; Fang, Y.-F.; Lagenaur, C.F.; Gresham, H.D.; Lindberg, F.P. Role of CD47 as a Marker of Self on Red Blood Cells. *Science* **2000**, *288*, 2051–2054. [CrossRef]
25. der Jeught, K.V.; Xu, H.-C.; Li, Y.-J.; Lu, X.-B.; Ji, G. Drug Resistance and New Therapies in Colorectal Cancer. *World J. Gastroenterol.* **2018**, *24*, 3834–3848. [CrossRef]
26. Belgiovine, C.; D'Incalci, M.; Allavena, P.; Frapolli, R. Tumor-Associated Macrophages and Anti-Tumor Therapies: Complex Links. *Cell. Mol. Life Sci.* **2016**, *73*, 2411–2424. [CrossRef]
27. Shmelkov, S.V.; Butler, J.M.; Hooper, A.T.; Hormigo, A.; Kushner, J.; Milde, T.; St. Clair, R.; Baljevic, M.; White, I.; Jin, D.K.; et al. CD133 Expression Is Not Restricted to Stem Cells, and Both CD133+ and CD133– Metastatic Colon Cancer Cells Initiate Tumors. *J. Clin. Invest.* **2008**, *118*, 2111–2120. [CrossRef]
28. Fan, Z.; Duan, J.; Wang, L.; Xiao, S.; Li, L.; Yan, X.; Yao, W.; Wu, L.; Zhang, S.; Zhang, Y.; et al. PTK2 Promotes Cancer Stem Cell Traits in Hepatocellular Carcinoma by Activating Wnt/β-Catenin Signaling. *Cancer Lett.* **2019**, *450*, 132–143. [CrossRef]
29. Luo, F.; Li, J.B.; Liu, J.H.; Liu, K.P. Stabilizing and Upregulating Axin with Tankyrase Inhibitor Reverses 5-Fluorouracil Chemoresistance and Proliferation by Targeting the WNT/Caveolin-1 Axis in Colorectal Cancer Cells. *Cancer Gene Ther.* **2022**, *29*, 1707–1719. [CrossRef]
30. Johnson, D.E.; O'Keefe, R.A.; Grandis, J.R. Targeting the IL-6/JAK/STAT3 Signalling Axis in Cancer. *Nat. Rev. Clin. Oncol.* **2018**, *15*, 234–248. [CrossRef]
31. Zhang, T.; Liu, L.; Lai, W.; Zeng, Y.; Xu, H.; Lan, Q.; Su, P.; Chu, Z. Interaction with Tumor-associated Macrophages Promotes PRL-3-induced Invasion of Colorectal Cancer Cells via MAPK Pathway-induced EMT and NF-κB Signaling-induced Angiogenesis. *Oncol. Rep.* **2019**, *41*, 2790–2802. [CrossRef]
32. Schiavoni, G.; Gabriele, L.; Mattei, F. The Tumor Microenvironment: A Pitch for Multiple Players. *Front. Oncol.* **2013**, *3*, 90. [CrossRef]

33. Buhrmann, C.; Kraehe, P.; Lueders, C.; Shayan, P.; Goel, A.; Shakibaei, M. Curcumin Suppresses Crosstalk between Colon Cancer Stem Cells and Stromal Fibroblasts in the Tumor Microenvironment: Potential Role of EMT. *PLoS ONE* **2014**, *9*, e107514. [CrossRef]
34. Wang, D.; Feng, F.; Ma, Y. Tumor-Associated Macrophages as Treatment Target in Colorectal Cancer. *Front. Med. Sci. Res.* **2022**, *4*, 12–18. [CrossRef]
35. Pikarsky, E.; Porat, R.M.; Stein, I.; Abramovitch, R.; Amit, S.; Kasem, S.; Gutkovich-Pyest, E.; Urieli-Shoval, S.; Galun, E.; Ben-Neriah, Y. NF-KB Functions as a Tumour Promoter in Inflammation-Associated Cancer. *Nature* **2004**, *431*, 461–466. [CrossRef]
36. Wang, B.-D.; Kline, C.L.B.; Pastor, D.M.; Olson, T.L.; Frank, B.; Luu, T.; Sharma, A.K.; Robertson, G.; Weirauch, M.T.; Patierno, S.R.; et al. Prostate Apoptosis Response Protein 4 Sensitizes Human Colon Cancer Cells to Chemotherapeutic 5-FU through Mediation of an NFκB and MicroRNA Network. *Mol. Cancer* **2010**, *9*, 98. [CrossRef]
37. Fu, J.; Xu, Y.; Yang, Y.; Liu, Y.; Ma, L.L.; Zhang, Y.Y. Aspirin Suppresses Chemoresistance and Enhances Antitumor Activity of 5-Fu in 5-Fu-Resistant Colorectal Cancer by Abolishing 5-Fu-Induced NF-κB Activation. *Sci. Rep.* **2019**, *9*, 16937. [CrossRef]
38. Shakibaei, M.; Kraehe, P.; Popper, B.; Shayan, P.; Goel, A. Curcumin Potentiates Antitumor Activity of 5-Fluorouracil in a 3D Alginate Tumor Microenvironment of Colorectal Cancer. *BMC Cancer* **2015**, *15*, 250. [CrossRef]
39. Ji, M.; Li, W.; He, G.; Zhu, D.; Lv, S.; Tang, W.; Jian, M.; Zheng, P.; Yang, L.; Qi, Z.; et al. Zinc-A2-Glycoprotein 1 Promotes EMT in Colorectal Cancer by Filamin A Mediated Focal Adhesion Pathway. *J. Cancer* **2019**, *10*, 5557–5566. [CrossRef]
40. Wei, C.; Yang, C.; Wang, S.; Shi, D.; Zhang, C.; Lin, X.; Xiong, B. M2 Macrophages Confer Resistance to 5-Fluorouracil in Colorectal Cancer through the Activation of CCL22/PI3K/AKT Signaling. *OncoTargets Ther.* **2019**, *12*, 3051–3063. [CrossRef]
41. Lu, Y.; Zhang, R.Z.; Zhang, X.J.; Zhang, B.; Yao, Q.H. Curcumin May Reverse 5-Fluorouracil Resistance on Colonic Cancer Cells by Regulating TET1-NKD-Wnt Signal Pathway to Inhibit the EMT Progress. *Biomed. Pharmacother.* **2020**, *129*, 110381. [CrossRef]
42. Koga, N.; Hu, Q.; Sakai, A.; Takada, K.; Nakanishi, R.; Hisamatsu, Y.; Ando, K.; Kimura, Y.; Oki, E.; Oda, Y.; et al. Clinical Significance of Signal Regulatory Protein Alpha (SIRPα) Expression in Esophageal Squamous Cell Carcinoma. *Cancer Sci.* **2021**, *112*, 3018–3028. [CrossRef]

Disclaimer/Publisher's Note: The statements, opinions and data contained in all publications are solely those of the individual author(s) and contributor(s) and not of MDPI and/or the editor(s). MDPI and/or the editor(s) disclaim responsibility for any injury to people or property resulting from any ideas, methods, instructions or products referred to in the content.

marine drugs

Article

Marine Bromophenol Bis(2,3,6-Tribromo-4,5-Dihydroxybenzyl) ether Inhibits Angiogenesis in Human Umbilical Vein Endothelial Cells and Reduces Vasculogenic Mimicry in Human Lung Cancer A549 Cells

Songtao Dong [1,2], Zhongyuan Chen [1], Li Wang [1], Yankai Liu [1], Dimitrios Stagos [3], Xiukun Lin [4] and Ming Liu [1,2,*]

1 Key Laboratory of Marine Drugs, Ministry of Education of China, School of Medicine and Pharmacy, Ocean University of China, 5 Yushan Road, Qingdao 266003, China; 21190831116@stu.ouc.edu.cn (S.D.); 21190831021@stu.ouc.edu.cn (Z.C.); 21190811062@stu.ouc.edu.cn (L.W.); liuyankai@ouc.edu.cn (Y.L.)
2 Laboratory for Marine Drugs and Bioproducts of Qingdao National Laboratory for Marine Science and Technology, Qingdao 266237, China
3 Department of Biochemistry and Biotechnology, School of Health Sciences, University of Thessaly, Biopolis, 41500 Larissa, Greece; stagkos@med.uth.gr
4 Department of Pharmacology, School of Pharmacy, Southwest Medical University, 319 Zhongshan Road, Jiangyang, Luzhou 646000, China; xiukunlin@swmu.edu.cn
* Correspondence: lmouc@ouc.edu.cn; Tel.: +86-532-8203-1980

Abstract: Angiogenesis, including the growth of new capillary blood vessels from existing ones and the malignant tumors cells formed vasculogenic mimicry, is quite important for the tumor metastasis. Anti-angiogenesis is one of the significant therapies in tumor treatment, while the clinical angiogenesis inhibitors usually exhibit endothelial cells dysfunction and drug resistance. Bis(2,3,6-tribromo-4,5-dihydroxybenzyl)ether (BTDE), a marine algae-derived bromophenol compound, has shown various biological activities, however, its anti-angiogenesis function remains unknown. The present study illustrated that BTDE had anti-angiogenesis effect in vitro through inhibiting human umbilical vein endothelial cells migration, invasion, tube formation, and the activity of matrix metalloproteinases 9 (MMP9), and in vivo BTDE also blocked intersegmental vessel formation in zebrafish embryos. Moreover, BTDE inhibited the migration, invasion, and vasculogenic mimicry formation of lung cancer cell A549. All these results indicated that BTDE could be used as a potential candidate in anti-angiogenesis for the treatment of cancer.

Keywords: anti-angiogenesis; bromophenols; tube formation; vasculogenic mimicry

Citation: Dong, S.; Chen, Z.; Wang, L.; Liu, Y.; Stagos, D.; Lin, X.; Liu, M. Marine Bromophenol Bis(2,3,6-Tribromo-4,5-Dihydroxybenzyl)ether Inhibits Angiogenesis in Human Umbilical Vein Endothelial Cells and Reduces Vasculogenic Mimicry in Human Lung Cancer A549 Cells. *Mar. Drugs* **2021**, *19*, 641. https://doi.org/10.3390/md19110641

Academic Editors: Celso Alves and Marc Diederich

Received: 28 September 2021
Accepted: 12 November 2021
Published: 16 November 2021

Publisher's Note: MDPI stays neutral with regard to jurisdictional claims in published maps and institutional affiliations.

Copyright: © 2021 by the authors. Licensee MDPI, Basel, Switzerland. This article is an open access article distributed under the terms and conditions of the Creative Commons Attribution (CC BY) license (https://creativecommons.org/licenses/by/4.0/).

1. Introduction

Angiogenesis, the growth of new capillary blood vessels from existing ones and capillary venules, involves vascular endothelial cell proliferation, migration, matrix degradation, and branching to form new tubes [1]. It has been recognized as a proven sign in tumor growth and metastasis on account of the functional blood supply [2]. Therefore, targeting angiogenesis is a valid strategy for tumor treatment [3]. In recent years, anti-angiogenic agents have been used clinically [4,5]. For example, bevacizumab, the recombinant humanized monoclonal antibody, playing obvious anti-angiogenesis effect, has been used clinically to treat various malignant tumors through binding with VEGF [6]. Another anti-tumor drug ENDOSTAR, inhibits cancer angiogenesis through targeting vascular EGFR, has been used in clinical tumor treatment [7]. However, these anti-angiogenesis agents usually bring about endothelial cells dysfunction and exhibit drug resistance [8]. Safer and more valid approaches and agents in anti-tumor angiogenesis are required.

Besides the classical angiogenesis, Maniotis et al. firstly propose the concept of vasculogenic mimicry, which is a spontaneous and endothelial cell-independent tube-forming procedure [9]. Vasculogenic mimicry is regarded as an important blood supply system in tumor development for providing nutrients and oxygen [10]. Vasculogenic mimicry is an alternative angiogenesis happened to metastatic and aggressive tumors such as pancreatic cancer [11], melanoma [12], breast cancer [13], and non-small cell lung cancer (NSCLC) [14]. When vasculogenic mimicry occurs, tumor cells have significant extent of plasticity [15] and epithelial-mesenchymal transition (EMT) process [16]. Moreover, various extracellular matrix remodeling factors such as hypoxia inducible factor 1 alpha (HIF-1α) and vascular endothelial cadherin (VE-cadherin) are involved in these processes. The powerful metastasis ability of lung cancer accounts for high incidence and mortality, and vasculogenic mimicry not only leads to lung cancer metastasis but also increases the difficulty of anti-angiogenesis treatment [17]. Therefore, inhibitors targeting both endothelial angiogenesis and vasculogenic mimicry will be a new strategy in the treatment of NSCLC.

Marine compounds are reported to have anticancer therapeutic and prophylactic activities [18–21], among them, marine bromophenols mainly distributing in the algae have attracted much attention in function[nal food and pharmaceutical drugs area. Previous studies have shown that bromophenols have a variety of biological activities, such as anti-tumor, anti-oxidation, anti-diabetic, and anti-viral activities [22,23]. Interestingly, the ability of bromophenols in anti-angiogenesis has also been widely reported. For example, BD-DPM, a bromophenol from marine red alga *Rhodomela confervoides*, shows anti-angiogenesis properties by targeting multiple receptor tyrosine kinases [24]. Another bromophenol compound BDDE, obtained from *L. nana and Rhodomela confervoides*, exhibits anti-angiogenesis effect both in vivo and in vitro through acting on VEGF signaling pathway [25]. Bis(2,3,6-tribromo-4,5-dihydroxybenzyl)ether (BTDE, Figure 1a), a typical bromophenol compound first derived from marine red alga *Symphyocladia latiuscula* [26], has a variety of biological activities, such as antioxidant [27,28], antidiabetic [29], anti-neurodegenerative diseases [30], and multiple enzyme inhibitory activity [31,32]. However, its effects in tumor angiogenesis have yet to be illustrated. In the present study, in order to investigate the anti-angiogenesis activity of BTDE both in vitro and in vivo, we evaluated the effects of BTDE on the migration, invasion, tube formation, and matrix metalloproteinases 9 (MMP9) activity on HUVECs model, and also on the growth of intersegmental blood vessel (ISV) in vivo using zebrafish embryos model. Furthermore, the effect of BTDE on the vasculogenic mimicry formation ability of A549 cells was also estimated.

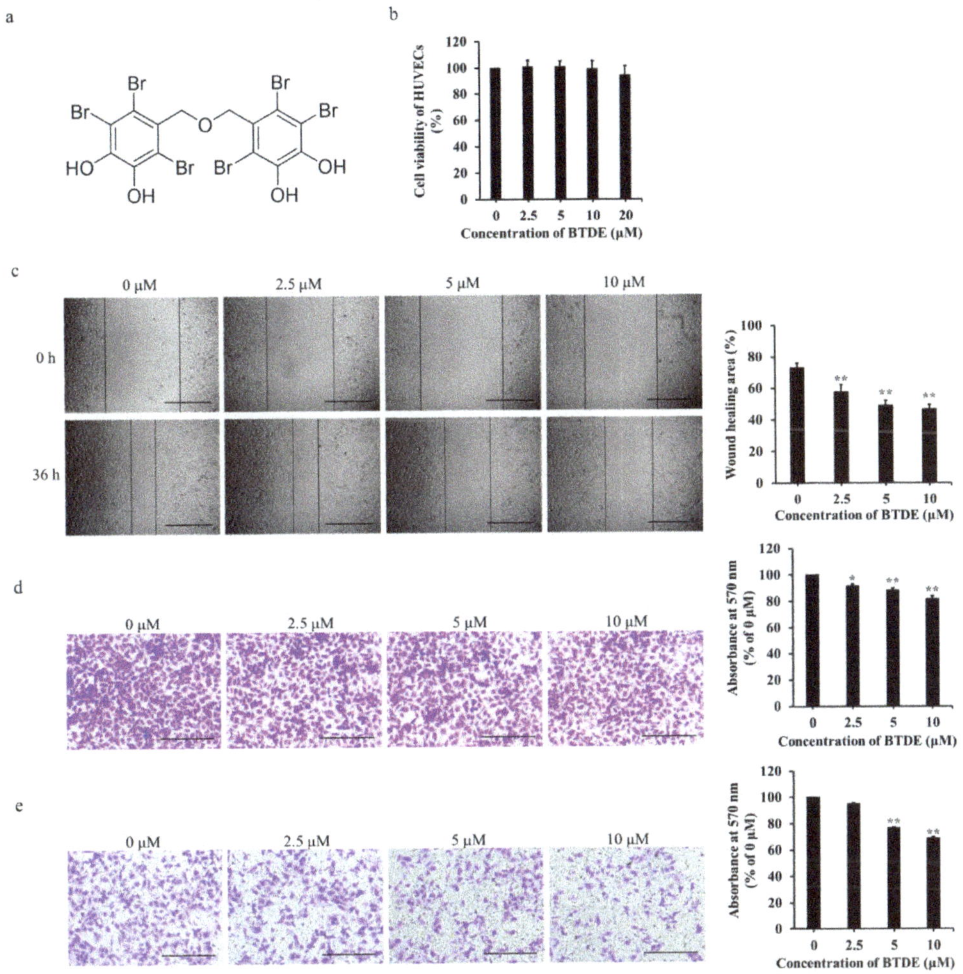

Figure 1. Bis(2,3,6-tribromo-4,5-dihydroxybenzyl)ether (BTDE) inhibits the migration and invasion of HUVECs. (**a**) Chemical structure of BTDE. (**b**) HUVECs was incubated in absence or presence of certain concentrations of BTDE at 37 °C for 36 h, cell viability was determined by MTT assay. (**c**) Wound healing of HUVECs after 36 h treatment with BTDE was reported by inverted microscope (original magnification, 4×; scale bar: 600 μm) and the wound-healing area was measured by Image J software. Migration (**d**) and invasion (**e**) abilities of HUVECs were examined by transwell assay. Photos of HUVECs traveled through membrane after incubation with BTDE for 24 h were recorded by inverted microscope (original magnification, 10×; scale bar: 300 μm) and OD values at 570 nm were measured. Data are represented as mean ± SD of three independent experiments. * $p < 0.05$, ** $p < 0.01$ versus control.

2. Results

2.1. BTDE Inhibits the Migration and Invasion of HUVECs

HUVECs is widely used in vitro to detect the ability of angiogenesis. MTT assay was applied first to measure the effect of BTDE on HUVECs proliferation. As shown in Figure 1b, BTDE had no cytotoxicity effect on HUVECs at 2.5–20 μM concentrations, indicating BTDE could not affect the proliferation of HUVECs under these experimental conditions. Endothelial cells migration is one of the crucial steps in blood vessels formation. To investigate the influence of BTDE on HUVECs migration, scratch-wound cell migration assay and transwell migration assay were used. As shown in Figure 1c, the migration area of HUVECs was inhibited after 36 h treatment by 2.5−10 μM BTDE with the wound healing percentage of 57.6, 49.1, and 46.8%. Moreover, in the transwell migration assay, the number of HUVECs traveling through the membrane was significantly reduced with the increased concentrations of BTDE (Figure 1d). Similarly, endothelial cells invasion is a pivotal step promoting HUVECs migration and neovascularization through degrading extracellular matrix [33]. Transwell invasion assay was used to investigate the invasion ability of HUVECs, and as shown in Figure 1e, the number of HUVECs degrading matrigel and traveling through the membrane was decreased with the treatment of BTDE. The above results proved that BTDE could inhibit the migration and invasion of HUVECs.

2.2. BTDE Reduces HUVECs Tube Formation and MMP9 Activity

Tube formation assay is a valid method to examine the effect of angiogenesis using matrigel to simulate endothelial cell growth and tube formation in vitro [34]. To further evaluate the effect of BTDE on vessel formation, tube formation assay was used with or without BTDE treatment on matrigel. As shown in Figure 2a, the endothelial tubes were significantly decreased and the total length of tubes dropped to 58.1, 36.3, and 4.9% when treated with 2.5−10 μM BTDE. These results illustrated that BTDE could restrain the tube formation of HUVECs. To further investigate whether BTDE has an impact on preformed vascular tubes, different concentrations of BTDE were added after tubes had already formed for 8 h, and incubated for another 6 h. The result showed that BTDE had no effect on the preformed tubes (Figure 2b). The above results exhibited that BTDE inhibited the tube formation but not the preformed vascular tubes of HUVECs.

MMPs are the important enzymes secreted by cells to degrade the extracellular matrix, and they play a significant role in endothelial cells migration, invasion, and angiogenesis [35,36]. Our results have confirmed that BTDE inhibited HUVECs migration, invasion, and tube formation, to further explore whether BTDE affects the activity of MMPs in HUVECs, gelatin zymography assay was used. HUVECs culture medium treated with different concentrations of BTDE were separated by SDS-PAGE containing gelatin, and incubated for 48 h. As shown in Figure 2c, BTDE inhibited the activity of MMP9 in HUVECs compared with control group which had obvious negative staining bands.

VEGF is a crucial pro-angiogenic factor which plays an important role in promoting tumor angiogenesis, moreover, AKT and ERK as its downstream signaling molecules participate in the regulation of angiogenesis [37–39]. HIF-1α as a significant transcriptional factor acts on Wnt/β-catenin pathway and regulates expression of genes that promote angiogenesis such as VEGF [40]. Therefore, we examined whether BTDE influences these molecules. As shown in Figure 2d, BTDE did not affect expression level of VEGF, HIF-1α, β-catenin, AKT, ERK, as well as the phosphorylation levels of AKT and ERK in HUVECs. The above experiments indicated that BTDE inhibits HUVECs tube formation and MMP9 activity, while did not affect the VEGF, HIF-1α, β-catenin expression.

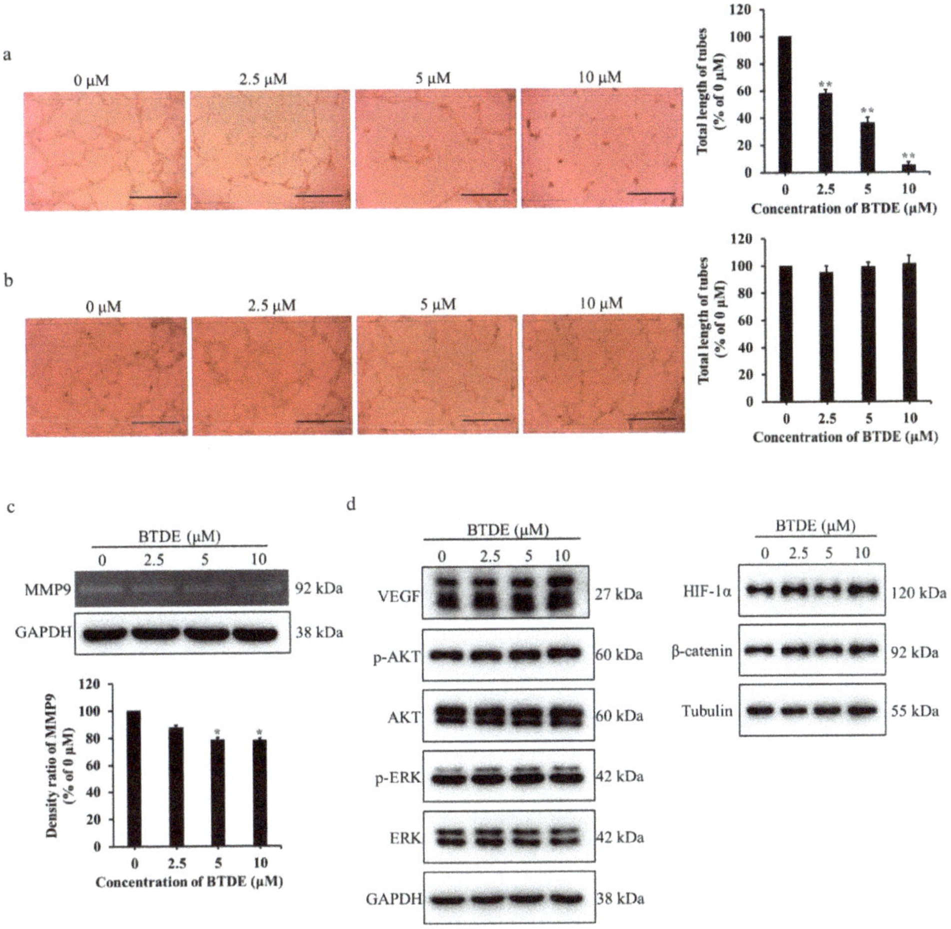

Figure 2. BTDE reduces HUVECs tube formation and MMP9 activity. (**a**) HUVECs was pretreated with BTDE for 24 h, then seeded on matrigel for 20 h, capillary-like structures of HUVECs were recorded by inverted microscope (original magnification, 4×; scale bar: 600 μm) and total length of tubes was measured by Image J software. (**b**) Different concentrations of BTDE were added after tubes have established on matrigel for 8 h, and incubated for another 6 h. Tubular structures were observed by inverted microscope (original magnification, 4×; scale bar: 600 μm) and total length of tubes compared with 0 μM was measured by Image J software. (**c**) Gelatin zymography experiment was used to detect the MMP9 activity of HUVECs after 24 h treatment of BTDE, GAPDH was used as an internal control. (**d**) Western blot was used to measure the VEGF, HIF-1α, β-catenin, AKT, and ERK as well as their phosphorylation levels in HUVECs treated with BTDE for 24 h. Data represent mean ± SD of three independent experiments. * $p < 0.05$, ** $p < 0.01$ versus control.

2.3. BTDE Blocks Intersegmental Vessel Formation in Zebrafish Embryos

Zebrafish is an ideal model for evaluating the effects of compounds on angiogenesis. It can sprout from dorsal arteries to form interstitial neovascularization during embryonic development [41,42]. To further confirm the anti-angiogenesis effect of BTDE in vivo, the formation of ISV in zebrafish embryos was detected. As shown in Figure 3a and b, ISV formation in zebrafish embryos was significantly suppressed by 2.5–10 μM BTDE with the vessel growth of 90.1, 40.3, and 31.2%, respectively, illustrating that BTDE exerted well anti-angiogenesis effect in vivo. Besides, zebrafish toxicity assay showed that 2.5–20 μM

BTDE had no specific deformity and mortality effects on zebrafish embryos (Table 1), which indicated that BTDE was nontoxic at these concentrations.

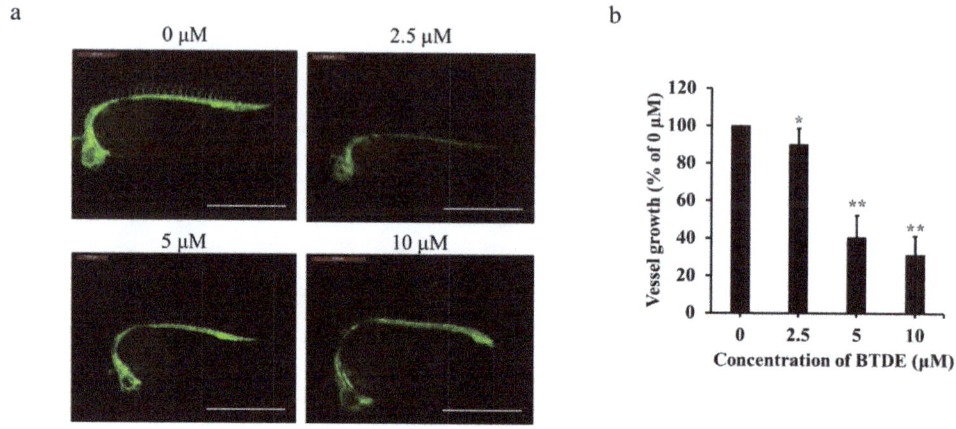

Figure 3. BTDE blocks intersegmental vessel formation in zebrafish embryos. (**a**) Lateral view of Tg (flk1: EGFP) zebrafish embryos at 16 hpf. Embryos were treated with different concentrations of BTDE. Vessels of zebrafish embryos were observed using a fluorescence microscope, photos were recorded by inverted fluorescence microscope (scale bar: 1.2 mm). (**b**) Quantification of intersegmental vessel growth induced by BTDE. Values represent the means ± SD of three independent experiments. * $p < 0.05$, ** $p < 0.01$ versus medium control.

Table 1. The effect of BTDE on zebrafish embryo deformity and mortality.

BTDE (μM)	Number of Embryos	Number of Deformities	Deformity Rate (%)	Number of Mortalities	Mortality Rate (%)
0	71	2	2.8	0	0
2.5	70	1	1.4	0	0
5	71	1	1.4	1	1.4
10	70	0	0	2	2.8
20	73	1	1.4	0	0

2.4. BTDE Decreases the Migration and Invasion of A549

In addition to study whether BTDE inhibited the endothelial angiogenesis, we next investigated the impact of BTDE on NSCLC vasculogenic mimicry. First, MTT assay related that 2.5–10 μM BTDE had no cytotoxicity effect on A549 and H1975 cells (Figure 4a,b). Considering migration of cancer cells are important for the formation of vasculogenic mimicry, we then detected the effects of BTDE on migration abilities of A549 and H1975 by using scratch-wound cell migration assay. Results showed that BTDE inhibited A549 migration with wound-healing area of 34.2, 26.5, and 17.5% under 36 h treatment of 2.5–10 μM BTDE (Figure 4c), and also restrained H1975 migration with wound-healing area of 12.6, 9.7, 5.9% with 72 h treatment of 2.5–10 μM BTDE (Figure 4d). Moreover, the number of A549 and H1975 migrated to the lower membrane was decreased with the increasing concentration of BTDE (Figure 4e,f). Transwell invasion assay illustrated that BTDE suppressed A549 to split matrigel and migrate to the lower surface of membrane (Figure 4g). The above results exhibited that BTDE inhibited A549, H1975 migration and invasion of A549.

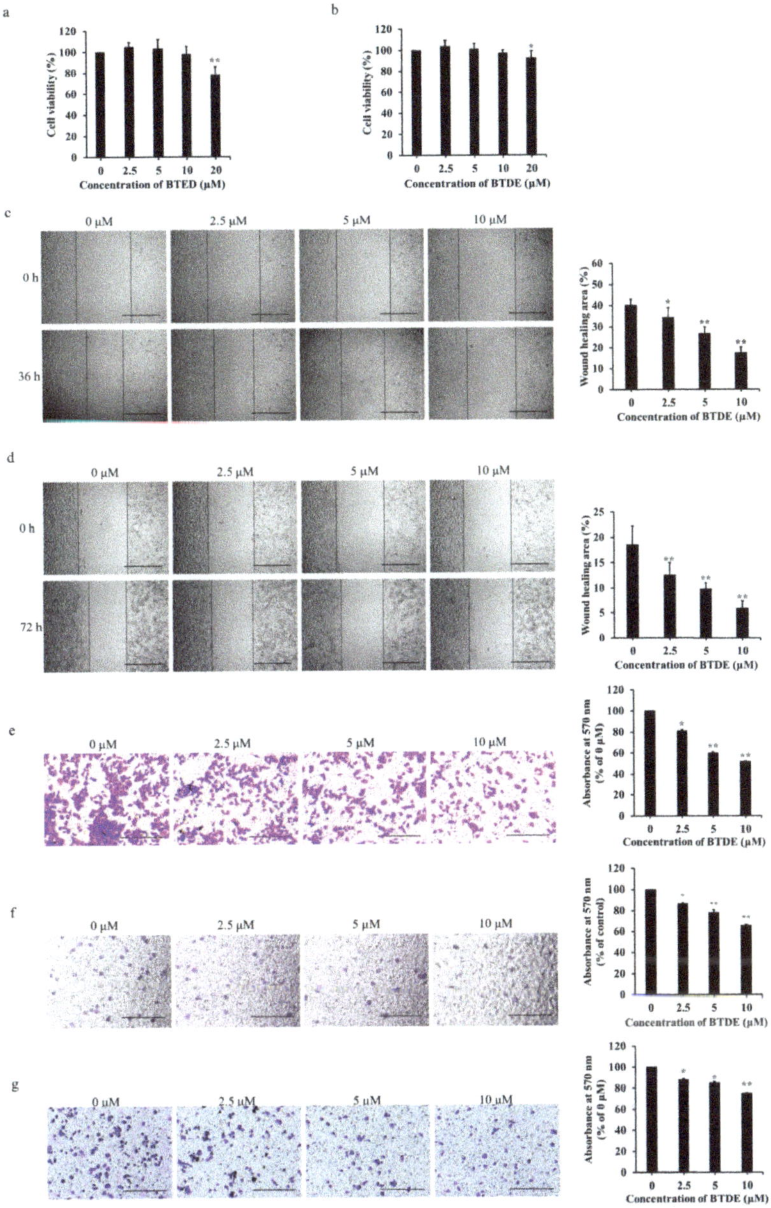

Figure 4. BTDE decreases the migration of A549, H1975 and the invasion of A549. The effect of BTDE on A549 (**a**) or H1975 (**b**) proliferation. A549 or H1975 was incubated with different concentrations of BTDE at 37 °C for 48 h, cell viability was determined by MTT assay. Wound healing of A549 after 36 h (**c**) or H1975 after 72 h (**d**) treatment with 0–10 μM BTDE was recorded with inverted microscope (original magnification, 4×; scale bar: 600 μm) and the wound healing area was measured by Image J software. Migration ability of A549 (**e**) or H1975 (**f**), invasion ability of A549 (**g**) treated with 0–10 μM BTDE for 24 h, photos were obtained by inverted microscope (original magnification, 10×; scale bar: 300 μm) and OD values of 570 nm were measured. Data are represented as mean ± SD of three independent experiments. * $p < 0.05$, ** $p < 0.01$ versus control.

2.5. BTDE Decreases the Vasculogenic Mimicry of A549 Cells

Vasculogenic mimicry is the endothelial cell independent vascularization pretend the plasticity of tumor cells. In the above study, we have already proved that BTDE inhibited the migration of NSCLC cells, considering the stronger migration ability of A549 cells, we next explored if BTDE affects A549 vasculogenic mimicry formation ability using vasculogenic mimicry assay. A549 was pretreated with different concentrations of BTDE for 24 h and then seeded on matrigel for 30 h. As shown in Figure 5a, the control group formed reticular vessel-like structures while 5 and 10 μM BTDE treated group formed a loose network structure with total length of tubes dropped to 73.3 and 63.1%. To further evaluate whether BTDE had an impact on the preformed vascular tubes, different concentrations of BTDE were added after tubes had already formed for 6 h, and incubated for another 20 h. The result showed that BTDE had no effect on the preformed tubes compared with control group (Figure 5b). These results illustrated that BTDE could inhibit the vasculogenic mimicry formation ability of A549 while did not affect the preformed vessels. To further explore the specific mechanism of BTDE inhibiting vasculogenic mimicry formation of A549, Western blot assay was used to detect the influence of BTDE on HIF-1α, β-catenin, VEGF, and its downstream AKT, ERK signaling pathways. We found that BTDE did not affect the expression of these molecules in A549 (Figure 5c). This was different from the previous study that bromophenol BOS-102 exhibited valid cytotoxic effects on A549 through ROS-mediated inhibition of PI3K/Akt and activation of p38/ERK signaling pathways [43], which may be caused by the difference of molecular structure and suggesting a novel mechanism. These results indicated that BTDE inhibited the vascular mimicry formation of A549 but had no effect on the preformed blood vessels of A549.

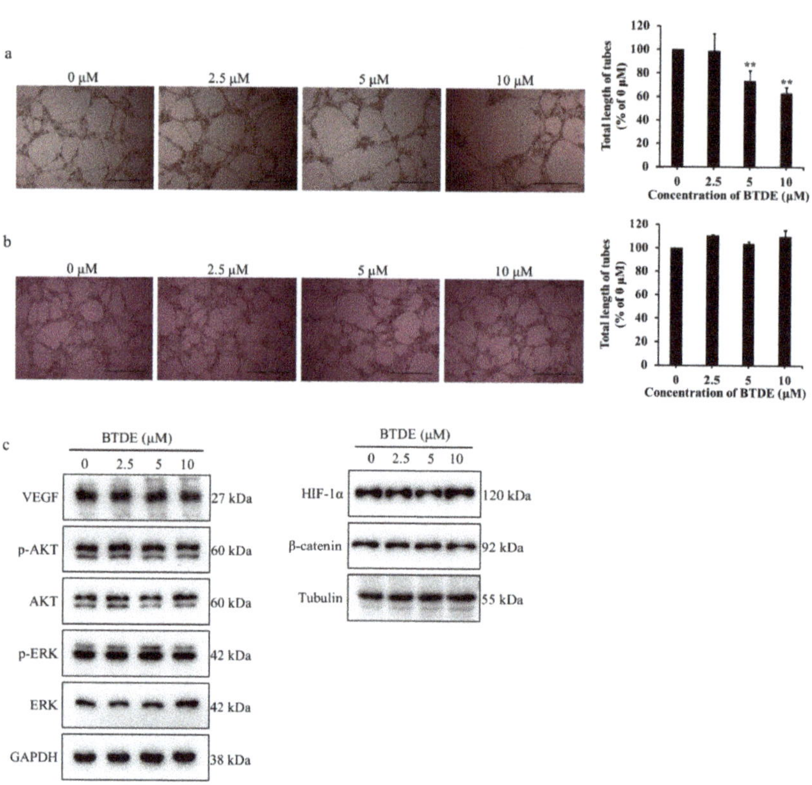

Figure 5. BTDE decreases the vasculogenic mimicry of A549 cells. (**a**) A549 was pretreated with BTDE

BTDE for 24 h, then seeded on matrigel for 30 h, capillary-like structures of A549 were recorded by inverted microscope (original magnification, 4×; scale bar: 600 μm) and total length of tubes was measured by Image J software. ** $p < 0.01$ versus control. (**b**) Different concentrations of BTDE were added after tubes were established on matrigel for 6 h, and incubated for another 20 h. Tubular structures were observed by inverted microscope (original magnification, 4×; scale bar: 600 μm) and total length of tubes compared with 0 μM was measured by Image J software. (**c**) Western blot was used to measure the VEGF, HIF-1α, β-catenin, AKT, and ERK as well as their phosphorylation levels in A549 treated with BTDE for 24 h. Data are represented as mean ± SD of three independent experiments. ** $p < 0.01$ versus control.

3. Discussion

Endothelial cells-mediated angiogenesis has been considered as a crucial process in angiogenesis because of the powerful abilities to migrate, invade, and degrade extracellular matrix to form new blood vessels [1]. Blood vessels play an important role in material exchange and pathological angiogenesis becomes a significant factor of cancer, therefore anti-angiogenesis is a common adjuvant strategy in tumor treatment [2]. Seeking novel drug candidates from natural products especially from marine resources has been implemented for many years, a number of marine bromophenols with significant anti-angiogenesis activity were found such as BDDPM [24] and BDDE [25]. Marine bromophenol BTDE illustrated various bioactivities including antioxidant [27] and antidiabetic [29], however, its anti-angiogenesis effect has not been explored. In the present study, we demonstrated first that BTDE potentially inhibited angiogenesis both in vitro and in vivo, and could be used as a promising candidate in cancer therapy. BTDE suppressed multiple angiogenesis process in endothelial cells, including the migration, invasion, and tube formation, which were consistent with some anti-angiogenesis drugs used clinically such as Bevacizumab [44]. BTDE showed no cytotoxicity on HUVECs proliferation in a short period, suggesting that the ability of BTDE to reduce HUVECs movement and angiogenesis did not include the influence on its proliferation. The in vivo zebrafish embryos assay also proved the anti-angiogenic effect of BTDE. MMPs are important enzymes secreted by endothelial cells, which promotes the cells migration and sprout to form new blood vessels by degrading extracellular matrix [36]. We found that BTDE indeed inhibited the activity of MMP9 in HUVECs thereby exerting a migration, invasion, and tube formation inhibitory effect. The stimulation of HIF-1α regulates the expression of angiogenic genes such as VEGF. As the crucial molecule in Wnt/β-catenin pathway, β-catenin, has a pivotal effect on cell migration and angiogenesis when receiving upstream gene regulation including HIF-1α [40,45]. However, our results suggested that BTDE had no effect on the expression of these molecules on HUVECs, which was different from BDDE, a bromophenol through inhibiting VEGF signaling plays an anti-angiogenesis effect [25]. Nevertheless, both of them were found to reduce HUVECs migration and tube formation, indicating that BTDE exerts the anti-angiogenesis effect through other signaling and the mechanisms still needs to be further explored.

In addition to the endothelial cell-dependent angiogenesis, another important factor for tumor blood supply is the diverse tumor vessels composition [46]. Vasculogenic mimicry is the microcirculation channel consisting of the aggressive tumor cells connection and extracellular matrix [9]. Many studies have confirmed the existence of vasculogenic mimicry in solid tumors such as melanoma, ovarian cancer, and lung cancer, and the poor prognosis of advanced cancer patients is significantly related with tumor vascular mimicry [47]. All these indicate that targeting vasculogenic mimicry therapy is a crucial strategy in tumor treatment. In our study, it is noteworthy that BTDE had a significant migration inhibitory effect on A549, H1975 cells. Moreover, BTDE also restrained the vasculogenic mimicry formation ability of A549 while had no impact on HIF-1α, β-catenin, VEGF, and the downstream signaling molecules. BTDE may target on other possible mechanisms such as EMT process [16], VE-cadherin [48], and wnt5a which are involved in the activation of Wnt signaling, and participated in cells proliferation, migration, adhesion, and vascularization [49,50]. The clear mechanism by which BTDE works remains to be further explored.

The anti-angiogenic activity of cancer chemopreventive agents is usually through inhibiting or retarding the development of tumor blood vessels [51]. For example, clinical antioxidant compound Nacetyl-L-cysteine is able to restrain the migration ability of melanoma cells, and to suppress endothelial cell invasion through inhibiting MMPs activity [52,53]. Similarly, our previous study has also showed the antioxidant effect of BTDE on HaCaT cells [28]. In the present studies, we revealed that BTDE inhibited the migration, invasion, and vasculogenic mimicry of A549 cells, as well as reducing HUVECs tube formation, MMP9 activity, and zebrafish embryo angiogenesis. All these investigations showed BTDE had valid anti-angiogenesis function and could be developed as potential angioprevention agent.

4. Materials and Methods

4.1. Drugs and Reagents

BTDE (purity > 98%) was provided by School of Medicine and Pharmacy. Antibodies against HIF-1α were purchased from Affinity (Canal Fulton, OH, USA), against β-catenin were purchased from Santa Cruz Biotechnology (Dallas, TX, USA), against VEGF, GAPDH, Tubulin were purchased from HuaAn Biotechnology (Hangzhou, China). Antibodies against AKT, p-AKT, ERK, p-ERK were purchased from Cell Signaling Technology (Boston, MA, USA). Transwell inserts (8 μm) were purchased from Corning company (Corning Costar, Cambridge, MA, USA). Matrigel was the product of BD company (Becton Dickinson, Bedford, MA, USA).

4.2. Cell Lines and Cell Culture

Human umbilical vein endothelial cells line HUVECs was from American Type Culture Collection (Gaithersburg, Maryland), human lung cancer cell lines A549 and H1975 were from Shanghai Cell Bank (Shanghai, China), Chinese Academy of Science. HUVECs was cultured in Dulbecco's modified Eagle's medium (DMEM, GIBCO, Grand Island, NY, USA). Human lung cancer cell lines A549 and H1975 were kept in RPMI-1640 medium (Gibco-BRL). All mediums were supplemented with 10% fetal bovine serum (FBS) and 1% penicillin/streptomycin. Cells were cultivated in a humidified incubator containing 5% CO_2 at 37 °C.

4.3. Cell Viability Assay

The proliferation effects of BTDE on differentiated HUVECs, A549, and H1975 cells were determined by 3-(4,5-dimethylthiazol-2-yl)-2,5-diphenyl-2H-tetrazolium bromide (MTT) assay. In brief, cells were plated in 96-well plate overnight to adhere, then 0–20 μM BTDE were administrated and incubated for 36 or 48 h. Total of 5 mg/mL MTT solution (20 μL per well) was added and incubated for another 4 h at 37 °C, discarding the supernatant and using dimethyl sulfoxide (DMSO) to dissolve products for 10 min at 37 °C. Microplate reader (BioTek, Winooski, VT, USA) was used to measure the 96-well plate at 570 nm, and the cell viability (%) was calculated by OD values.

4.4. Scratch-Wound Cell Migration Assay

HUVECs, A549, and H1975 were plated in 96-well plate and cultivated to reach 90% confluence. Then scratch-wounds were made by 10 μL pipette tip. After washing twice with PBS, the cells were treated with fresh DMEM or RPMI-1640 (1% FBS) with 0–10 μM BTDE. After incubation for 36 or 72 h, images of wound in each well were recorded by inverted microscope (NIB-100, Novel Optics, Ningbo, China, original magnification, 4×). Image J was used to measure the area of each wound, and the migration rate was calculated as follows:

$$\text{Wound healing area (\%)} = (\text{Area}_{\,0\,\text{h}} - \text{Area}_{\,t\,\text{h}})/\text{Area}_{\,0\,\text{h}} \times 100\%$$

4.5. Transwell Migration and Invasion Assay

Transwell chamber with 8 μm pore size was used to evaluate the migration of cells. Briefly, differentiated HUVECs, A549, and H1975 cells suspended in 1% FBS medium with 0−10 μM BTDE were seeded into the upper chamber of transwell 24-well plates. Then the lower chamber was added with complete medium and different 0−10 μM BTDE. After treatment for 24 h, the chambers were fixed with methanol, stained with 0.1% crystal violet, and the upper surface of the membrane containing non-migrating cells was gently wiped off with cotton swab. Random visual fields were calculated using inverted microscope (NIB-100, CHN, original magnification, 10×), chambers were decolorized with 33% acetic acid, then each group of decolorizing solutions was transferred to a new 96-well plate. A microplate reader (BioTek, Winooski, VT, USA) was used to measure OD values of the plate at 570 nm.

To investigate the invasion ability of HUVECs and A549, transwell invasion assay was conducted similarly with transwell migration assay except that the upper side of the chambers was spread with diluted matrigel (200 μg/mL).

4.6. HUVECs Tube Formation and A549 Vasculogenic Mimicry Assay

The ability of HUVECs or A549 to form capillary-like structures when treated with 0−10 μM BTDE was measured on matrigel. Briefly, pre-cooled matrigel was layered in 96-well plate and allowed to solidify at 37 °C for 45 min. HUVECs or A549 that has been treated with BTDE for 24 h was seeded on matrigel, after 20 h incubation for HUVECs or 30 h for A549, tube structure was recorded by inverted microscope (NIB-100, Novel Optics, Ningbo, China, original magnification, 4×) from randomly chosen fields. For investigating the effect of BTDE on performed vascular tubes, same concentrations of BTDE were added with HUVECs or A549 after tubes had already formed for 8 or 6 h, and incubated for another 6 h for HUVECs and 20 h for A549. Total length of tubes was measured by Image J software (version 1.48, National Institutes of Health, Rockville Pike, Maryland).

4.7. Zebrafish Embryo Assay

For intersegmental vessel formation assay, Tg (flk1: EGFP) zebrafish embryos were generated by natural pairwise mating. Healthy, hatched zebrafish were picked out at 16 h post-fertilization and distributed into a 24-well plate (10 embryos per well). Embryos were treated with 0−10 μM BTDE for 24 h at 28.5 °C and then observed for intersegmental blood vessel (ISV) under inverted fluorescence microscope (DM6000, Leica, Wetzlar, Germany). Vessel growth was measured by Image J software.

For toxicity assay, zebrafish embryos were picked out at 4 h post-fertilization and distributed into a 24-well plate (about 17 embryos per well). Embryos were treated with 0−20 μM BTDE for 24 h at 28.5 °C and then observed for morphologic changes under stereo microscope (SMZ645, Nikon, Tokyo, Japan). The deformity and mortality rates were recorded.

4.8. Gelatin Zymography Assay

Gelatin zymography assay was used to determine the activity of MMP9. HUVECs was treated with different concentrations of BTDE in serum free DMEM for 24 h, then culture supernatants were collected and centrifuged at 1200 rpm for 5 min, and then 12,000 rpm for 5 min to remove cellular components. Proteins existed in supernatants and were separated by 8% SDS-PAGE containing 1 mg/mL gelatin under non-reducing condition and then subjected to electrophoresis. Gels were washed twice for 40 min each time in washing buffer (2.5% Triton X-100/50 mM Tris/5 mM $CaCl_2$/1 μM $ZnCl_2$, pH 7.6), and washed twice for 40 min each time in rinse buffer (50 mM Tris/5 mM $CaCl_2$/1 μM $ZnCl_2$, pH 7.6), then incubated 48 h at 37 °C in renaturation solution containing 50 mM Tris/0.15 M NaCl/5 mM $CaCl_2$/1 μM $ZnCl_2$ and 0.02% Brij-35, pH 7.6). Gels were finally stained with 0.05% Coomassie Blue R250 for 30 min and decolorized with decolorizing liquid (10%

acetic acid and 30% methanol) until negative staining bands appear. Gels were recorded by Bio-Red Gel Imaging Analysis System (bio-rad GelDoc XR, Hercules, CA, USA).

4.9. Western Blotting

HUVECs and A549 were treated with different concentrations of BTDE (0−10 μM) for 24 h. Cells were centrifuged, then washed twice with PBS and lysed with loading buffer for 45 min in 4 °C. Then, the cell lysate was boiled for 10 min and stored at −80 °C. Protein samples were resolved by 8–10% SDS-PAGE, transferred to nitrocellulose filter membranes (Millipore, Billerica, MA, USA). The nitrocellulose filter membranes were blocked with 5% skimmed milk and then incubated with the primary antibodies overnight at 4 °C. Subsequently, the membranes were incubated with HRP-secondary antibody at 25 °C for 1 h. Finally, the image was detected by Tanon 5200 (Tanon, Beijing, China).

4.10. Statistical Analysis

Statistical analysis was performed using one-way ANOVA with Tukey's post-hoc test, and values were expressed as mean ± SD. Differences of $p < 0.05$ were considered statistically significant.

5. Conclusions

The present study illustrated for the first time that BTDE inhibited HUVECs migration, invasion, tube formation, and the activity of MMP9 in vitro. In zebrafish embryo, BTDE also restrained the growth of zebrafish embryo intersegmental blood vessel. In addition, BTDE suppressed A549, H1975 migration and A549 invasion, as well as the vasculogenic mimicry of A549 cells. These results definitely revealed that marine bromophenol compound BTDE was a potential agent for future cancer therapy due to its valid anti-angiogenesis effect.

Author Contributions: Conceptualization, S.D. and M.L.; methodology, S.D. and Z.C.; software, S.D.; validation, M.L.; formal analysis, S.D.; investigation, S.D., Z.C. and L.W.; resources, Y.L. and L.W.; data curation, S.D.; writing—original draft preparation, S.D.; writing—review and editing, M.L. and D.S.; visualization, S.D.; supervision, M.L.; project administration, M.L.; funding acquisition, M.L. and X.L. All authors have read and agreed to the published version of the manuscript.

Funding: This research was funded by National Key Research and Development Program of China (2017YFE0195000), Key Research and Development Program of Shandong Province (2017YFE0195000), and Qingdao Science and Technology Development Plan (21-1-6-gjxm-46-gx).

Institutional Review Board Statement: Not applicable.

Informed Consent Statement: Not applicable.

Conflicts of Interest: The authors declare no conflict of interest.

References

1. Ellis, L.M.; Liu, W.; Ahmad, S.A.; Fan, F.; Jung, Y.D.; Shaheen, R.M.; Reinmuth, N. Overview of angiogenesis: Biologic implications for antiangiogenic therapy. *Semin. Oncol.* **2001**, *28*, 94–104. [CrossRef]
2. Carmeliet, P.; Jain, R.K. Angiogenesis in cancer and other diseases. *Nature* **2000**, *407*, 249–257. [CrossRef]
3. Chan, L.; Daruwalla, J.; Christophi, C. Selective targeting of the tumour vasculature. *ANZ J. Surg.* **2008**, *78*, 955–967. [CrossRef] [PubMed]
4. Deplanque, G.; Harris, A.L. Anti-angiogenic agents: Clinical trial design and therapies in development. *Eur. J. Cancer* **2000**, *36*, 1713–1724. [CrossRef]
5. Taraboletti, G.; Margosio, B. Antiangiogenic and antivascular therapy for cancer. *Curr. Opin. Pharmacol.* **2001**, *1*, 378–384. [CrossRef]
6. Simons, M.; Gordon, E.; Claesson-Welsh, L. Mechanisms and regulation of endothelial VEGF receptor signalling. *Nat. Rev. Mol. Cell Biol.* **2016**, *17*, 611–626. [CrossRef] [PubMed]
7. Xiao, L.; Yang, S.C.; Hao, J.; Yuan, X.; Luo, W.; Jiang, L.; Hu, Y.; Fu, Z.; Zhang, Y.; Zou, C. Endostar attenuates melanoma tumor growth via its interruption of b-FGF mediated angiogenesis. *Cancer Lett.* **2015**, *359*, 148–154. [CrossRef]
8. Loges, S.; Schmidt, T.; Carmeliet, P. Mechanisms of resistance to anti-angiogenic therapy and development of third-generation anti-angiogenic drug candidates. *Genes Cancer* **2010**, *1*, 12–25. [CrossRef]

9. Maniotis, A.J.; Folberg, R.; Hess, A.; Seftor, E.A.; Gardner, L.M.; Peter, J.; Trent, J.M.; Meltzer, P.S.; Hendrix, M.J. Vascular channel formation by human melanoma cells in vivo and in vitro: Vasculogenic mimicry. *Am. J. Pathol.* **1999**, *155*, 739–752. [CrossRef]
10. Hendrix, M.; Seftor, E.A.; Hess, A.R.; Seftor, R. Molecular plasticity of human melanoma cells. *Oncogene* **2003**, *22*, 3070–3075. [CrossRef]
11. Yang, J.; Zhu, D.M.; Zhou, X.G.; Yin, N.; Zhang, Y. HIF-2α promotes the formation of vasculogenic mimicry in pancreatic cancer by regulating the binding of Twist1 to the VE-cadherin promoter. *Oncotarget* **2017**, *8*, 47801–47815. [CrossRef]
12. Van Beurden, A.; Schmitz, R.F.; Van Dijk, C.M.; Baeten, C.I.M. Periodic acid Schiff loops and blood lakes associated with metastasis in cutaneous melanoma. *Melanoma Res.* **2012**, *22*, 424. [CrossRef]
13. Liu, T.J.; Sun, B.C.; Zhao, X.L.; Zhao, X.M.; Sun, T.; Gu, Q.; Yao, Z.; Dong, X.Y.; Zhao, N.; Liu, N. CD133+ cells with cancer stem cell characteristics associates with vasculogenic mimicry in triple-negative breast cancer. *Oncogene* **2013**, *32*, 544–553. [CrossRef]
14. Wu, S.; Yu, L.; Wang, D.; Zhou, L.; Cheng, Z.; Chai, D.; Ma, L.; Tao, Y. Aberrant expression of CD133 in non-small cell lung cancer and its relationship to vasculogenic mimicry. *BMC Cancer* **2012**, *12*, 535. [CrossRef] [PubMed]
15. Zhang, X.; Zhang, J.; Zhou, H.; Fan, G.; Li, Q. Molecular mechanisms and anticancer therapeutic strategies in vasculogenic mimicry. *J. Cancer* **2019**, *10*, 6327–6340. [CrossRef] [PubMed]
16. You, X.; Liu, Q.; Wu, J.; Wang, Y.; Lian, Y. Galectin-1 promotes vasculogenic mimicry in gastric cancer by upregulating EMT signaling. *J. Cancer* **2019**, *10*, 6286–6297. [CrossRef] [PubMed]
17. Williamson, S.C.; Metcalf, R.L.; Trapani, F.; Mohan, S.; Antonello, J.; Abbott, B.; Leong, H.S.; Chester, C.; Simms, N.; Polanski, R. Vasculogenic mimicry in small cell lung cancer. *Nat. Commun.* **2016**, *7*, 13322. [CrossRef] [PubMed]
18. Mayer, A.; Guerrero, A.; Rodríguez, A.; Taglialatela-Scafati, O.; Nakamura, F.; Fusetani, N. Marine pharmacology in 2016–2017: Marine compounds with antibacterial, antidiabetic, antifungal, anti-inflammatory, antiprotozoal, antituberculosis and antiviral activities; affecting the immune and nervous systems, and other miscellaneous mechanisms of action. *Mar. Drugs* **2021**, *19*, 49.
19. Dyshlovoy, S. Recent updates on marine cancer-preventive compounds. *Mar. Drugs* **2021**, *19*, 558. [CrossRef]
20. Yue, Z.; Jie, Z.; Li, Y.; Xu, D.P.; Li, S.; Chen, Y.M.; Li, H.B. Natural polyphenols for prevention and treatment of cancer. *Nutrients* **2016**, *8*, 515.
21. Newman, D.; Cragg, G. Natural products as sources of new drugs over the nearly four decades from 01/1981 to 09/2019. *J. Nat. Prod.* **2020**, *83*, 770–803. [CrossRef]
22. Liu, M.; Hansen, P.E.; Lin, X. Bromophenols in marine algae and their bioactivities. *Mar. Drugs* **2011**, *9*, 1273–1292. [CrossRef] [PubMed]
23. Dong, H.; Dong, S.; Hansen, P.E.; Stagos, D.; Lin, X.; Liu, M. Progress of bromophenols in marine algae from 2011 to 2020: Structure, bioactivities, and applications. *Mar. Drugs* **2020**, *18*, 411. [CrossRef] [PubMed]
24. Wang, S.; Wang, L.J.; Bo, J.; Wu, N.; Shi, D. Anti-angiogenic properties of BDDPM, a bromophenol from marine red alga rhodomela confervoides, with multi receptor tyrosine kinase inhibition effects. *Int. J. Mol. Sci.* **2015**, *16*, 13548–13560. [CrossRef]
25. Qi, X.; Liu, G.; Qiu, L.; Lin, X.; Liu, M. Marine bromophenol bis(2,3-dibromo-4,5-dihydroxybenzyl) ether, represses angiogenesis in HUVEC cells and in zebrafish embryos via inhibiting the VEGF signal systems. *Biomed. Pharmacother.* **2015**, *75*, 58–66. [CrossRef]
26. Kurata, K.; Amiya, T. Bis(2,3,6-tribromo-4,5-dihydroxybenzyl) ether from the red alga, *Symphyocladia latiuscula*. *Phytochemistry* **1980**, *19*, 141–142. [CrossRef]
27. Duan, X.J.; Li, X.M.; Wang, B.G. Highly brominated mono- and bis-phenols from the marine red alga *Symphyocladia latiuscula* with radical-scavenging activity. *J. Nat. Prod.* **2007**, *70*, 1210–1213. [CrossRef]
28. Dong, H.; Liu, M.; Wang, L.; Liu, Y.; Lu, X.; Stagos, D.; Lin, X.; Liu, M. Bromophenol bis (2,3,6-tribromo-4,5-dihydroxybenzyl) ether protects HaCaT skin cells from oxidative damage via Nrf2-mediated pathways. *Antioxidants* **2021**, *10*, 1436. [CrossRef]
29. Paudel, P.; Seong, S.H.; Park, H.J.; Jung, H.A.; Choi, J.S. Anti-diabetic activity of 2,3,6-tribromo-4,5-dihydroxybenzyl derivatives from *Symphyocladia latiuscula* through PTP1B downregulation and α-glucosidase inhibition. *Mar. Drugs* **2019**, *17*, 166. [CrossRef]
30. Paudel, P.; Park, S.; Seong, S.; Jung, H.; Choi, J. *Symphyocladia latiuscula* bromophenols from target human monoamine oxidase and dopaminergic receptors for the management of neurodegenerative diseases. *J. Agric. Food Chem.* **2020**, *68*, 2426–2436. [CrossRef]
31. Paudel, P.; Wagle, A.; Seong, S.H.; Park, H.J.; Jung, H.A.; Choi, J.S. A new tyrosinase inhibitor from the red alga *Symphyocladia latiuscula* (harvey) yamada (rhodomelaceae). *Mar. Drugs* **2019**, *17*, 295. [CrossRef]
32. Mikami, D.; Kurihara, H.; Ono, M.; Kim, S.M.; Takahashi, K. Inhibition of algal bromophenols and their related phenols against glucose 6-phosphate dehydrogenase. *Fitoterapia* **2016**, *108*, 20–25. [CrossRef] [PubMed]
33. Sobierajska, K.; Ciszewski, W.M.; Sacewicz-Hofman, I.; Niewiarowska, J. Endothelial cells in the tumor microenvironment. *Adv. Exp. Med. Biol.* **2020**, *1234*, 71–86. [PubMed]
34. Kubota, Y. Role of laminin and basement membrane in the morphological differentiation of human endothelial cells into capillary-like structures. *J. Cell Biol.* **1988**, *107*, 1589–1598. [CrossRef] [PubMed]
35. Coussens, L.M.; Fingleton, B.; Matrisian, L.M. Matrix metalloproteinase inhibitors and cancer: Trials and tribulations. *Science* **2002**, *295*, 2387–2392. [CrossRef]
36. McCawley, L.J.; Matrisian, L.M. Matrix metalloproteinases: They're not just for matrix anymore! *Curr. Opin. Cell Biol.* **2001**, *13*, 534–540. [CrossRef]
37. Miriam; Martini; Maria; Chiara; De; Santis; Laura; Braccini; Federico; Gulluni. PI3K/AKT signaling pathway and cancer: An updated review. *Ann. Med.* **2014**, *46*, 372–383. [CrossRef]

38. Ruchika, S.; Tahera, Z.; Huang, H.; Zhang, J.; Parul, G.; Soledad, F.; Colleen, K.J.; Landreth, G.E.; Gustavo, L.; Ostrowski, M.C. Erk1 and Erk2 regulate endothelial cell proliferation and migration during mouse embryonic angiogenesis. *PLoS ONE* **2009**, *4*, e8283.
39. Carmeliet, P. VEGF as a key mediator of angiogenesis in cancer. *Oncology* **2005**, *69*, 4–10. [CrossRef]
40. Bai, X.; Zhi, X.; Zhang, Q.; Liang, F.; Chen, W.; Liang, C.; Hu, Q.; Sun, X.; Zhuang, Z.; Liang, T. Inhibition of protein phosphatase 2A sensitizes pancreatic cancer to chemotherapy by increasing drug perfusion via HIF-1α-VEGF mediated angiogenesis. *Cancer Lett.* **2014**, *355*, 281–287. [CrossRef]
41. Cross, L.M.; Cook, M.A.; Lin, S.; Chen, J.N.; Rubinstein, A.L. Rapid analysis of angiogenesis drugs in a live fluorescent zebrafish assay. *Arterioscler. Thromb. Vasc. Biol.* **2003**, *23*, 911–912. [CrossRef] [PubMed]
42. Childs, S.; Chen, J.N.; Garrity, D.M.; Fishman, M.C. Patterning of angiogenesis in the zebrafish embryo. *Development* **2002**, *129*, 973–982. [CrossRef]
43. Guo, C.L.; Wang, L.J.; Yue, Z.; Liu, H.; Li, X.Q.; Bo, J.; Jiao, L.; Guo, S.J.; Wu, N.; Shi, D.Y. A novel bromophenol derivative BOS-102 induces cell cycle arrest and apoptosis in human A549 lung cancer cells via ROS-mediated PI3K/Akt and the MAPK signaling pathway. *Mar. Drugs* **2018**, *16*, 43. [CrossRef] [PubMed]
44. Papadopoulos, N.; Martin, J.; Qin, R.; Rafique, A.; Rosconi, M.P.; Shi, E.; Pyles, E.A.; Yancopoulos, G.D.; Stahl, N.; Wiegand, S.J. Binding and neutralization of vascular endothelial growth factor (VEGF) and related ligands by VEGF Trap, ranibizumab and bevacizumab. *Angiogenesis* **2012**, *15*, 171–185. [CrossRef] [PubMed]
45. Sui, H.; Zhao, J.; Zhou, L.; Wen, H.; Deng, W.; Li, C.; Ji, Q.; Liu, X.; Feng, Y.; Chai, N.; et al. Tanshinone IIA inhibits beta-catenin/VEGF-mediated angiogenesis by targeting TGF-beta 1 in normoxic and HIF-1 alpha in hypoxic microenvironments in human colorectal cancer. *Cancer Lett.* **2017**, *403*, 86–97. [CrossRef]
46. Vasudev, N.S.; Reynolds, A.R. Anti-angiogenic therapy for cancer: Current progress, unresolved questions and future directions. *Angiogenesis* **2014**, *17*, 495–497. [CrossRef]
47. Cao, Z.; Shang, B.; Zhang, G.; Miele, L.; Zhou, Q. Tumor cell-mediated neovascularization and lymphangiogenesis contrive tumor progression and cancer metastasis. *BBA Rev. Cancer* **2013**, *1836*, 273–286. [CrossRef]
48. Yeo, C.; Lee, H.J.; Lee, E.O. Serum promotes vasculogenic mimicry through the EphA2/VE-cadherin/AKT path-way in PC-3 human prostate cancer cells. *Life Sci.* **2019**, *15*, 267–273. [CrossRef]
49. Masckauchan, T.N.H.; Agalliu, D.; Vorontchikhina, M.; Ahn, A.; Parmalee, N.L.; Li, C.M.; Khoo, A.; Tycko, B.; Brown, A.M.C.; Kitajewski, J. Wnt5a signaling induces proliferation and survival of endothelial cells in vitro and expression of MMP-1 and Tie-2. *Mol. Biol. Cell* **2006**, *17*, 5163–5172. [CrossRef]
50. Yang, D.H.; Yoon, J.Y.; Lee, S.H.; Bryja, V.; Andersson, E.R.; Arenas, E.; Kwon, Y.G.; Choi, K.Y. Wnt5a is required for endothelial differentiation of embryonic stem cells and vascularization via pathways involving both Wnt/beta-catenin and protein kinase Calpha. *Circ. Res.* **2009**, *104*, 372–379. [CrossRef]
51. Tosetti, F.; Ferrari, N.; De Flora, S.; Albini, A. Angioprevention: Angiogenesis is a common and key target for cancer chemopreventive agents. *FASEB J.* **2002**, *16*, 2–14. [CrossRef] [PubMed]
52. Albini, A.; D'Agostini, F.; Giunciuglio, D.; Paglieri, I.; Balansky, R.; De Flora, S. Inhibition of invasion, gelatinase activity, tumor take and metastasis of malignant cells byN-acetylcysteine. *Int. J. Cancer* **1995**, *61*, 121–129. [CrossRef] [PubMed]
53. Cai, T.; Fassina, G.F.; Morini, M.; Aluigi, M.G.; Albini, A. N-acetylcysteine inhibits endothelial cell invasion and angiogenesis. *Lab. Investig. J. Tech. Methods Pathol.* **1999**, *79*, 1151–1159.

MDPI
St. Alban-Anlage 66
4052 Basel
Switzerland
Tel. +41 61 683 77 34
Fax +41 61 302 89 18
www.mdpi.com

Marine Drugs Editorial Office
E-mail: marinedrugs@mdpi.com
www.mdpi.com/journal/marinedrugs

www.ingramcontent.com/pod-product-compliance
Lightning Source LLC
Chambersburg PA
CBHW061454210926
51850CB00008B/1714

9783036575681